A CLINICAL HANDBOOK ON
child development
paediatrics

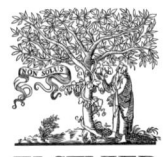

Churchill Livingstone
is an imprint of Elsevier

Elsevier Australia. ACN 001 002 357
(a division of Reed International Books Australia Pty Ltd)
Tower 1, 475 Victoria Avenue, Chatswood, NSW 2067

This edition © 2012 Elsevier Australia. Reprinted 2014.
eISBN: 9780729580892

This publication is copyright. Except as expressly provided in the Copyright Act 1968 and the Copyright Amendment (Digital Agenda) Act 2000, no part of this publication may be reproduced, stored in any retrieval system or transmitted by any means (including electronic, mechanical, microcopying, photocopying, recording or otherwise) without prior written permission from the publisher.

Every attempt has been made to trace and acknowledge copyright, but in some cases this may not have been possible. The publisher apologises for any accidental infringement and would welcome any information to redress the situation.

This publication has been carefully reviewed and checked to ensure that the content is as accurate and current as possible at time of publication. We would recommend, however, that the reader verify any procedures, treatments, drug dosages or legal content described in this book. Neither the author, the contributors, nor the publisher assume any liability for injury and/or damage to persons or property arising from any error in or omission from this publication.

National Library of Australia Cataloguing-in-Publication Data

---

Author: Johnson, Sandra Lucille.
Title: A clinical handbook on child development paediatrics / Sandra Johnson.
ISBN: 9780729540896 (pbk.)
Subjects: Child development–Handbooks, manuals, etc.
           Pediatrics–Australia–Handbooks, manuals, etc.
Dewey Number: 612.65

Publishing Director: Luisa Cecotti
Developmental Editor: Neli Bryant
Project Manager: Nayagi Athmanathan
Project Coordinators: Lisa Shillan, Liz Malcolm
Edited by Brenda Hamilton
Proofread by Sarah Newton-John
Cover and internal design by Toni Darben
Index by Robert Swanson
Typeset by Toppan Best-set Premedia Limited
Printed in China by China Translation & Printing Services Limited.

Contents

Foreword	vii
The author	ix
Contributors	ix
Reviewers	xi
Dedication	xiii
Preface	xv
Acknowledgements	xvii

1 NORMAL DEVELOPMENT — 1
Sandra Johnson

2 DEVELOPMENTAL ASSESSMENT IN THE YOUNG CHILD — 25
Natalie Silove

3 MOTOR AND COORDINATION PROBLEMS — 40
Sandra Johnson with Manoj Menezes

4 HEARING AND VISION LOSS — 50
Shirley Russ

5 AUTISM SPECTRUM DISORDERS — 88
Natalie Silove

6 SPECIFIC LEARNING DISORDERS — 113
Sandra Johnson

7 LANGUAGE DISORDERS — 127
Sandra Johnson

8 ATTENTION DEFICIT HYPERACTIVITY DISORDER — 145
Sandra Johnson

9 BEHAVIOUR DIFFICULTIES — 173
Sandra Johnson

10 SCHOOL REFUSAL AND TRUANCY — 185
Sandra Johnson

11 MOOD DISORDERS IN CHILDREN AND ADOLESCENTS — 194
Kenneth Nunn

12	**CEREBRAL PALSY** Sandra Johnson with Mary-Clare Waugh	**212**
13	**DEVELOPMENTAL AND INTELLECTUAL DISABILITY** Jacqueline Small	**232**
14	**CHILD ABUSE AND NEGLECT** Paul Tait	**247**
15	**LEGAL ISSUES** Sandra Johnson	**273**

Index **287**

Foreword

One of my teachers at medical school remarked that 'when parents order a baby, they order a perfect one'. That piece of wisdom has stayed with me through forty years of paediatric practice and was reinforced by watching my own children and grandchildren grow up. Parents learn about child development from observation, from their own parents and, in the modern era, from a huge range of books, TV and radio and the internet. They are now much better informed than previous generations, but this increased knowledge comes at a price. Their expectations are greater, they are conscious of the pressure for their child to succeed in an increasingly competitive world and they worry more if their child's development seems to be slower than that of their peers, or is atypical in some way.

In response to these changes, paediatricians have recognised over the past half century that their brief is no longer confined to physical health and illness. They are now expected to be competent in assessing a child's developmental progress, their behaviour and their personality. The body of research and knowledge needed to do this comes from many areas of enquiry – not just medical paediatrics, but neurology and neuroscience, psychology and psychiatry, linguistics, genetics, orthopaedics and orthotics. Furthermore, children with developmental disabilities often have more than one problem, including, for example, growth disturbances, epilepsy, cardiac disorders, facial malformations and many more.

When parents consult a health professional with concerns about their child's development or behaviour, they do not necessarily know whether there is a problem at all, let alone whether it is due to a brain disorder, a psychological disturbance or misguided parenting. The paediatrician working in this field has to unravel these complex problems, often supported by a team of colleagues working in other disciplines, and advise on appropriate therapy or treatment. Indeed, the paediatrician is often conductor of an orchestra consisting of many ultra-specialised colleagues, and has to ensure that amidst all this high-level expertise the best interests of the child and the family remain at the centre. Sometimes they must also address the challenging issues of possible child abuse or consider whether the child's problems are the result of medical error or accident.

Considering the importance of these topics in modern paediatric practice, there are surprisingly few comprehensive texts on child development and disability. This is partly because the field has to draw on the expertise of so many other disciplines, and perhaps also because it is only quite recently that child development and disability has become a recognised area of specialisation.

Dr Sandra Johnson, like all successful paediatricians working in this field, is clearly a team player and has recruited an expert group of colleagues to contribute to this excellent book, *A Clinical Handbook on Child Development Paediatrics*. The titles of the chapters indicate the breadth of knowledge that such specialists require. The team members have of course drawn heavily on their own extensive clinical experience but they have also provided a concise overview of the recent research literature, which indicates how this subject is rapidly developing a much more robust evidence base than was the case in the past.

The various forms of developmental disorder discussed in *A Clinical Handbook on Child Development Paediatrics* have one thing in common – the parents have to come to terms with the fact that their child may not be perfect. The task for the paediatrician's team includes guiding parents through the emotions of grief, anger and acceptance as well as helping them to formulate a plan of action, often in partnership with education and social service authorities as well as health professional colleagues. Dr Johnson's book should be available to, and be used by, paediatricians in many parts of the world.

David Hall
Emeritus Professor of Community Paediatrics, University of Sheffield, England
Honorary Professor of Paediatrics, University of Cape Town, South Africa

The author

Sandra Johnson MBChB, DPAED, FRACP, FRCPCH, FACLM
Clinical Senior Lecturer, Discipline of Paediatrics and Child Health, Faculty of Medicine, University of Sydney, New South Wales
Consultant Developmental Paediatrician, Child Development Paediatrics (Private Practice Clinic), Pennant Hills, Sydney, New South Wales

Contributors

Manoj Menezes MBBS, FRACP
Neurogenetics Fellow, Institute for Neuroscience and Muscle Research, The Children's Hospital at Westmead, New South Wales

Kenneth Nunn MBBS (Hons), FRANZCP, FRCPsych, PhD
Senior Staff Specialist, The Children's Hospital at Westmead, New South Wales

Shirley Russ MD, MPH, FRACP
Clinical Professor of Pediatrics, Cedars-Sinai Medical Center
Faculty Researcher, UCLA Center for Healthier Children, Families and Communities, Los Angeles, California

Natalie Silove MBBCh, MMed, FCP(SA)Paeds, FRACP
Head of the Child Development Unit, Senior Staff Specialist, The Children's Hospital at Westmead
Senior Clinical Lecturer Sydney University, New South Wales

Jacqueline Small MBBS, FRACP, MPH(Hons)
Senior Staff Specialist, The Children's Hospital at Westmead
Clinical Lecturer, University of Sydney, New South Wales

Paul Tait MBBS, FRACP
Senior Staff Specialist, Child Protection Unit, The Children's Hospital at Westmead, New South Wales

Mary-Clare Waugh MBBS, FRACP, MRCP and CH (UK), FAFRM
Head, Cerebral Palsy and Movement Disorder Service
Head, Spinal Cord Injury Service, Kids Rehab, The Children's Hospital at Westmead, New South Wales

Reviewers

Andrew Biggin BSc, PhD, MBBS(Lon)
Clinical Lecturer, University of Sydney
Honorary Research Fellow, Marfan Research Group
Medical Registrar, The Children's Hospital at Westmead, New South Wales

Margot Bosanquet FRACP, MBBS, BSc(Hons)
Royal Children's Hospital Foundation Clinical Fellow in Cerebral Palsy and Rehabilitation, Royal Children's Hospital, Brisbane, Queensland

Chamanthi Nanayakkara MBBS, MRCPCH
Staff Specialist Paediatrics, Toowoomba and St Vincent's Hospital, Toowoomba, Queensland

Kim Oates AM, MD, DSc, MHP, FRACP, FRCP, FAFHPM
Emeritus Professor, University of Sydney, New South Wales

Kate Rodwell MBBS
Cerebral Palsy Fellow, Royal Children's Hospital, Queensland

Dedication

This book is dedicated to the memory of my parents, Arthur and Deborah Johnson, who inspired and encouraged me in my career and my work.

Preface

This book is written primarily for paediatric registrars who want a practical, clinical approach to the specialty of child development. Apart from developmental trainees it will also assist general paediatricians, general practitioners and allied health professionals who are interested in this field of work. The aim is to give the busy practitioner a quick overview with extensive references in each chapter and recommended reading at the end of chapters to allow in-depth exploration of the topic.

I was inspired to write *A Clinical Handbook on Child Development Paediatrics* because there was no specific pathway for child development training in Australia in the mid-1980s, when I first began my training in the field. I searched for textbooks that covered child development in a concise and comprehensive way, and found a number of helpful, detailed textbooks, many of which are referenced in this book. However, I could not find a stand-alone handbook to use as a quick reference that covered a range of subjects in the field of child development, hence came the notion to write such a book.

A Clinical Handbook on Child Development Paediatrics is written as a practical guide that covers the more common conditions encountered in the management of children with developmental problems. It provides a logical progression in terms of approach to each subject, with many aspects given in lists to allow the reader to move through various stages quickly and access information without the need to read large volumes of text to extract pertinent details. Lists and tables throughout the book continue the easy access approach to information about management, investigations and treatment. Each chapter provides sufficient detail on important aspects like prevalence, aetiology and new research, and in some instances, controversies in the literature are discussed. The reader is encouraged to delve more deeply into the subject by using the extensive references and resources for each chapter.

In addition, the book has an online module covering clinical cases in common conditions to provide an opportunity for study of case management in relation to specific problems, using a question-and-answer format. This is intended to allow revision of the topics and to give the reader a 'handle' on how these cases might present and how they are dealt with in clinical practice.

There are topics that I would like to have included, particularly adolescent medicine and genetics, but it was not possible to cover additional material in the time frame of 12 months for bringing this book to completion. Instead all chapters address genetics and transition to adulthood; both being important aspects of this field of specialty.

To my readers, I trust that you will find this to be a practical, relevant and useful book in the management of your patients, and that it will help to enhance your understanding of and appreciation for this very special branch of Paediatrics.

Sandra Johnson

Acknowledgements

I held the notion for some time that I would write a book for the paediatric trainee. This intention was encouraged by Patrina Caldwell and a group of registrars at the RACP meeting in Melbourne in 2010, who suggested that I write a book to assist registrars in the field of child development. Sophie Kalinecki's warm reaction to the idea with the subsequent positive response by Elsevier to my book proposal led to commencement of the work. I am very grateful to the team at Elsevier for their support while the book was being written. A special thank you to Neli Bryant.

I particularly wish to thank Professor Sir David Hall, who has been my mentor in the field of child development while I worked in the United Kingdom and also in recent times, for reading all my chapters for *A Clinical Handbook on Child Development Paediatrics*. He generously provided extensive critique that gave me an objective view of the work. Many colleagues gave their time to read and comment on my work and I am very grateful to all. Elizabeth Elliott and Manoj Menezes read Chapter 1 Normal development; Paul Hutchins provided helpful comment to Chapter 6 Specific learning disorders and particularly to the medication section of Chapter 8 Attention deficit hyperactivity disorder; Simon Clarke read Chapter 8 Attention deficit hyperactivity disorder; Frank Oberklaid read Chapter 7 Language disorders; and Eve Blair read and commented on Chapter 12 Cerebral palsy. Patrina Caldwell read and commented on most chapters of this book. I would also like to thank Debbie Perkins for giving me an update on developmental assessments in young children.

My acknowledgements extend beyond my paediatrician friends and colleagues to friends and colleagues in allied health. Andrew Martin, psychologist, gave extensive support and comment to Chapter 10 School refusal and truancy and also to Chapter 6 Specific learning disorders; Judith Middleton and Michael Berger, UK psychologists, provided comment to Chapter 9 Behaviour difficulties; and Jacqui Roberts, speech pathologist, provided comment and overview to Chapter 7 Language disorders.

Chapter 15 Legal issues as the final chapter was an addition that I felt would be helpful to the paediatric trainee, as doctors rarely have exposure to Law in their medical careers. I am grateful for the helpful feedback to this chapter provided by my colleague Roy Beran, a physician with legal qualifications and president of the Australasian College of Legal Medicine.

I also wish to thank the peer reviewers, whose rigorous feedback was readily taken on board thereby ensuring that the content of the book is valid and up to date.

My thanks and appreciation extend to my contributing authors for their dedicated work and time in providing chapters to *A Clinical Handbook on Child Development Paediatrics*: Natalie Silove, Jacki Small, Ken Nunn, Paul Tait, Shirley Russ, Mary-Clare Waugh and Manoj Menezes. I am grateful that they have shared their extensive knowledge with me as well as the reader.

Finally, my gratitude goes to my husband, John Lock, for his patience and loving support during the period when a large proportion of my time and energy was taken up with writing this book.

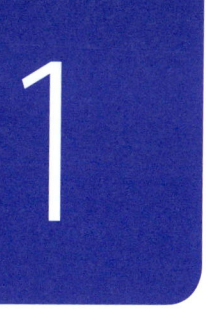

Normal development

Sandra Johnson

DEFINITION

Normal development refers to the development pathway that is followed by the majority of children within a population group. There is a time range during which the majority of children acquire particular developmental skills defined by the 3rd and 97th percentile. Beyond this range development might still be following a normal path for the child's family or cultural group within the general population so that 6 per cent, representing 2 standard deviations from the mean, occurs outside these percentiles. Therefore it is important to follow the progress of the individual child's development over time before diagnosing developmental delay with respect to achieving milestones.

Delayed development implies that the child's development is slower than that of other children of the same age and that skills are acquired at a later stage, but in these children development will not necessarily be permanently delayed or impaired. This term 'developmental delay' should only be used in retrospect when it becomes clear at follow-up that milestones have been delayed but that 'catch up' has occurred. The paediatrician should be cautious about using this term early in the assessment process as parents might infer from 'delay' that 'catch up' will occur and this cannot be guaranteed.

'Developmental disability' refers to significant delay and impairment, where skills are acquired beyond at least two standard deviations from the mean. The term implies a permanent condition with high morbidity with respect to the child's social, language, sensory, motor, self-help and cognitive abilities[1] (see Chapter 13 Developmental and intellectual disability). In children with language disorder, cognitive skills may be within the typical range for age but language and communicative skills may be delayed or deviant (see Chapter 7 Language disorders and Chapter 5 Autism spectrum disorders.)

WHY ASSESS A CHILD'S DEVELOPMENT?

The trainee paediatrician working in acute paediatrics, where organic pathology is often clearly evident, might ask 'why assess a child's development' and 'why have a specialty in paediatrics dedicated to this work?' These are good questions that deserve a thoughtful response.

Children are our young compatriots and by investing in their health and wellbeing we invest in the future of our culture and our society. Parents have concern for the health, education and prosperity of their children and seek support in providing for their children in many ways. Apart from their health, parents have concern about their children's development and want them to achieve to the best of their ability in their chosen area of interest. There are many conditions that can impact on a child's development and hinder the achievement of this goal. The paediatrician should play an active role in ensuring that such conditions are addressed thoroughly and be a long-term partner with parents/carers in the management, treatment, intervention and advocacy for children with developmental problems. This partnership approach is taken throughout this book and the role of the paediatrician is listed below.

The role of the paediatrician in assessing a child's development

The role of the paediatrician is to:
- Respectfully address parental concerns regarding the child's development and to give them the time to express their concerns
- Address the concerns of others involved with the child, e.g. allied health professionals, teachers, community leaders
- Thoroughly examine and assess the child with respect to physical, emotional, education and cognitive ability
- Support parents when they learn that the child's development is delayed or disordered
- Ensure that the delay/disorder is not due to a treatable condition and, when this is the case, to treat the condition or refer to other specialists promptly
- Empower parents/carers with evidence-based information, so that they can understand, cope with and make decisions about their child's condition
- Support the child and family in an empowering and non-judgemental manner
- Carefully listen to the parents and encourage them to raise all of their concerns, even those parents who may initially feel reluctant to ask
- Approach the diagnosis with an open mind
- Communicate findings clearly with other professionals involved in management of the child's problems to enhance collaboration in treatment and intervention.

In order to achieve these aims it is important to have an understanding of 'normal' development and to detect problems early that fit into particular 'diagnostic categories', so that specific treatments and interventions can be instituted.

THEORIES OF DEVELOPMENT

Besides early learning and cognitive skills, normal development also refers to the development of emotional and social skills.

Psychoanalytic theories of development provide the views of Freud in the early 1900s, Klein in the 1940s, Erikson in the 1950s and Winnicott in the late 1950s. DW Winnicott, a paediatrician who did psychoanalytic work with children and adults, discussed the importance of nurturing and 'attachment'. He also postulated 'the good enough' mother who provides for her infant's physical and emotional needs to the best of her ability within her particular circumstance.[2]

Melanie Klein, a psychoanalyst who was faithful to Sigmund Freud's ideas about emotional development and who influenced psychoanalysis in United Kingdom, was the first person to use traditional psychoanalysis methods with children following World War 1. John Bowlby was supervised by Klein in his psychoanalytic training but his psychoanalytic methods were essentially different to those of Klein. He was interested in real-life events and not unconscious fantasies in children. As a psychoanalyst, he provided a different approach and published extensively on 'Attachment and Loss' in the late 1960s to 1980.[3]

Mary Ainsworth, Bowlby's student, devised 'A Strange Situation' in the 1970s which examines the response of young children when caregivers and strangers enter a room where they are playing. She observed and described types of attachment; secure, anxious-resistant insecure, anxious-avoidant insecure and subsequently disorganised/disorientated attachment. She believed that there are 'adverse development effects' when the child lacks a mother figure.[4] The importance of attachment is now widely accepted but the assessment of attachment in the clinical setting is difficult.

Jean Piaget, a Swiss psychologist, influenced thinking in 1930 to the 1940s on education and child development. His theory described four stages of development: the sensorimotor stage from birth to 2 years (exploration and learning through senses and movement); pre-operational stage, 2–7 years (magical thinking, acquisition of motor skills and egocentricity); concrete operational stage, 7–11 years (logical thinking begins but concrete, less egocentric); and formal operational stage, 11–16 years and beyond (abstract reasoning and logical thinking).[5]

Lev Vygotsky, a Russian psychologist, pioneered work on human cognitive development and the influence of thought and language. In his treatise on communication in the early 1960s he emphasised the interrelationship between thought and word and its impact on learning, which subsequently influenced ideas on education and school instruction. His theory about the 'zone of proximal development' (ZPD) has been incorporated in research studies on memory, problem solving and intelligence testing.[6] ZPD refers to the range of tasks that a child will complete independently versus those that are done with the assistance and guidance of adults or more skilled peers. Essentially the ZPD relates to the process of maturation of the child's cognitive skills with the help of a more skilled person.

FACTORS THAT INFLUENCE DEVELOPMENT

Intrinsic

Genetic or hereditary
Genes code for growth, development and behaviour. It is difficult to determine the extent to which this influences development in a particular child, but there is a significant effect. Consequently, familial factors with a genetic basis may affect development. For example, there may be a familial tendency to bottom shuffle and walk late; there may a familial tendency to talk late despite having a normal developmental profile in other skills; or there may be a familial tendency to slow physical growth, also referred to as constitutional growth delay, despite normal cognitive progress.

As a result of progress in genetics and mapping of the human genome, there has been an increase in identification of regions that code for specific diseases affecting development. These include muscular dystrophy, fragile X syndrome, Rett syndrome, Down syndrome and many others.

Twin studies provide the best evidence for genetic influence on the development of language, learning and attention skills.[7]

Conditions that impact on development

Congenital abnormalities affecting vision, hearing and/or motor development may adversely affect development in other areas.

Sensory impairments are significant in this regard. The deaf child will have delayed speech and language development and the vision-impaired child might display caution when moving about or bumping into objects. Children with total or near total blindness may also exhibit a variety of apparently odd behaviours and even developmental regression (see Chapter 4 Hearing and vision loss). There is evidence of developmental setback in children with visual impairment, especially where impairment is severe to profound.[8]

Children who have significant disease affecting major organs are likely to show delay in their development. The extent of the delay will depend on the degree to which the medical condition affects the child's ability to explore and learn from the environment, as well as the extent of brain and cognitive involvement.

Motor impairment, e.g. in quadriplegic cerebral palsy, limits the child's ability to move effectively thereby affecting play and exploration of the environment. It is notable that some immobile children have normal intelligence and have an amazing ability to learn even without physically exploring their environment.

Gender

Twin studies support clinical findings that some developmental conditions are more common in males, particularly ADHD (attention deficit hyperactivity disorder) and SLI (specific language impairment)[9] (see Chapter 7 Language disorders and Chapter 8 Attention deficit hyperactivity disorder).

We often observe that girls in general attain language milestones earlier than boys in preschool years, and boys tend to attain spatial perception skills earlier than girls, but there are many exceptions to this rule.

Prenatal factors

Babies born prematurely will appear to acquire milestones at a later stage compared with full-term babies. The deficit in the premature infant's milestone attainment needs correction corresponding to the degree of prematurity until two years of age. As expected, premature babies are significantly smaller than full-term babies at the same postnatal age.

Low and very low birth weight babies, and babies who are small for gestational age, are at greater risk for developmental problems such as learning, language and cognitive difficulties.[10,11] Low birth weight babies are more likely to have had an adverse intrauterine environment associated with intrauterine growth retardation (IUGR), such as maternal infections, hypertension or other maternal conditions that cause placental insufficiency.

Extrinsic

Environment

There is no doubt that both the prenatal and postnatal environments influence a child's development.

Prenatal

It is acknowledged that there are sensitive or critical periods in brain development and that the effects of nutrition, social adversity and parental stress are all relevant.

Factors in the prenatal environment including maternal stress, depression and anxiety mediated through HPA (hypothalamic–pituitary–adrenal) pathways have been studied and the effect of maternal stress on fetal heart rate has also been examined. Findings suggest a significant affect of maternal psychological health on fetal neurobehavioural development.[12] High salivary cortisol on waking, used as a marker of adrenal function, was associated with lower birth weight in a small sample of newborn infants, leading to the conclusion that high levels of cortisol in pregnancy may be a risk factor for low birth weight. However high cortisol levels could not be correlated with maternal perception of distress in this study and further work using a larger sample size was recommended.[13]

Optimal nutrition is required for optimal fetal growth and development. This is particularly true for twins who are at greater risk of low birth weight, prematurity and IUGR. Micronutrient supplementation in pregnancy has been examined. The authors in a review of twin pregnancies recommend nutrient supplementation for multiple pregnancy because of accelerated depletion of maternal nutrient reserves and the increased risk of intrauterine growth restriction in twin pregnancy.[14] Animal studies show that maternal nutrition affects fetal development via insulin-like growth factors IGF-1 and IGF-2 that are believed to influence fetal and placental growth.[15] Maternal undernutrition affects placental transport capacity and vasculogenesis, consequently impacting on nutrient delivery to the fetus with implications for optimal fetal development and long-term adult health.[16]

The effect of alcohol in the developing infant is well known. Even brief exposure of rodent infants to alcohol impairs the neurogenesis process through which new neurons are formed.[17] Some studies show alterations in neuronal proliferation and migration, and decreased neurogenesis as a result of alcohol exposure. One study examined the effect of ethanol on fetal brain-derived stem and progenitor cells in tissue samples. They showed altered differentiation of progenitor and stem cells with abnormal cell adhesion in the presence of ethanol. They infer that alcohol can affect neuronal migration, proliferation and cell differentiation.[18] There appears to be no safe level for drinking alcohol in pregnancy. In embryonic stem cell research, even low concentrations of ethanol showed altered gene expression for CHRNA5 subunit of the nicotinic acetylcholine receptor. Changes in CHRNA5 expression is linked to altered GABA and NMDA receptor expression and abnormal development of the frontal cortex.[19] These effects in turn have implications for long-term neuropsychological function with respect to learning, cognition and behaviour. (See further reading on this subject at the end of this chapter.)

Postnatal

Early experiences in the first few years of life are significant. Social disadvantage, poverty, parenting issues, family dynamics and cognitive factors have an impact on the child's development.[20]

Apart from physical health and wellness, the child's emotional health and later behaviour can be influenced by the quality of attachments with parents and caregivers.[21] Children thrive and progress in their development when they are in secure, safe environments where their needs for comfort, warmth, nutrition and nurturing are met.

The interactional process between the young child and their environment is particularly noticeable in language development: when the mother makes eye contact and talks to her baby, the baby in turn makes sounds to which she responds, and the progressive interaction enhances further language development. The baby through this early process learns over time that they have an effect on those around them, and positive responses to their attempts lead to repetition of the behaviour so that learning is enhanced.

Children are given toys along with activities that stimulate their curiosity about the environment through play. As young children explore and learn about their environment, their experience of the environment is enriched. Through continued exploration and positive experiences, new activities are tried and new skills develop.

Where the environment is lacking in parental or carer response, where there is a paucity of stimulation within the environment, and where children are not encouraged to play or explore for a variety of reasons, their development is at risk. Parenting styles have a significant influence, e.g. the warm and engaging versus the detached and harsh responses to the child. The relationship between weight problems in first grade children and parenting styles was examined in one study that showed authoritarian parenting style was associated with a greater risk of being overweight in first grade children.[22]

Siblings can influence development but the extent is difficult to quantify. The child with older siblings to observe and imitate will have different experiences in relation to sharing, turn-taking and sense of adventure compared with the single child. The young child with older siblings might be more adventurous and undertake activities that older siblings have already mastered. However, learned behaviour also depends on temperament because the timid child is less likely to follow boisterous siblings. The influence of siblings is complex and possibly the presence of siblings influences the capacity for emotional closeness, conflict resolution and ability to deal with life events. Siblings can act as sources of support for each other, particularly in disharmonious family environments.[23]

Nutrition is an important environmental factor. Children who are malnourished show significant delay in developmental skills compared with those who have a healthy balanced diet. Many socioeconomic factors impinge on diet and nutrition and need to be taken into account when assessing the child's development. Severe chronic malnutrition can irreversibly affect brain growth. Poverty and social disadvantage have an enormous impact on children's development, as shown in many studies.[24]

Feinstein examined data from the 1970 United Kingdom Birth Cohort Survey for the effect of socioeconomic status (SES) on educational achievement. His results showed that the effect of SES was evident even before children attended school. In children of low SES that were in the bottom quartile of a developmental index at 22 months, 60 per cent were still at this level by age 10 years, compared with children of high SES in the bottom quartile at 22 months who were more likely to be in the top quartile by 10 years. This work showed that SES impacts on children's development even after they enter school, which has implications for inequality in the education system.[25]

We cannot ignore the negative impact of civil unrest and war on the development of young children. Fear for children's safety might mean that parents are more protective of their children and therefore these children are less likely to play outside, run about and interact with other children in the neighbourhood. Consequently, their development is negatively impacted by unhealthy and stressful circumstances. Pearn writes about the impact of war on children, which challenges paediatricians to advocate against war.[26]

Culture
Cultural factors also affect development. Children who spend a large amount of time in the outdoors are usually more adept at physical and motor skills at an earlier age than those who grow up in city apartments.

One study showed that Black African children acquire motor skills earlier than Causasian infants of the same age, and while this difference is likely to be genetic in part, cultural factors also play a significant role.[27]

Cultural attitudes about child-rearing are worth noting. For example, respect for elders taught to African, Asian and Australian Aboriginal children versus the attitudes in Western countries significantly affects the interaction and behaviour of young children in the company of adults and older relatives. The children in the former group may at first appear shy and reticent in the company of adults, which could mistakenly be assumed to indicate social interaction difficulty.

Children who are expected to be quiet and who are discouraged from participating in adult conversation may be less skilled at listening and interacting in conversation with others. It is also possible that children raised in boisterous families where adults display poor listening skills could develop similar conversation styles due to poor modelling.

Children raised in modern cities might learn to read and write sooner than those raised in a tribal culture, where understanding the land and learning to survive on the land is of greater importance. Consequently the culture places value and emphasis on aspects of learning and development that can influence the development of particular skills in young children within that culture. In addition, limited access to educational services for indigenous children can have a significant impact on their learning and development.

Transactional and biopsychosocial models
The transactional model suggests interplay between the intrinsic and extrinsic determinants of development, which can also be referred to as interplay between 'nature' and 'nurture'. The influence of temperament on the individual's interaction with his environment is also relevant. For example, a teenager with risk-taking genes may impulsively perform risky acts under peer pressure, whereas another teenager without similar genes might avoid the situation altogether. The reader is encouraged to read more about the interactions and effects of genes, temperament and personality on development.[28-30]

The biopsychosocial model extends the transactional model to include the broader impact of socioeconomic factors like poverty, education and cultural influences.

Further discussion about the effect of temperament can be found in Chapter 9 Behaviour difficulties and Chapter 11 Mood disorders in children and adolescents.

Epigenetics: the link between the environment and gene expression
The term 'epigenetics' essentially means 'outside or beyond genetics'. In epigenomics the interaction between the environment and genes is examined. Scientific

work with animal models suggests a plausible link between the environment and alterations in gene expression that can ultimately lead to disease phenotypes. Changes to DNA and chromatin; mainly DNA methylation in the former, and histone modifications that lead to changes in chromatin packaging in the latter, appear to be mechanisms that impact on gene expression. Studies show that the developing organism in early life adapts to environmental signals that can have an impact on later disease occurrence. This expanding science allows research on the impact of diet, toxins, etc, on the developing organism, and findings in animal models suggest 'trans-generational inheritance of environmentally induced epigenetic changes', which potentially has enormous impact on the study of human diseases.[31,32]

In addition to DNA methylation and histone modification, non-coding or interference RNA, including microRNA (miRNA), maintain or change transcription of DNA in a manner that is heritable, thereby modifying gene expression. miRNA also modifies epigenetic pathways that are involved in methylation and histone modifications. This emerging field of study provides mounting evidence for the influence of environmental factors on the genome, which changes the way we understand diseases and potentially provides a window of opportunity for positive interventions.[33]

Research findings suggest that environmental enrichment can promote structural changes in the brains of rodents, which leads to enhanced learning. Mice raised in an enriched environment showed changes in the expression of genes involved in the formation of new synapses and the number of genes associated with NMDA receptor function, which affects synaptic plasticity and learning.[34] These studies could enhance current understanding of brain development and brain recovery after trauma.

IMPACT OF EARLY EXPERIENCES

Despite the positive outcomes described in some research, it is essential to recognise the negative impact of child maltreatment and neglect on the developing brain. Children who are neglected perform poorly in academic tasks compared to non-neglected children, and neglected children are more likely to exhibit developmental, emotional and behavioural problems.[35] (See Chapter 14 Child abuse and neglect.)

It has long been suggested that early experiences affect development and that there may be critical periods for the development of skills and competencies. Animal studies with rodents and non-human primates demonstrate that changes occur in the number of neural connections, synaptic density and subsequent neuronal pruning in relation to experience and quality of stimulation. Fox and Rutter reviewed studies that examined the effects of maternal smoking, maternal antenatal depression and cortisol levels on the developing fetus. Neurotoxins, such as alcohol and exposure to drugs in pregnancy, can affect fetal development by affecting neuronal migration and enrichment.[36]

In the Romanian Adoptees study, Rutter et al report evidence that there may be long-term sequelae of adverse early experiences, that individual cognitive processing of these experiences can have a determining role and that adverse experiences cause effects on somatic structure and function of the neuroendocrine system. The findings of this study showed a strong association between cognitive impairment and institutional deprivation, particularly length of institutionalisation. However, there was measurable recovery for many adopted children once they were placed in normal family environments.[37]

Prenatally, the maternal mental state in pregnancy can potentially have an impact on the fetus. A link has been demonstrated between maternal antenatal depression, especially when depression is severe, and later child psychiatric problems.[38] Adverse effect is thought to be mediated through direct exposure of the infant to the mother's depressive state, parenting difficulties associated with being depressed, and maternal social adversity such as marital discord, poverty and overcrowding. Postnatally, the mental state of the parent can also have an impact on a child's development. The effect of postnatal maternal depression on infant development has been examined in a number of studies, showing that there is an adverse effect on growth and development, particularly when depression is severe.[39,40] Boys appear to show greater vulnerability to maternal postnatal depression.[41]

Resilience

Resilience refers to the 'ability to bounce back' despite emotional adversity for whatever reason. Positive early experience, attachments, temperament and self-concept all influence resilience in some way or other.

Children who have been institutionalised show individual differences in cognitive and social functioning: some children show few measurable deficits despite experiencing prolonged deprivation as noted in the Romanian Adoptees study, suggesting that resilience, as yet unexplained, is contributing.[37]

Infants from extremely negative environmental circumstances show improvement or recovery to some extent if they are placed in positive and healthier environments at a later period in time.[42] Sameroff and Chandler discuss 'self-righting tendencies' in development following early trauma or deficits in the environment, which again supports the notion of resilience.[43]

Research using data from the United Kingdom's Millennium Cohort Study suggests that resilience in young children is located in the cognitive domain and that neither parenting nor temperament buffer the effect of cumulative risk on young children's emotional and behavioural adjustment.[44]

Further work on resilience is found in scientific literature on adults where factors like hope, belonging and ability to make sense of negative factors all play a part in coping with adversity.[45]

Brain development and neuroplasticity

Brain development is complex and continues well after birth. Prenatally, neurons migrate from the germinal lining of the lateral and third ventricles to their eventual destinations in the cerebral cortex where differentiation, proliferation and increasing complexity of the architecture occur. Cerebellar neurons develop from the sub-ventricular region of the fourth ventricle. Neurological dysfunction and/or abnormality can occur if there is disruption to any part of this process.[46]

Neuroimaging studies have identified linear increases in white matter through to early adulthood and nonlinear changes in cortical grey matter over time. These changes are measurable by volumetric studies on standard magnetic resonance imaging (MRI) and newer MRI techniques such as magnetisation transfer imaging (MTI), magnetic resonance spectroscopy (MRS) and diffusion tensor imaging (DTI). White matter volume in various lobes increases linearly with age in 4 to

22-year-old subjects, while grey matter volume in the frontal lobes increases during pre-adolescence followed by decline in post adolescence.[47,48] The latter is of particular relevance to child development because it suggests a critical period where activities and learning in pre-teen years could impact on later synapse elimination, or 'pruning', in later adolescence. Further research provides interesting MRI findings of brain changes with maturity.[49,50]

Research also supports learning-induced plasticity of the brain. Plasticity of auditory pathways has been noted in studies with functional MRI (fMRI) and electrical neuroimaging, where repetition-induced plasticity is noted in auditory spatial representations and encoding of sounds.[51] MRI study of grey matter volume in parts of Broca's area (pars opercularis) in musicians shows volume increase with years of musical performance, suggesting use-dependent modification of brain structures.[52] Further research in these aspects of brain development is continuing.

Neuroplasticity of the brain following injury is also being studied. Animal studies using gene microarray data show molecular responses in growth, development and metabolism that may play a role in brain injury recovery.[53] A case report of cortical activation with near-infrared spectroscopy (NIRS) of an infant following hemispherectomy for intractable seizures showed that reorganisation of brain pathways occurred, resulting in gradual recovery from hemiplegia following a period of neuro-rehabilitation.[54]

It appears that the brain is not static and pathways may change and develop over time, even in adults.[55] This notion has implications for intervention, particularly in the absence of structural abnormalities, where early intervention might have an impact on neural pathways and the development of skills in young children. As research in this area continues, further support is given to the importance of assessment and intervention in childhood developmental problems.

Despite new research to support plasticity of the brain, emphasis on the importance of early intervention is paramount, particularly as most learning and cognitive development occurs in early childhood.

STAGES OF NORMAL DEVELOPMENT: MILESTONES

When the stages of normal or typical development are considered, the above factors need to be taken into account. For ease of recall, the stages and milestones are given in Tables 1.1, 1.2 and 1.3. The stages provided give the mean age, so there is a range of normal above and below this mean.

The stages of development are considered in relation to the functional skills that children acquire over time. These include vision, hearing, language, social, fine and gross motor skills. Each function relates to and influences the development of others, so that healthy 'normal' development requires that all the skills develop in concert, with one skill building upon the next. At a physiological level this progression is better understood when we think about neural pathways maturing together with increasing synaptic connections between them, so that the child's skills emerge over time as the brain develops and matures.

Milestones are achieved at varying rates, and periods of plateau in development can be followed by bursts of skill attainment. Typical development is non-linear and does not occur at a constant rate, and variability occurs both within one child and across many children. This intra-individual variability has implications for developmental screening. Inter-individual and across-domain variability

CHAPTER 1 Normal development   11

TABLE 1.1 Stages 6 weeks to 6 months

Mean age	Vision	Hearing	Motor	Social
Newborn	Pupils react to light	Baby startles to loud sound	Primitive reflexes are present	Baby makes eye contact
6 weeks	Fixes and follows face or bright light	Baby stills to sound at 15 cm from ear Baby responds to mother's voice	Able to support head when held upright	Smiling
3 months	Baby looks at own fingers		Head in midline Will raise head off bed in prone position	Vocalisations
4 months	Hand regard Fixes and follows through 180°	Baby turns to sound at level of own head	Reaching for toy Primitive reflexes disappear Begins to roll over at 4.5 months Infant begins to weight bear with 'buckling' at the knee	Two-way vocalisations
6 months	Watches others and will follow them as they move around the room		Achieves sitting position Palmar grasp Transfer across the midline from one hand to other Stands when held to weight bear, less 'buckling at knee'	Loud vocalisations and will blow raspberries Shows distress when mother leaves the room

is also noted in typically developing children.[56] Consequently, assessments or screening done at a single point in time does not give an accurate indication of the child's developmental profile and monitoring with review assessments is recommended.[57]

The variability described for general development is also noted for language development. In The Early Language in Victoria Study, the language development profiles of preschool children revealed accelerated development, followed by slow development and then catch-up periods. This study also found that high maternal education, maternal vocabulary level and socioeconomic status was more common in groups showing improving language profiles over time in children aged between 8 months and 4 years.[58] This work also supports the notion that early development

TABLE 1.2 Stages 7 to 20 months

Mean age	Vision	Hearing	Motor/ performance	Language/ social
7 months	Visual attention to 1 m Picks up tiny objects	Locates sound at 1 m on level of ear	Object permanence begins Raking action to attain raisin off surface	Baby uses double sounds
8 months			Intermediate grasp Sits well unsupported	
10 months	Visual attention to 3 m	Locates sounds above and below head	Infant stands to weight bear well Not voluntary release of toy held in hand Parachute reflex	Says 'mumma' and 'dada' Exhibits shyness
12 months			Bang 2 cubes together Pincer grasp Cruising around furniture Casting of objects Can release toy held in hand	Pointing gesture Single words
15 months			Walking with wide-based gait	Recognises names of body parts
18–20 months			Tower of 2 cubes Hand dominance emerges, but not definitive Drinks from a cup Walking well, gait less wide based Will crawl up stairs	Can name 4–6 familiar objects Can understand names of up to 20 familiar objects

CHAPTER 1 Normal development **13**

TABLE 1.3 Stages at 21 months to 4.5 years

Mean age	Vision	Hearing	Motor/performance	Language/social
21 months			Shape recognition	4–5 single words
24 months			Uses spoon to feed self Hand dominance consistent Goes up stairs two feet at a time, down two feet each stair holding hand or rail	2-word combinations Can understand more complex sentences Begins to follow 2-part simple instruction
2½ years			Tower of 4 cubes Scribbles on page	Can name at least one object from picture book
3 years	Can use E chart	Can repeat words whispered in ear	Has an early tripod pencil grasp Copies a line Begins to copy circle Jumps well Copies a 3-cube bridge Goes up stairs one foot at a time, down two feet each stair	Knows plural Puts on items of clothing with help Speaks intelligibly within family unit 3-word combinations Begins to follow 3-part simple instruction Colour recognition
3½ years			Draws circle well Begins to draw a person Copies a 4-cube train Can balance on one leg	
4 years			Copies a cross Emerging ability to copy a square Begins to do buttons Up and down stairs one foot at a time	Can name shapes Puts on items of clothing with less help
4½ years			Copies 6-cube steps Copies a recognisable square Immature drawing of a person	Intelligible speech and better grammar

can be slow in poorer children and improve in prosperous children so that socioeconomic factors should be kept in mind when assessing children.

Recall of developmental milestones is easier when considered in stages. This approach is based on the work of Dorothy Egan, who wrote extensively on the subject of child development.[59] The stages are:
1. 6 weeks to 6 months
2. 7 to 20 months
3. 21 months to $4\frac{1}{2}$ years.

Tables 1.1, 1.2 and 1.3 summarise the stages of development and are a modified version of tables produced by Dorothy Egan (with permission from Mac Keith Press, UK).

IMPORTANCE OF THE HISTORY AND THE EXAMINATION

Taking a thorough history from the parents or carers is paramount. When parents are concerned about an issue related to their child's development, attention must be given to their concerns especially when examining the child. It is unwise to give false reassurance if parental concerns have not been fully addressed. The converse is not always true. Some parents are not worried when perhaps they should be, and are not well informed about development or may have very low expectations, for instance if they live in an deprived area where their concept of 'normal' development may be a long way below the national norms. For this reason, the PEDS (Parents' Evaluation of Developmental Milestones)[60] approach that taps into parents' knowledge of their child is helpful with most parents, but must be used with caution with families from poor backgrounds.

The complete paediatric history includes the family, social, obstetric/perinatal and past medical history. When taking the obstetric history any concerns that the parents have about the pregnancy is important: difficulties with conception, previous stillbirths, multiple miscarriages or other history that might alert the clinician to potential problems related to the child's development, e.g. multiple miscarriage indicating possible genetic or haematological problems. Refer to Chapter 12 Cerebral palsy.

The developmental assessment of the young child is discussed in Chapter 2. It is important to ask why the assessment is being done: who is most concerned and what is the concern? The assessment may be part of a routine well-baby check, or part of an evaluation of a primarily medical condition (such as asthma), or part of an in-depth assessment where the parent is concerned and where the child has been referred to the paediatrician. The paediatrician who does the complete assessment needs to decide whether the problem is a developmental one, which will need the implementation of a management plan and include involvement of allied health and/or education, or whether the child needs referral to another specialist, for example a paediatric neurologist. Referral to another specialist for a second opinion might also allay anxiety about the child's development, particularly where concern is unfounded due to misunderstanding.

While taking the history the doctor should observe the child's behaviour and interaction with their parents. This point is emphasised throughout this book. Interaction with the younger child in play or with the older child on a topic of interest to them before commencing any formal examination or assessment is advisable. Including the child in the assessment process means that they are more likely to cooperate with the assessment.

Medical assessment requires time and the full attention of the examiner to ensure that subtle signs are not missed. The physical examination is performed as for any child presenting with a medical problem. Growth parameters with height, weight and head circumference measurements must always be done and checked on growth charts. See Chapter 2 for the assessment of the young child, including a list of formal and informal assessment tools; the paediatric approach in Table 6.4 of Chapter 6 on Specific learning disorders; and assessment outlines in Chapter 8 on Attention deficit hyperactivity disorder and Chapter 10 on School refusal.

THE IMPORTANCE OF LANGUAGE AND CULTURE

When assessing children's development the clinician must remain aware of the importance of language. When interviewing non-English speaking families many nuances of conversation are lost even when an interpreter is used to assist the interviewer. Body language, which gives the clinician an indescribable 'feel' for the situation and for parental concerns while the history is being reported, may also be lost. Thus it can be difficult to obtain a true picture of the child's skills and level of development based on the history alone. The involvement of a family or community member, who is able to speak English well and who knows the child and family intimately, is a valuable informant in the interview process.

It is worth remembering that when families do not speak English, or whichever language is used in the clinical setting, they might appear to understand what is being said to them in order to be agreeable, yet have little true understanding of the implications of what they are being told.

The clinician must remain aware of the cultural influences in child-rearing that might affect presentation, e.g. in some Asian, African and Australian Aboriginal cultures direct eye contact by young children with adults is viewed as disrespectful, yet we might regard this behaviour as significant when autism spectrum disorder is being considered.

Language assessment of children in a cross-cultural society is challenging, particularly when resource allocation is based on assessment. The clinician needs to remain sensitive to the values, beliefs, codes of conduct and communication styles inherent in a culture. Validity and bias with regards to assessment and treatment programs must be taken into consideration.[61]

Assessment of children's development is fraught with difficulty when their upbringing and experience is different to what many expect or experience. Aboriginal children might perform less well than their Caucasian peers on developmental tools, especially when tools have been designed specifically for non-Aboriginal children. There is the risk that some aspects of the diagnostic or screening tool will not be relevant in aboriginal communities, whether in Australia, Africa or elsewhere. It has been legitimately suggested by many that developmental tools need to be modified and adapted for use in these settings.[62]

The Universal Nonverbal Intelligence Test (UNIT; Bracken & McCallum 1998) and the Leiter International Performance Scale-Revised (Leiter-R; Roid & Miller 1997)[63] were designed for use without language-based skills to overcome bias when testing children from diverse cultural and linguistic backgrounds. The validity of these tests was examined concurrently. While both tests are multidimensional in assessing skills and both use non-verbal instructions, the UNIT uses more standardised sets of gestures than the Leiter-R and the tasks remain the same for all ages on the UNIT, whereas the tasks on the Leiter-R vary with different ages.[63]

The reader might find an article on Universal Intelligence interesting with respect to defining intelligence, measurement of human intelligence and using mathematical constructs to measure intelligence across a wide range of systems like animals and machines, such as computers and robots.[64]

IMPORTANCE OF THE NEUROLOGICAL EXAMINATION IN THE INFANT AND YOUNG CHILD

The neurological examination is essential in the assessment of the child's development. As the brain matures, new skills develop and the emergence of these skills is dependent on proficiency attained in prior skills. Good core knowledge and competency in neurology is essential when assessing the development of children. As mentioned, growth parameters are essential and head circumference can provide clues to early brain development.

Aspects of the neurological examination relating to development are mentioned here in brief and the reader is encouraged to refer to neurology textbooks for more detail.[65,66]

General appearance and behaviour

- Note the presence of dysmorphic features or neurocutaneous stigmata that might provide a clue to an underlying congenital syndrome, e.g. Down syndrome, Noonan syndrome, fragile X syndrome, tuberous sclerosis.
- Observe the baby's interaction and response to their mother or parent, their temperament and general physical condition.

Primitive reflexes in the infant

- Moro reflex: Support the baby's head with one hand and the baby's back in the midline with the other hand. Drop the baby's head slightly in relation to their back and observe the response of their arms and hands. The arms fling out symmetrically to the side of their body in the normal response. Importantly, the Moro reflex should be complete and symmetrical by 34 weeks gestation. Absence is abnormal and an asymmetrical reflex may suggest hemiplegia, brachial plexus palsy or clavicular fracture. The Moro reflex should not be present after 3–4 months of age.
- Grasp reflex: Place your thumb or finger in the baby's palm to promote a grasp response. Usually present in the neonate and may persist up to 6 months.
- Placing/stepping reflex: Stimulate the dorsum of the baby's foot with the edge of a horizontal surface, for example a table, while holding them upright. The baby flexes at the knee and places the foot on top of the surface. Typically this neonatal reflex disappears after 6 weeks.
- Asymmetric tonic neck reflex (ATNR): Place the baby on their back and turn their head slowly to one side and hold it there. The baby assumes a 'fencing posture' with extension of the arm to the same side as the face and flexion of the opposite arm. This position is adopted for a few seconds only and then the baby's posture returns to normal. An obligatory fixed ATNR beyond 4 months of age is abnormal and precludes the ability to roll over.

- Side protective reflex: emerges after 5 months of age. Baby in sitting position will put a hand out to the side to prevent falling when gently pushed to the same side.
- Parachute reflex: emerges at 7–8 months and is well developed by 10–12 months. Baby held at the trunk and propelled towards a lower surface with their head held slightly downward will thrust arms and hands forward in a protective manner, which ultimately prevents falling on their face once walking. Note that an asymmetrical parachute response can be an early sign in hemiplegia.

Tone

As the infant matures motor tone and control improves. When the newborn baby is pulled to the sitting position by their hands from supine position, there will be significant head lag. Head control improves over time and by 3 months there is no head lag when the baby pulled to sitting position.

Notice how the baby feels when they are held upright with your hands held below the axillae. The hypotonic infant feels as if they will slip through your hands. Alternatively, the baby under 6 months old with increased tone might tend to arch backwards or have stiffness in their legs, such that when held in the standing position there is no 'buckling' at the knees. Instead the baby might feel fairly hypertonic. These findings may occur in spastic cerebral palsy as well as in other neurological conditions. Standing position while being held without buckling at the knees typically occurs at around 8 months of age.

> **Practice Point**
>
> It is important to note here that infants who are advanced in their development might hold the standing posture at an earlier age, for example native African babies are often advanced in development of their motor milestones. Therefore the paediatrician needs to be very careful about over-interpreting signs in isolation. Take all factors regarding the infant's development and the physical examination into account.

RED FLAGS: WHEN TO BE CONCERNED

As mentioned, whenever the parent or carer is concerned about the child's development the paediatrician should pay careful attention. The child might be brought for assessment because of the concerns of other carers, early childhood teachers, school teachers, allied health professionals or doctors. It is important to establish who is most concerned, why they are concerned and what the concern is about.

Red flags are signs in the developmental history and examination that warrant further investigation.

Vision

When the mother reports that the baby does not look at her, it is of concern. The absence of a fixing and following response at 4–5 weeks using a bright red ball is a significant sign and may be due to vision impairment or brain damage/

dysfunction. Special attention must be given to the history and other neurological findings on examination because this infant will require further investigations. Inspect the eyes carefully for abnormal size (microphthalmia, buphthalmos) and appearance.

The presence of abnormal eye movements, e.g. nystagmus, might indicate severe vision, developmental or neurological problems.

The absence of the red reflex when the pupil is viewed through an ophthalmoscope might indicate cataract or retinoblastoma. (Sometimes parents will report a white instead of red eye in flash when taking photographs.) This baby's vision needs to be assessed urgently by a paediatric ophthalmologist.

Newborn infants might appear to have a squint due to the position of the epicanthic folds. The cover test can help to determine if there is a true squint, but this is difficult to execute in young infants. Best practice is to refer the infant to paediatric ophthalmology if there is any doubt in relation to squint. (See Chapter 4 Hearing and vision loss.)

Hearing

The parent might mention that the infant seems unresponsive to loud sounds. Infants who are born deaf do not respond to their mother's voice or environmental sounds but are very alert to visual cues, such as their mother's face or gesture. Deaf infants will babble at the same time as normal hearing infants, but babbling fails to develop further or become richer in expression.

Hearing impairment can be related to many causes. (See Chapter 4 Hearing and vision loss.) Those below are mentioned in relation to infants and young children.

Congenital deafness
- Congenital sensorineural deafness is a significant impairment and may be associated with other developmental problems as discussed in Chapter 4.
- Consider syndromes that may be associated with deafness, e.g. mitochondrial encephalopathies, cytomegalovirus or rubella during pregnancy, Pendred syndrome, Waardenburg syndrome and many others.[65,66]

Deafness secondary to infections
- Systemic: infections such as meningitis (bacterial or viral) or mumps can lead to unilateral or bilateral deafness.
- Local: otitis media (middle ear infection) is not uncommon and can result in reduced hearing, particularly when chronic as in serous otitis media (glue ear). In this case the parent might not suspect the reduced hearing because the child will be able to hear some but not all sounds. Chronic suppurative otitis media with perforated drum will significantly affect hearing.

Deafness secondary to drugs
- Not common and epidemiological evidence reveals weak associations between drugs and hearing loss (see Chapter 4).

Deafness secondary to toxins
- Bilirubin encephalopathy where exposure to high serum bilirubin levels in the neonatal period might lead to deafness.

Practice Point
Recognising that deaf infants will babble is important as doctors sometimes wrongly reassure parents that a baby who babbles cannot be deaf.

Speech and language
The following findings should alert the paediatrician that further assessment is indicated:
- Infant that does not vocalise: typically starts around 6 weeks; concern if none by 4 months
- No babble (two or more word-like sounds): usually starts around 7 months; concern if none by 8–10 months
- No single words by age 18 months: usually starts at 10–12 months
- No word combinations or two-word phrases by the age of 2 years: usually starts at around 18 months
- The child under age 2 years who does not respond to simple requests
- No simple sentences or phrases at 3 years
- Persistent dysfluency at 4 years (persistent stutter)
- Speech sound errors at 7 years.

There are many causes for delayed language development. The more common are deafness, developmental disability (mental handicap), specific language disorders, severe deprivation and neglect. (See Chapter 7 Language disorders.)

Other less common causes include autism, visual impairment, cerebral palsy and orofacial abnormalities that impede speech development. (See Chapter 7 Language disorders and Chapter 5 Autism spectrum disorders.)

Social interaction
These findings may indicate that the child's social development is delayed or impaired:
- No smile at 6–8 weeks
- Little or no eye contact with mother when being nursed
- No interactive vocalisation (typically the infant responds to mother's voice and to her verbal interaction with him)
- No reaching for objects or interest in surroundings
- No pointing to objects at around 12 months
- No interest in play or interaction with other children at 2 years
- No turn taking behaviour in play at 3 years
- Older child that seems to be 'in own world' and showing little desire to interact with others.

Gross and fine motor skills
Fine motor
Reaching for objects (around 3–4 months), banging objects together, casting and pointing to objects (the latter at around 12 months) indicate normal development, so that the infant who does not show this behaviour may be developmentally delayed. The subsequent development of the pincer grip at 1 year, leading to early pencil control at 3 years is also an indication of fine motor development.

Early development of hand dominance might indicate weakness on the opposite side, e.g. hemiplegia. Handedness should not develop before 12 months of age and consistent hand dominance typically occurs at around 2 years of age.

Gross motor

Delay in sitting alone at 6–8 months, not crawling by 10–12 months and no cruising at 12–15 months should alert the paediatrician to the likelihood of delayed development and/or motor impairment, e.g. cerebral palsy. With respect to walking, the upper limit is about 18 months and delay beyond this time might indicate neuromuscular problems.

Be aware that 18 months for walking is on about the 97th percentile, so that a minority of 'normal' children might not be walking at this time. This is often associated with bottom shuffling and a positive family history of late walkers, with no other neurological problems. Bottom shufflers often dislike being in the prone position in infancy.

Creatine kinase estimation is recommended for boys not walking by 18 months of age, but the paediatrician needs to be aware that a percentage of boys with Duchenne muscular dystrophy may in fact be walking by 18 months of age.[67] (Refer to Chapter 3 Motor and coordination problems.)

Persistence of primitive reflexes beyond the stages mentioned above could indicate neurological problems with dysfunction or pathology of central neural pathways, e.g. the child with spastic cerebral palsy might show persistent Moro reflex well beyond 5 to 6 months of age.

EARLY INTERVENTION

Early intervention is discussed throughout this book with respect to various childhood developmental problems. As clinicians we need to be aware of the importance of intervention in facilitating the development of the young brain. While doctors walk a balance between not providing false hope, we can encourage parents to play some part in the development of their young children. Hope is an important survival tool for parents when they discover that their child has developmental delay or disorder. The notion of intervention and 'doing something' to help their child is a common and natural parental response, which the paediatrician does well to respect.

CONCLUSION

While the need for early intervention is recognised, the clinician is challenged to maintain a balanced perspective based on clinical knowledge, up-to-date research and experience about variations in development. A wise approach is to monitor the child's progress without feeling the need to rush to diagnosis, to empower parents in their care for their developing child, and to avoid medicalisation of what might merely be part of the broader range of normal or typical development.

REFERENCES

1 Batshaw M. The child with developmental disabilities. The Pediatric Clinics of North America June 1993;40(3)

CHAPTER 1 Normal development   21

2   Dare C. Psychoanalytic theories of development, ch12. In: Rutter M, Hersov L, editors. Child and Adolescent Psychiatry. 2nd ed. Oxford: Blackwell Scientific; 1985
3   Bowlby J. Online. Available: http://en.wikipedia.org/wiki/John_Bowlby; 16 Feb 2012
4   Rutter M. Clinical implications of attachment concepts: retrospect and prospect. J Child Psychol Psychiatry 1995;36:549–71
5   Hobson RP. Piaget: On the ways of knowing in childhood, ch 11. In: Rutter M, Hersov L, editors. Child and Adolescent Psychiatry. 2nd ed. Oxford: Blackwell Scientific; 1985
6   Vygotsky LS. The development of scientific concepts in childhood. In: Vygotsky L, Hanfmann E, editors. Thought and language: Studies in communication. Cambridge MA: MIT Press; 1962. p. 82–118
7   Dale PS, Simonoff E, Bishop DVM, et al. Genetic influence on language delay in two year old children. Nature Neuroscience 1998;1(4):324–8
8   Dale N, Sonksen P. Developmental outcome, including setback, in young children with severe visual impairment. Developmental Medicine and Child Neurology 2002;44: 613–22
9   Bishop DVM. Genetic and environmental risks for specific language impairment in children. International Congress Series 2003;1254:225–45
10 Stanton-Chapman TL, Chapman DA, Bainbridge NL, et al. Identification of early risk factors for language impairment. Research in Developmental Disabilities 2002;23: 390–405
11 Potter NL. Examining speech of very low birth weight children during everyday activities. Developmental Medicine Child Neurology 2010;52:502–7
12 Kinsella MT, Monk C. Impact of maternal stress, depression and anxiety on fetal neurobehavioral development. Clinical Obstetrics and Gynaecology 2009;52:425–40
13 Bolten MI, Wurmser H, Buske-Kirschbaum A, et al. Cortisol levels in pregnancy as a psychobiological predictor for birth weight. Arch Women's Mental Health 2011;14: 33–41
14 Goodnight W, Newman R. Optimal nutrition for improved twin pregnancy outcome. Obstetrics and Gynaecology 2009;114(5):1121–34
15 Igwebuike UM. Impact of maternal nutrition on ovine foetoplacental development: A review of the role of insulin-like growth factors. Animal Reproduction Science 2010;121:189–96
16 Belkacemi L, Nelson DM, Desai M, et al. Maternal undernutrition influences placental–fetal development. Biology of Reproduction 2010;83:325–31
17 Farber NB, Creeley CE, Olney JW. Alcohol-induced neuroapoptosis in the fetal macaque brain. Neurobiology of Disease 2010;40:200–6
18 Vangipuram SD, Lyman WD. Ethanol alters cell fate of fetal human brain-derived stem and progenitor cells. Alcoholism: Clinical and Experimental Research 2010;34:1574–83
19 Krishnamoorthy M, Gerwe BA, Scharer CD, et al. Low ethanol concentration alters CHRNA5 levels during early human development. Reproductive Toxicology 2010;30:489–92
20 Maggi S, Irwin LJ, Siddiqi A, et al. The social determinants of early child development: An overview. Journal of Paediatrics and Child Health 2010;46:627–35
21 Rees CA. Thinking about children's attachments. Archives of Disease in Childhood 2005;90:1058–65
22 Rhee KE, Lumeng JC, Appugliese DP, et al. Parenting styles and overweight status in first grade. Pediatrics 2006;117:2047–54
23 Dunn J, McGuire S. Sibling and peer relationships in childhood. Journal Child Psychol Psychiatry 1992;33:67–105
24 Hertzman C, Siddiqi A, et al. Bucking the inequality gradient through early child development. BMJ 2010;340:c468
25 Feinstein L. Very early evidence. CentrePiece Summer 2003:24–30
26 Pearn J. Children and War. Journal of Paediatrics and Child Health 2003;39:166–72
27 Kelly Y, Sacker A, et al. Ethnic differences in achievement of developmental milestones by 9 months of age: the Millennium Cohort Study. Developmental Medicine & Child Neurology 2006;48:825–30

28 Fulchiero Gordon M. Normal child development, ch 32.2. In: Kaplan and Sadock's Comprehensive Textbook of Psychiatry. 8th ed. Philadelphia: Lippincott Williams & Wilkins; 2005
29 Kagan J. The temperamental thread: how genes, culture, time and luck make us who we are. New York: Dana Press; 2010
30 Shiner R, Caspi A. Personality differences in childhood and adolescence: measurement, development and consequences. Journal Child Psychol Psychiarty 2003;44:2–32
31 Jirtle RL, Skinner MK. Environmental epigenomics and disease susceptibility. Nature Reviews/Genetics 2007;8:253–62
32 Jaenisch R, Bird A. Epigenetic regulation of gene expression: how the genome integrates intrinsic and environmental signals. Nature Genetics Supplement 2003;33:245–54
33 Groom A, Elliott HR, Embleton ND, et al. Epigenetics and child health: basic principles. Archives of Disease in Childhood 2011;96:863–9
34 Rampon C, Jiang CH, Dong H, Tang Y, et al. Effects of environment enrichment on gene expression in the brain. Proceedings of the National Academy of Sciences (PNAS) 2000;97:12880–4
35 Dubowitz H. Tackling child neglect: a role for pediatricians. Pediatric Clinics of North America 2009;56:363–78
36 Fox N, Rutter M. Introduction to the special section on the effects of early experience on development. Child Development 2010;81(1):23–7
37 Rutter M, O'Connor T, et al. Are there biological programming effects for psychological development? findings from a study of Romanian adoptees. Developmental Psychology 2004;40(1):81–94
38 Hay D, Pawlby S, Waters CS, et al. Mother's antenatal depression and their children's antisocial outcomes. Child Development 2010;81:149–65
39 Murray L, Cooper PJ. Effects of postnatal depression on infant development. Arch Dis Child 1997;77:99–101
40 Avan B, Richter LM, Ramchandani PG, et al. Maternal postnatal depression and children's growth and behaviour during the early years of life: exploring the interaction between physical and mental health. Arch Dis Chil 2010;95:690–5
41 Essex MJ, Klein MH, Cho E, Kraemer HC. Exposure to maternal depression and marital conflict: gender differences in children's later mental health symptoms. J Am Acad Child Adolsec, Psychiatry 2003;42(6):728–37
42 Emde R N. Changing Models of infancy and the nature of early development: remodeling the foundation. J American Psychoanalytic Assocn 1981;1:179–219
43 Sameroff AJ, Chandler M. Reproductive risk and the continuum of caretaking casualty. Review of Child Development Research, No 4. Chicago: Univ of Chicago Press; 1975. p. 187–244
44 Flouri E, Tzavidis N, Kallis C. Adverse life events, area socioeconomic disadvantage, and psychopatholgy and resilience in young children: the importance of risk factors' accumulation and protective factors' specificity. European Child Adolesc Psychiatry 2010;19:535–46
45 Eggerman M, Panter-Brick C. Suffering, hope and entrapment: resilience and cultural values in Afghanistan. Social Science and Medicine 2010;71:71–83
46 Barkovich AJ. Formation, maturation and disorder of brain neocortex. American Journal of Neuroradiology 1992;13(2):423–46
47 Giedd JN, Blumenthal J, Jeffries N, et al. Brain development during childhood and adolescence: a longitudinal MRI study. Nature Neuroscience 1999;2(10):861–3
48 Wozniak JR, Lim KO. Advances in white matter imaging: a review of in vivo magnetic resonance methodologies and their applicability to the study of development and aging. Neuroscience and Biobehavioral Reviews 2006;30:762–74
49 Suzuki M, Hagino H, Nohara S, et al. Male-specific volume expansion of the human hippocampus during adolescence. Cerebral Cortex 2005;15:187–93
50 Yang F, Shan ZY. Mapping developmental precentral and postcentral gyral changes in children on magnetic resonance images. Journal of Magnetic Resonance Imaging 2010;33:62–70
51 Spierer L, De Lucia M, Bernasconi F, et al. Learning-induced plasticity in human audition: objects, time and space. Hearing Research 2011;271:88–102

52 Abdul-Kareem IA, Stancak A, Parkes LM, et al. Increased gray matter volume of left pars opercularis in male orchestral musicians correlates positively with years of musical performance. Journal of Magnetic Resonance Imaging 2011;33(1):24–32
53 Babikian T, Prins ML, Cai Y, et al. Molecular and physiological responses to juvenile traumatic brain injury: focus on growth and metabolism. Developmental Neuroscience 2010;32(5–6):431–41
54 Honda N, Matuoka T, Sawada Y, et al. Reorganization of sensorimotor function after functional hemispherectomy studied using near-infrared spectroscopy. Pediatric Neurosurgery 2010;46(4):313–17
55 Doidge N. The brain that changes itself. Carlton North, Melbourne: Scribe, 2007
56 Darrah J, Hodge M, Magill-Evans J, et al. Stability of serial assessments of motor and communication abilities in typically developing infants – implications for screening. Early Human Development 2003;72:97–110
57 Darrah J, Senthilselvan A, Magill-Evans J. Trajectories of serial motor scores of typically developing children: Implications for clinical decision making. Infant Behavior and Development 2009;32:72–8
58 Ukoumunne OC, Wake M, Carlin J, et al. Profiles of language development in pre-school children: a longitudinal latent class analysis of data from the Early Language in Victoria Study. Child Care, Health and Development. 24 Mar 2011. doi:10.1111/j.1365-2214.2011.01234.x
59 Egan DF. Developmental examination of infants and preschool children. Clinics in Developmental Medicine, ch 1 Normal development. London: Mac Keith Press; 1990
60 Wright M, Oberklaid F. Child development – issues in early detection. Community Paediatric Review 2003;12:1–3
61 Carter JA, Lees JA, Murira GM, et al. Issues in the development of cross-cultural assessments of speech and language for children. International Journal of Language and Communication Disorders 2005;40(4):385–401
62 D'Aprano AL, Carapetis JR, Andrews R. Trial of a developmental screening tool in remote Australian Aboriginal communities: a cautionary tale. Journal of Paediatrics and Child Health 2011;47:12–17
63 Hooper VS, Bell SM. Concurrent validity of the Universal Nonverbal Intelligence Test and the Leiter International Performance Scale-Revised. Psychology in Schools 2006;43(2):143–8
64 Legg S, Hutter M. Universal Intelligence: A definition of machine intelligence. Minds and Machines 2007;17:391–444. DOI 10.1007/s11023-007-9079-x
65 Ronald B David. Pediatric neurology for the clinician. Norwalk, Connecticut: Appleton & Lange; 1992
66 John H Menkes. Textbook of child neurology. 3rd ed. Philadelphia: Lea & Febiger; 1985
67 Fenton-May J, Bradley DM, et al. Screening for Duchenne muscular dystrophy. Archives of Disease in Childhood 1994;70:551–2

FURTHER READING

Gesell A. The mental growth of the preschool child. New York: Macmillan; 1925. (The work of Gesell in 1925 emphasised the acquisition of milestones as indicators of neurologic integrity.)
Brazelton TB. Neonatal behavioral assessment scale. Clin Child Dev Med 1973;50
Dubowitz L, Dubowitz V. The neurological assessment of the preterm and full-term newborn infant. Philadelphia: JB Lippincott; 1981. (Brazelton in 1973 [b] and Dubowitz in 1981 [c] used the combination of psychological and neurological items to indicate progress when examining newborn infants.)
David RB. Child and adolescent neurology. 2nd ed. Massachusetts: Blackwell; 2005
Rosenberg MJ, Wolff CR, El-Emawy A, et al. Effects of moderate drinking during pregnancy on placental gene expression. Alcohol 2010;44:673–90

Fetal Alcohol Spectrum Disorders: extending the range of structural defects. American Journal of Medical Genetics, Part A 2010;152A(11):2731–5

Burns H. Properly functioning families are the key to making Scotland healthier, 20/12/2009 (Commentary on social disadvantage, parenting and health). Online. Available: http://news.scotsman.com/health/Harry-Burns-39Properly-functioning-families.5926334.jp; 16 Feb 2012

2 Developmental assessment in the young child

Natalie Silove

The vision of a paediatrician crawling on all fours on the floor, making strange noises, flashing a light with a piggy on the top of it, playing peekaboo and waving bye-bye with an over-the-top grin, always comes into mind when considering a developmental assessment of a young child. As a result we never video record ourselves doing an assessment, but these strange behaviours are mostly for good reasons, other than an opportunity to have fun and play!

DEFINITIONS AND BASIC CONCEPTS

- Child development goes through definitive stages and phases that are constant for all typically developing children, although there is significant variability among them.
- 'Typical' or 'normal' development refers to development that occurs in the expected order and time frame, while 'atypical' development refers to development that is significantly different from that expected as compared to peers of the same age, sex and background.
- Development infers change. Each developmental phase has a past and a future. An assessment of the present phase allows for a prediction of the next one.
- Development includes a physical increase in size.
- There is psychological growth seen with an increase in function and ability.
- Development and maturity take time.
- Motor development occurs in a cephalo–caudal route (from head to toe) and from proximal to distal (face to fingers).
- Development moves from the general to the specific, e.g. pincer grasping of an object (by one year of age) develops into pencil control and handwriting skills (preschool years).
- Development has a compound interest effect. Each developmental phase builds on the previous ones and allows for further broader aspects of development. For example, the ability to move (crawl or walk) opens up further opportunities for exploring and learning.[1]
- *Delayed* developmental milestones are achieved in the 'typical' order but with an increase in the length of time between achieved milestones, e.g. instead of sitting, crawling and standing at 6, 8 and 10 months, the infant achieves these milestones at 12, 18 and 24 months respectively.
- *Disordered* development refers to achieving milestones not in the expected sequence, e.g. some children with autism may rote learn chunks of language

consisting of many sentences before they are able to generate their own spontaneous two-word phrases.
- Development can be both delayed and disordered.

WHY MONITOR DEVELOPMENT?

It is estimated that 16 per cent of children have a developmental and/or behavioural disorder. Only 30 per cent of these children are identified before school entrance. The opportunity to participate in early intervention programs, shown to have significant benefits, is therefore missed.[2] The National Health and Medical Research Council Report on Screening and Surveillance in Children concluded that the early identification of developmental delay/disability (or of significant risk factors for their occurrence) and subsequent early intervention can improve developmental and other social outcomes.[3]

Developmental domains

It is best to clearly separate the developmental domains to ensure they are all considered.

Communication

Both verbal and non-verbal communication should be taken into consideration.

Verbal communication
- Expressive language: early feeding history includes latching, sucking, transition to solids (the muscles used for feeding are the same as those used for speech). In broad terms the child is expected to have single specific words by 12 months (dad, mum, dog, bottle), two-word spontaneous combinations by two years (bottle please, pick up), and three-word combinations (including a verb) by three years of age (I go out?).
- Receptive language refers to the understanding (semantics) of language. In general terms young children will follow one-step instructions by one year of age, two-step instructions by two years and three-step instructions by three years.
- Articulation refers to the motor aspects of producing expressive language (i.e. how much of what the child is saying is intelligible).
- Prosody refers to the musicality and expression of the expressive language (i.e. is the language used with intonation or is the voice monotonous, staccato and unusual in pitch or accent?).
- Pragmatics refers to the social appropriateness of the language used (e.g. when asked 'how old are you?' the answer ' Thomas is red' is inappropriate and unrelated).

Non-verbal communication
This refers to the combination of gestures and facial expression that the child uses to communicate with others. Many children who have English as a second language express their needs and thoughts using appropriate gestures and expressions. Smiling appropriately, pointing to request with coordinated eye contact (under one year of age), waving bye-bye socially and spontaneously by 1 year of age, giving gestural 'instructions' such as 'go away' or 'come here' by 2 years of age, and descriptive gestures such as 'big' and 'little' by three years. Facial expressions

directed to others to impart feelings are very effective means of communication not to be overlooked during assessment.

Gross motor skills
Gross motor skills refer to movement involving the larger muscle groups. Motor development occurs in a cephalo–caudal route (from head to toe). In practical terms, the baby will attain head control by three months (neck control), sit independently by 6 months (truncal control), crawl by 8 months (hip control), stand by 10 to 12 months and walk by 18 months (lower limb control). In addition, motor development occurs from 'proximal to distal', i.e. facial (lips, tongue, eyes), neck, shoulders, arms, hands and fingers. As this development occurs it is clear that primitive neurological reflexes need to be inhibited before the next skill can be acquired. Examples would include the sucking reflex, which requires inhibition and must be under voluntary control for the infant to be able to chew rather than suck; the asymmetric tonic neck reflex (ATNR) that requires inhibition to allow the infant to roll. The emergence of new reflexes is essential, such as the parachute reflex where the arms come out to prevent one falling on one's face!

Fine motor skills (eye–hand coordination)
Fine motor development evolves with control of the hand, fingers and thumb, and ultimately is aimed towards the skills of handwriting and typing. Gross motor development occurs first and fine motor skills become increasingly developed once the child is able to adopt the upright position. Fine motor development is very dependent on adequate vision, so any delay in fine motor development should alert to a formal visual assessment, and vice versa.

Personal–social skills
These skills refer to the development of independence in a practical sense such as self-help skills, but also the development of personality and awareness of 'separateness' from others. Adaptive functioning includes the ability to feed, toilet, dress and eventually be able to live independently in all aspects. Social skill development evolves from the awareness of others and develops towards meaningful relationships. Relationships begin with the infant and primary carer, move to include other family members and then extend towards peers and the community.

Cognitive skills
This refers to thinking, reasoning and problem-solving skills. Testing of these skills 'in isolation' in the young child is difficult as most tests involve either fine motor (e.g. building with blocks, drawing) or language skills. These skills can be tested using puzzles, block designs and understanding of concepts, such as money and time.

Play skills
Play is often described as 'children's work' as it is such an important part of their learning, development and understanding of the world around them. Play milestones can be broadly described as below.

Social
- Solitary: child plays alone with no interest in engaging others
- Parallel: child will play alongside others but not 'chat' or interact with them (2–2½ yr)

- Spectator: child observes others play but does not engage (2½–3 yr)
- Associative and leading into cooperative play: child shares ideas in groups (+3 yr).

Functional
- Exploratory: child explores the object by shaking, licking, touching the toy
- Functional: child uses the toy for its intended use, e.g. a spoon used to eat
- Symbolic: child uses the object for a function it was not intended for, e.g. a spoon used as a flying broomstick.

Attention and behaviour

Attention and behaviour impact on learning and development, and vice versa. Attention to goal-directed tasks, such as 'reading' a book, listening to a story, completing a puzzle, is vital for learning. Watching television is not a goal-directed task as it is very passive, and is often confused by parents as they report that 'Charlie's attention is excellent when he is interested and wants to, he can watch 2 hours of television straight!'

OFFICE-BASED DEVELOPMENTAL ASSESSMENT

Screening tools

In order to identify atypical development, it is essential to know what typical development is.

It is important to be familiar with significant milestones in each area of development. Please refer to Chapter 1 for reference to normal milestones.

The use of a developmental screening tool as a routine can be a helpful addition to alert that there may be a concern (see Table 2.1).[4]

> **Practice Point**
>
> **Formal screening tools** such as the Denver II can be useful as a guide to expected 'evolution' of milestones, monitoring ongoing development, and contributing to a comprehensive history and physical examination. However the Denver II, while accurately identifying 80 per cent of children with developmental delay, also only identifies approximately 40 per cent of typically developing children.[5]
>
> A helpful website to assist in choosing the best screening tool for a particular practice or population can be found online at http://www.commonwealthfund.org/Content/Publications/Fund-Manuals/2008/Feb/Pediatric-Developmental-Screening--Understanding-and-Selecting-Screening-Instruments.aspx; 14 Feb 2012

Why do an office assessment?

Assessment implies that there should be specific outcomes. Ten questions to be answered are:
1. Is the development delayed, disordered or both?
2. Is the delay isolated to one area of development (isolated delay) or two or more areas of delay (global delay)?

TABLE 2.1 Tools for developmental screening

Name	Age range	Description	Scoring	Time frame	Availability
Parents' evaluation of developmental status	0–8 years	Ten questions eliciting parents' concerns. Written at a 5th grade reading level. Through the use of the PEDS Score and Interpretation Forms it advises when to refer, provide a second screen, provide patient education, or monitor development, behaviour and academic progress.	Identifies children as low, moderate or high risk	2 min	Centre for Community Child Health, Royal Children's Hospital, Parkville, Vic 3052 Ph: 03 9345 6150 Fax: 03 9345 5900 Email: enquiries.cch@rch.org.au
Ages and Stages Questionnaire, 3rd Edition (ASQ-3)	0–66 months	Parent report questionnaire. Clear drawings and simple directions help parents indicate child's skills. Separate reproducible forms of 25–35 items for each age range.	Single pass or fail score for each developmental domain and a summary score	7 min	MacLellan & Petty, Suite 405, 152 Bunnerong Road, Eastgardens, NSW 2036 Ph: 02 9349 5811 Fax: 02 9348 5911
Brigance Screens	0–90 months	Uses direct elicitation and observation. Four screening books are available with nine separate forms, one for each 12-month range. Taps speech–language, motor, readiness and general knowledge at younger ages and also reading and maths at older ages. In the 0–2 year age range, can be administered by parent report	Cut-off and age equivalent scores for motor, language, readiness and a summary score	10–15 min	Hawker Brownlow Education, 1123a Nepean Hwy, Highett, Vic 3190 Ph: 1800 334 603 Fax: 03 9553 4538

3 How significant is the delay, i.e. what impact does it have on the child's learning and daily life?
4 Is the child hearing impaired?
5 Is the child vision impaired?
6 Is the child dysmorphic?
7 Is there an identifiable cause for the delay?
8 What further assessments are required?
9 What intervention is required?
10 What follow up is required, and with whom?

Setting the stage

A number of important factors require consideration when setting the stage for a developmental assessment. Most important is to make sure the young child and their parent feel comfortable, relaxed and not rushed. A good rapport that is culturally sensitive should be established, so that parents feel valued and not 'judged'. The environment needs to be light, clean and spacious with sufficient room for the child to move and explore toys independently; and the toys on display should be appropriate for the developmental age (safe and interesting).

Have all your necessary equipment ready and easily accessible, so that it is easy to maintain the child's attention once you have their interest. Young children have a limited attention span, tend to move quickly from one activity to the next, and go from happy to irritable, tired and hungry very quickly. There's a need to be ready to engage and 'test' when the opportunity arises. Often a few attempts are necessary (over several visits), especially for children who may have difficulty separating from parents to sit at a table, run around, or become anxious in new and unfamiliar environments.

At times it may be best to assess in a familiar environment such as the home or the preschool. However while providing great opportunity for valuable observation, these environments are often very distracting making formal assessment difficult. The clinic is always preferable as the environment is more controlled.

History

As in any other area of medicine, history is vital and will often give you all the information required if the historian knows the child well and is reliable in their observation. History has proven to be so reliable that many questionnaires on development and adaptive behaviour are used for screening and diagnostic purposes and take into account the performance of the child in their own environment (see Table 2.1).

The history required is detailed and often takes 30–60 minutes depending on the complexity of the presentation and parental concerns. Always begin with asking what the parental concerns are, so that parents are immediately engaged and see the relevance of providing the history. If the concern is delayed speech and language, begin with communication and then enquire about the other areas of development.

Enquire how many languages the family speaks at home, whether English is the first or second language, which language the child speaks and understands best, and whether the family feel the child is developing appropriately in the primary language spoken at home.

When asking about a milestone, clarify whether the skill is fully established (present most of the time) rather than a skill that the child demonstrates on occasion. Regression refers to the loss of an established skill and occurs in up to 30 per cent of children with ASD, some neurological disorders (aphasic epileptic syndromes), neurodegenerative disorders and inborn errors of metabolism.

History includes: method of conception, pregnancy, maternal health, gestation, birth, Apgar scores, neonatal progress, medication, chronic illness or hospitalisation, head injuries, seizure disorders, malnutrition, meningitis, spina bifida, physical or emotional abuse or neglect, lead poisoning, muscular dystrophies, infections such as acquired immune deficiency syndrome, genetic disorders, inborn errors of metabolism, sleep, diet, behaviour, hearing, vision and family history, including level of education achieved, occupation and mental health. (Refer to Chapter 6 Specific learning disorders, Chapter 8 Attention deficit hyperactivity disorder and Chapter 10 School refusal and truancy for assessment approach.)

It is best to clearly separate the developmental domains to ensure that they are all discussed. Different questionnaires and tools describe and combine these domains slightly differently, but the general concept is similar. Failure to do this in a structured organised way may lead to failure to recognise specific developmental delays or patterns in disordered development, e.g. autism spectrum disorder.

Domains:
- Speech and language
- Fine motor skills
- Gross motor skills
- Personal social skills
- Cognitive skills
- Play
- Behaviour
- Attention.

Observations

In no other area of medicine is observation more important. Observation begins when the child and family are first seen and greeted. Everything the child does (and doesn't do) needs to be noted. Observations include: how is the child *spontaneously* communicating, moving around, playing and responding to the people and environment.

Often once the child is aware that you are a doctor and you start examining them … the fun and games are over! That's when you need to move quickly and complete the physical and neurological examination as well as possible.

Helpful 'props'
- Light
- Interesting small toy that does not make a noise
- Bell or rattle
- Hundreds and thousands
- Raisins or round cereal that dissolves quickly in the mouth
- Crayons, pencils and paper
- Ten 2.5 cm blocks (preferably in different colours so they can be used to test whether the child knows colours)

- Ball
- Toy cup, spoon and fork
- Tape measure, stethoscope and patella hammer.

Physical examination

How this occurs depends on the age of the child. A small child who is happy sitting on the parents lap could be left there to assess vision, hearing and language skills. However to assess fine motor and cognitive skills, it is important to have the child settled comfortably in front of a hard surface such as the floor or a table. Make sure the table and chair are an appropriate height and that the child's feet can reach the ground.

The method of testing **vision** depends on the age of the child. It is possible to test the ability to fix and follow using a light, toy or ball of red wool. Use a toy that does not make a noise, otherwise it is impossible to know if the child is following the sound or the visual cue. Placing hundreds and thousands on a hard surface for infants (1 year old), using Allen picture cards (or equivalent) or Stycar balls for older children can give an indication of visual acuity. Testing each eye separately using glasses with one eye patched can be trialled but may upset the child. *If there is any concern or difficulty in accurately assessing vision, it is important to refer to an ophthalmologist.*

Adequate **hearing** assessment is not possible in an office situation, but it is possible to assess whether the child can *localise* to sound. To do this, a helper is required. Someone needs to distract the child with a toy or book, while someone else stands behind the child and rings a bell or rattle and observes whether the child responds or not. This is done on both sides and repeated if necessary. *If there is any speech and language delay, formal hearing assessment is required regardless of the outcome of this office-based assessment.*

Fine motor skill is assessed while observing how the child grasps a small object, e.g. raisin or rattle, and holds a pencil while drawing. Once engaged in fine motor tasks it is easy to move onto the blocks and see how many the child can stack in a tower, then in a row on the table, build a 'gate' or copy 'stairs'. A pencil can then be introduced if appropriate and the child asked to copy the shapes drawn by the examiner. Thereafter the child is asked to draw their best picture of a person. (See Figure 2.2 Gesell figures[6] and Figure 2.3 Goodenough–Harris Drawing Test.[7,8])

During this process the child's use of **language** should be noted.

With regards **self-help skills**, take the opportunity to observe the child eat a snack and drink from a bottle or cup. Also observe how they indicate their toilet needs.

To assess **gross motor skills**, the child will need to be coaxed off the parent's lap to engage in running, jumping and ball skills. If stairs are available and are safe, observations can be made of how the child manages going up and down the stairs.

See Table 2.2 for physical examination and investigations.

Physical examination includes:
- Growth parameters (height, weight, head circumference)
- Dysmorphism
- Skin for hyper- and hypo-pigmented lesions (preferably using a Wood's lamp)

CHAPTER 2   Developmental assessment in the young child   ■   33

TABLE 2.2   Physical examination and investigations

Bayley Infant Neurodevelopmental screener (BINS)	3–24 m	Directly elicited items Neurology (reflexes tone) Neurodevelopmental skills (movement and symmetry) Milestones (object permanence, imitation, language)	Cut offs for low, moderate, high risk 10–15 min	http://psychcorp.com
Battelle Developmental Inventory Screening test (BDIST)	12–96 m	Discrete domains, receptive and expressive language, fine and gross motor, adaptive, personal–social, cognitive and academic	Provides age equivalents (1.5SD below the mean providing best sensitivity and specificity) 15–35 min	Riverside Publishing Company, 8420 Bryn Mawr Ave, Chicago, Illinois http://www.riverpub.com/
The Australian Developmental Screening Test (ADST)	6 m–5 y	Five domains of development: personal–social, language, cognitive, fine motor, gross motor	15–20 min	http://psychcorp.com

- Other neurocutaneous stigmata
- Cardiac
- Neurological examination including cranial nerves
- Vision
- Hearing.

Medical investigations[9]

Clinical diagnosis may be evident following physical examination, e.g. Down syndrome or neurofibromatosis. Subsequent medical investigations can then be targeted where global developmental delay is confirmed.

When organic cause for delay is not clinically obvious, the first-line investigations would include Array Comparative Genomic Hybridisation (ACGH). Other genetic investigations will need to be considered on a case by case basis, including standard cytogenetic examination, to exclude an apparently balanced rearrangement not detectable with CGH. Investigations include:
- DNA for Fragile X
- Electrolytes, urea, creatinine
- Creatine kinase
- Lead
- Thyroid function tests

- Urate
- Full blood count
- Ferritin
- Urine amino and organic screen plus mucopolysaccharide screen (MPS)
- Routine EEG and cranial imaging is not indicated.

Second-line investigations depend on the individual presentation and referral to a neurologist, metabolic or genetic specialist should be considered.

'Informal' assessment tools to use in the office[6]

Blocks

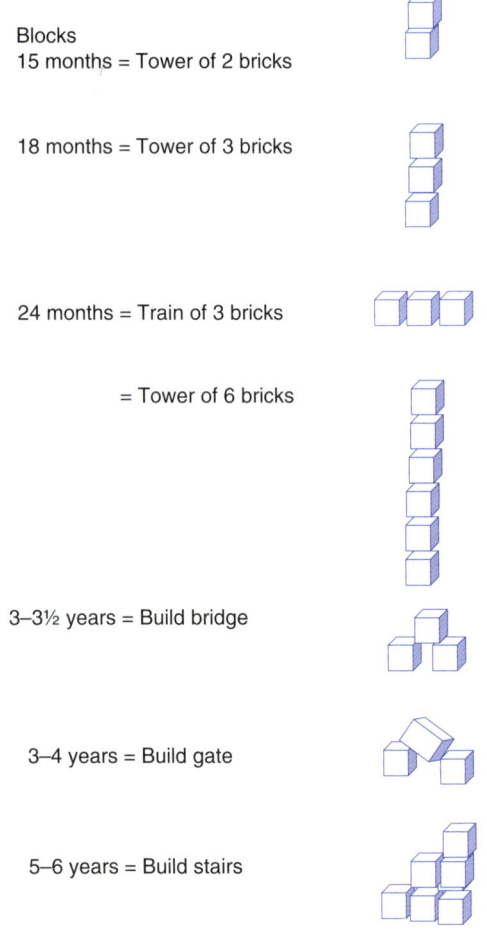

Blocks
15 months = Tower of 2 bricks

18 months = Tower of 3 bricks

24 months = Train of 3 bricks

= Tower of 6 bricks

3–3½ years = Build bridge

3–4 years = Build gate

5–6 years = Build stairs

FIGURE 2.1 Block assessment tool.

Pencil

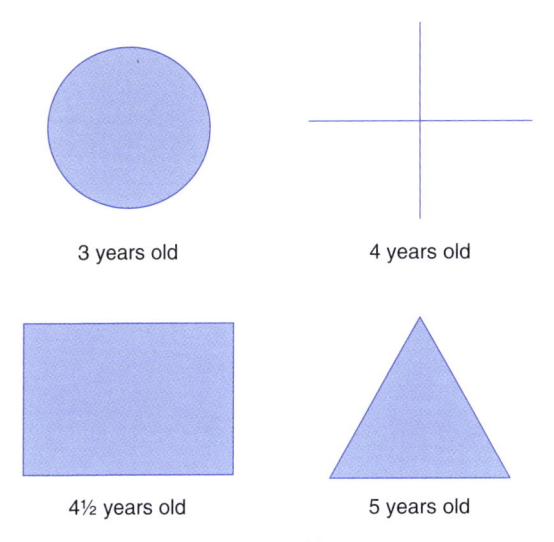

3 years old

4 years old

4½ years old

5 years old

FIGURE 2.2 Gesell figures for preschool age children.

Goodenough–Harris drawing test

Developed originally by Florence Goodenough in 1926, this test was first known as the Goodenough Draw-A-Man test. Dale B Harris later revised and extended the test, now known as the Goodenough–Harris Drawing Test. The child is asked to draw the best person they can draw. The starting point is a circle for the face at 3 years of age. An additional point is then given for each item drawn, with each point being worth an extra 3 months.

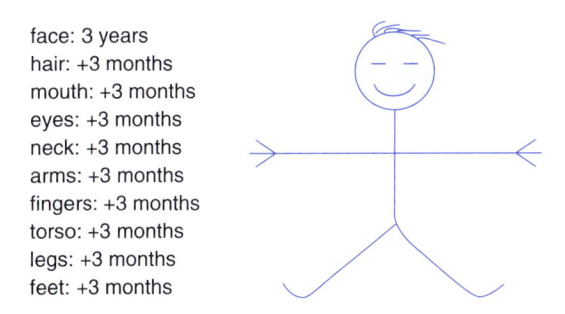

face: 3 years
hair: +3 months
mouth: +3 months
eyes: +3 months
neck: +3 months
arms: +3 months
fingers: +3 months
torso: +3 months
legs: +3 months
feet: +3 months

3 years + (9 × 3 months) = 5 years 3 months

FIGURE 2.3 Goodenough–Harris Drawing Test.

Multidisciplinary developmental assessment[10]

After the screening and office-based assessment, one should have an idea whether the young child's development is within the broad range of average expected for age or whether there remains concerns regarding development in one or more areas.

If the concern is regarding an isolated delay, referral to that specific professional is indicated, that is, speech and language pathologist (and hearing test), physiotherapist (motor and tone), occupational therapist (fine and gross motor coordination), clinical psychologist (behaviour, parenting) and formal vision assessment.

If there is concern regarding delay in two or more areas of development, referral to a multidisciplinary specialist unit or professional(s) is required for comprehensive diagnosis and assessment. Standardised developmental assessments require formal training that is costly and time consuming. It is advisable that professionals undertaking these formal assessments have in-depth understanding of child development and the issues that impact on development. At least two or more professionals may be involved in the comprehensive assessment (see Fig 2.4).

The multidisciplinary team may consist of a medical specialist (paediatrician or neurologist), psychologist, speech pathologist, occupational therapist (usually to assess toddlers and older children), physiotherapist (to assess the younger infants), with referrals made to other subspecialties as required.

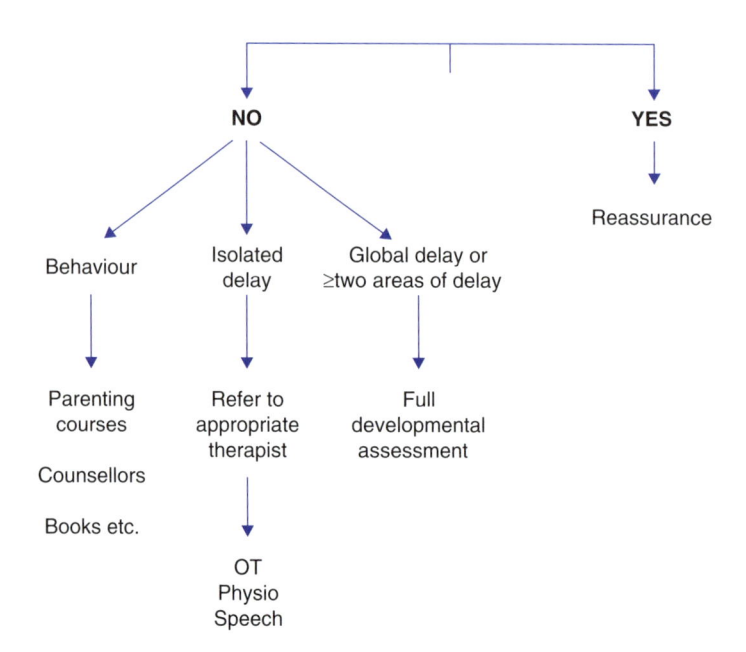

Note: If unsure, err on the side of caution and refer to a paediatrician

FIGURE 2.4 Is the development normal?

The process follows a similar pattern to that described above:
- Review of relevant information from parents, carers, teachers, therapists and all previous reports and assessments, which often requires a telephone call to preschools and day care centres so that their observations and concerns are also taken into consideration
- Detailed history from the parents
- Medical assessment as described above
- Observations may be required in a number of settings (office, home, preschool)
- Standardised testing of developmental domains
- Formulation of the clinical presentation, diagnosis and comorbidity
- Medical investigations as outlined in Table 2.2
- Discussion and feedback with parents
- Providing a written report of the findings and recommendations
- Follow up and review of progress and needs throughout childhood, adolescence and during transition to adulthood.

The assessment process may occur over several visits as the young child is usually only able to participate for relatively short periods of time.

Standardised assessments

These assessments include the following:
1. Developmental assessments
   Generally carried out for children under the age of four years. The Griffiths may be used when an older child has a significant developmental delay and items on the psychometric assessment are too difficult or not engaging enough. Paediatricians, psychologists and occupational therapists are able to administer the Bayley-III, while only paediatricians and psychologists can administer the Griffiths.
   - The Bayley Scales of Infant Development (Bayley-III): 0 to 3.6 years old
   - Griffiths Mental Development Scales, Revised: birth to 2 years
   - Griffiths Mental Development Scales, Extended Revised: 2 to 8 years
2. Psychometric assessments (by clinical psychologists)
   Some IQ assessments are normed for children as young as two years old, **but** intellectual assessment is not usually appropriate (not indicated nor accurate) in the preschool aged child. Intellectual assessment is performed usually from the age of four years in order to assess suitable school placement and to prioritise intervention. The intellectual assessment of choice depends on the verbal abilities of the child, sensory issues (vision and hearing) and behaviour.
   Commonly used psychometric tests include:
   - The Wechsler Preschool and Primary Scale of Intelligence, Third Edition (WPPSI III)
   - Differential Ability Scales II (DAS II)
   - Stanford–Binet Intelligence Scale, Fifth Edition
   - The Kaufman Assessment Battery for Children, Second Edition (KABC-II)
3. Adaptive functioning
   - Vineland Adaptive Behavior Scales, Second Edition (Vineland-II)
   - Adaptive Behavior Assessment System-Second Edition (ABAS-II)

4   Psychosocial Assessment and behaviour
5   Speech therapist: speech and language assessments
6   Occupational therapist: fine and gross motor, sensory processing

Follow-up and review

- Ongoing monitoring of development is important in all children
- Developmental issues and other concerns can arise at any time
- Having a developmental delay places the child at risk for future developmental or learning difficulties
- Transition periods (e.g. preschool to school, primary school to secondary school, and school to post-school options and adulthood) are critical times for development
- Medical review is required to monitor for expected problems associated with a specific condition, e.g. recurrent otitis media in Down syndrome. Conditions associated with developmental delay may increase the risk of other problems (epilepsy) and associated co-morbid conditions, e.g. attention deficit hyperactivity disorder, anxiety.

Family support

Raising children is challenging, expensive and can be anxiety generating for parents, even more so if a child has a developmental disability. As health professionals, supporting a child to develop and meet their potential requires forming a partnership with families and carers. This includes support for siblings, providing the necessary information to parents and advocacy with other institutions, such as the educational and social support systems.

CONCLUSION

In conclusion, developmental surveillance is important for all children. Often a number of visits are required to identify that a child's development is atypical and not following the expected developmental trajectory. Identifying a developmental disorder early allows for appropriate intervention to commence and provides the best opportunity for optimal outcomes. Monitoring development over a period of time and reviewing at critical periods of transition allows for identifying issues and better planning of needs into the future. Optimal care includes a multidisciplinary approach, good communication and working in partnership with families and carers.

REFERENCES

1. Pollak M. Textbook of Developmental Paediatrics. London: Churchill Livingstone; 1993
2. LaRosa A, Glascoe F. Developmental surveillance and screening in primary care. UptoDate 2011. Online. Available: http://www.uptodate.com; 21 March 2011
3. NHMRC Report on Screening and Surveillance in Children. Online. Available: http://www.nhmrc.gov.au/guidelines/publications/ch42; 22 Feb 2012
4. Wright M, Oberklaid F. Child development – issues in early detection. Community Paediatric Review April 2003;12(1)
5. Frankenburg WK, Dodds J, Archer P, et al. The Denver II: a major revision and restandardisation of the Denver Developmental Screening Test. Pediatrics 1992;89:91

6 Parry T. Assessment of developmental learning and behavioural problems in children and young people. MJA 2005;183(1):43–8
7 Goodenough F. Measurement of intelligence by drawings. New York: World Book Co; 1926
8 Harris DB. Children's drawings as measures of intellectual maturity. New York: Harcourt Brace & World; 1963
9 McDonald L, Rennie A, Tolmie J, et al. Investigation of global developmental delay. Arch Dis Child 2006;91:701–5
10 Shevell M, Ashwal S, Donley D, et al. Practice parameter: Evaluation of the child with global developmental delay: Report of the Quality Standards Subcommittee of the American Academy of Neurology and The Practice of the Child Neurology Society. Neurology 2003;60:367–80

3 Motor and coordination problems

Sandra Johnson with Manoj Menezes

INTRODUCTION

Appropriate electrical stimulation of the intact lower motor unit (anterior horn cell, peripheral nerve, neuromuscular junction and muscle) leads to muscle contraction. The resting tone, voluntary control of muscle contraction and coordination of movement is a complex process controlled by the upper motor unit (cortical neurons and descending motor tracts), cerebellum and basal ganglia. Coordination refers to the integrated functioning of various pathways to allow smooth and efficient movement.

The focus of this chapter is the motor and coordination problems that are seen in otherwise normally developing ambulant children. Previously referred to as 'motor dyspraxia', more recently the term 'developmental coordination disorder' has come to be widely accepted. Poorly recognised and often overlooked, these difficulties cause significant impairment in both academic achievement and activities of daily living.

The chapter does not discuss in detail movement disorders or inherited neuromuscular disorders, conditions that are best assessed and managed by paediatric neurologists. At the end of this chapter a list of textbooks that provide in-depth review of these disorders can be found.

Non-progressive motor impairment as a result of insult to the developing brain, usually within the first two years of life, is known as cerebral palsy and is discussed in Chapter 12.

DEVELOPMENTAL COORDINATION DISORDER (DCD) DEFINED

The DSM-V (proposed revisions) characterises DCD by the following criteria.[1]
A   Motor performance that is substantially below expected levels, given the person's chronologic age and previous opportunities for skill acquisition. The poor motor performance may manifest as coordination problems, poor balance, clumsiness, dropping or bumping into things; marked delays in achieving developmental motor milestones (e.g. walking, crawling, sitting); or in the acquisition of basic motor skills (e.g. catching, throwing, kicking, running, jumping, hopping, cutting, coloring, printing, writing).
B   The disturbance in Criterion A, without accommodations, significantly interferes with activities of daily living or academic achievement.
C   The disturbance is not due to a general medical condition (e.g. cerebral palsy, hemiplegia, or muscular dystrophy).

PREVALENCE AND COMORBIDITIES

The term 'developmental/motor dyspraxia' has commonly been used to describe children with motor coordination and motor planning problems.[2] Terms like 'the clumsy child syndrome', 'minor neurological dysfunction', 'minimal brain dysfunction', 'perceptio-motor dysfunction' and 'sensory motor dysfunction', have also been used. More recently, the term developmental coordination disorder has been used widely and criteria for the condition are outlined in DSM IV/V.

In the USA, it is estimated that 5–6 per cent of the population meets criteria for DCD.[3,4] Being born extremely premature and extremely-low-birth weight appears to be a risk factor for developing DCD, with a prevalence of DCD at 8 years of age – three times that in term born children.[5]

DCD represents a heterogenous group of children who have varying presentations related to their coordination skills. There is a high comorbidity with other developmental problems including ADHD (attention deficit hyperactivity disorder), autism spectrum disorder, specific learning disabilities and emotional disorders.[6–9]

In a Swedish community study of 409 seven-year-old children, approximately half of all the children with DCD had moderate to severe symptoms of ADHD.[10] A motor deficit is often identified in children with ADHD, and many will satisfy the criteria for DCD.[9] Learning with language difficulties and problems with speech and social communication skills may coexist in children with DCD, although they are less severe than the motor and coordination impairment.[2] Difficulties with empathy, social behaviour, and the presence of psychiatric disorders, particularly anxiety and depression, have also been reported.[11–13]

Consensus reached in Canada in 1995 and again in the UK in 2004 and 2006[14] agreed that:
- the core characteristic of DCD is marked impairment in motor skills
- the impairment has a significantly negative impact on activities of daily living like dressing, feeding, academic achievement and handwriting
- the condition is not due to general medical conditions like cerebral palsy or muscular dystrophy
- the diagnosis should not be given to individuals with IQ below 70
- it was recognised that comorbid conditions affecting attention, cognitive, language and social skills occur in DCD.

CLINICAL PRESENTATION

The preschool or school-aged child may present to the general practitioner or paediatrician because of parental or teacher concerns about their motor skills. The child might appear clumsy, bump into objects, have frequent falls and have difficulty with handwriting and pencil control. These difficulties may be associated with learning, attention and social interaction difficulties.

The history often reveals delay in acquisition of motor milestones and early awkwardness in motor coordination, and there may be a family history of similar motor difficulties. The clinician needs to ask about delayed walking or progressive weakness in a family member, which could indicate an inherited neuromuscular disorder.

Children with DCD show delay or difficulties with their gross and fine motor skills, but should have an otherwise normal neurological examination including normal muscle strength and reflexes. These difficulties may include:

- Problems with hopping, skipping, climbing and awkwardness when running
- Tendency to bump into objects and trip easily
- Poor pencil grip and control
- Poor letter formation and illegible handwriting
- Difficulty with doing buttons and shoelaces
- May struggle to speak in a clear and articulate way (verbal dyspraxia).

Occasionally 'soft' neurological signs such as mirror movements in one hand while doing precision finger movements with the other, finger agnosia (difficulty with copying the exact finger movements of the examiner) and some posturing of hands when performing complex tasks may be seen, and opinion varies about their relevance.

It is also important to recognise attention or concentration difficulties that may be consistent with a diagnosis of ADHD and children with DCD can often be:
- Fidgety and restless
- Poorly attentive and easily distracted
- Have difficulty with organising complex tasks
- Have short-term memory problems and poor retention of learned information.

PROGRESS AND OUTCOMES

Social interaction problems are not uncommon in children who have DCD, particularly in middle school years, where emphasis is placed on sport and physical prowess. These children can have poor self-esteem and may be the victims of bullying.[15]

Children who have DCD are often reluctant to participate in sport and physical activity because their clumsiness might then become more obvious to others. The result is that they withdraw from such activities, spend time in the school library during school breaks and display reluctance in attending school sport. As a result of this withdrawal, they run the risk of weight problems due to participation in only sedentary activities.

The motor difficulties may persist into adolescence and many children continue to perform poorly at school. Social and emotional difficulties also persist and may worsen.[16]

ASSESSMENT

Various normative-referenced tests are widely used to identify and monitor children with motor difficulties. These include:
- Griffiths Mental Development Scales (GMDS) measures five areas of development (gross motor skills, personal–social, hearing and language, eye and hand coordination and performance) in the 0–2 age group.
- Peabody Developmental Motor Scales, Second Edition, (PDMS–2) assesses both gross and fine motor development in children between 0–5 years and can be used to recommend specific interventions.
- Bruininks–Oseretsky Test of Motor Proficiency (BOTMP) assesses motor skills in children 4.5–14.5 years of age and is widely used for diagnostic testing and monitoring intervention programs.

Clinical assessment must include assessment of mental state where self-esteem and mood is a concern, particularly in view of comorbidity with anxiety and depression. The degree of motor impairment may correlate with anxiety in adolescents, particularly among males.[17]

> **Practice Point**
>
> There is a wide spectrum for motor coordination skills in the general population. Also, if the child has not had the opportunity to experience physical activities that enhance the development of motor skills, for reasons unrelated to a developmental problem, the child will be less able at physical tasks than his more experienced peers.
>
> The aim of assessment is to identify children who are having significant difficulties and not to 'medicalise' findings that the child does not perceive to be a problem, particularly where their motor functioning is not significantly outside the normal range for age.

EXCLUDING NEUROMUSCULAR DISORDERS

Before making the diagnosis of Developmental Coordination Disorder, it is necessary to confirm that the child has delay in gross motor milestones, and that language and social skills are preserved, although learning difficulties and language delay do not exclude a diagnosis of DCD.

Central (involving the brain and spinal cord) and peripheral or neuromuscular (involving anterior horn cell, peripheral nerve, neuromuscular junction or muscle) disorders may cause motor delay or abnormalities with motor coordination, and a detailed history and physical examination are essential to exclude them. A history of perinatal difficulties including fetal distress, the presentation and mode of delivery, Apgar scores and need for resuscitation and support in the neonatal period are important when considering the possibility of cerebral palsy. A family history of developmental delay, regression of milestones or a neuromuscular disorder, and the presence of consanguinity, indicate an inherited disorder and suggest the possible mode of inheritance. The age at which various developmental milestones were achieved should be accurately documented (refer to Chapter 1 and Tables 1.1, 1.2, 1.3 for a list of normal developmental milestones).

Children with DCD should have a normal neurological examination without weakness (focal or generalised), sensory loss, spasticity, cranial nerve abnormalities or cerebellar signs. Hypertonia, spasticity, brisk reflexes and a positive Babinski sign indicate a central disorder. Excessive ligamentous laxity may indicate a connective tissue disorder. Initial evaluation for a central disorder usually includes thyroid function tests, urine metabolic screen, serum lactate, cranial and spinal imaging, karyotype and a comparative genomic hybridisation (CGH) array.

Hypotonia and absent reflexes are indicative of a neuromuscular disorder. The commonly occurring neuromuscular inherited disorders presenting in childhood, and the level of lesion, are indicated in Table 3.1.

Identifying the level of the lesion and then achieving a specific genetic diagnosis requires an accurate clinical assessment followed by the appropriate

TABLE 3.1 Inherited neuromuscular disorders

Level of lesion	Common disorders
Anterior horn cell	Spinal muscular atrophy
Peripheral nerve	Charcot-Marie-Tooth disease (CMT)
Neuromuscular junction	Congenital myasthenic syndromes
	Juvenile myasthenia gravis
Muscle	Duchenne and Becker muscular dystrophy (DMD)
	Other limb–girdle dystrophies
	Congenital myopathies
	Congenital muscular dystrophies
	Myotonic dystrophy

investigations. The serum creatine kinase (CK) is significantly raised (>ten times the upper limit of normal) in muscular dystrophies, e.g. Duchenne muscular dystrophy, and is raised to a lesser extent with spinal muscular atrophy and other myopathies. Histopathological examination, electron microscopy and immuno-blotting on a muscle biopsy are required when the underlying gene mutation cannot be identified from the clinical phenotype alone.[18,19]

There is increasing interest in the use of muscle MRI to differentiate inherited neuromuscular disorders.[20] Nerve conduction studies and EMG help identify the presence of the neuropathy and define its characteristics, helping direct genetic screening accurately.[21] The 'muscle chip', a method of screening for multiple gene mutations at the same time, and 'exome sequencing', a method of sequencing all coding regions of the genome, are exciting new modalities that promise to revolutionise the diagnosis of inherited neuromuscular disorders.[22]

Fifty per cent of boys with Duchenne muscular dystrophy from families without other affected relatives present because of delayed motor milestones.[23] The other half will learn to walk independently before 18 months of age, and appropriately achieving this milestone does not exclude the diagnosis.[24] Presence of a Gowers' sign when asked to rise from the supine position and hypertrophied calves may be seen on examination. The serum creatine kinase (CK) is significantly raised in affected boys and may be mild to moderately raised in carrier mothers. The diagnosis is confirmed by identifying a mutation on the dystrophin gene on multiplex PCR, multiplex ligation-dependent probe amplification (MLPA), or sequencing. Consensus standards for the diagnosis and management of boys with DMD have recently been published.[25]

Children with Charcot-Marie-Tooth disease (CMT), a genetically heterogeneous group of inherited peripheral neuropathies, may present with poor fine motor skills and difficulties with motor coordination. With progression, distal weakness and wasting, foot deformity and distal sensory loss are seen. Deep tendon reflexes are absent or reduced on examination.[26] Nerve conduction tests are necessary to define the presence and pattern of peripheral nerve involvement, and to guide genetic screening.[27]

Identifying children with these inherited neuromuscular diseases is essential to start appropriate disease-specific therapy and rehabilitation. In children with Duchenne muscular dystrophy, glucocorticoids (prednisolone, deflazacort) improve muscle strength and prolong ambulation, reduce risk of progressive scoliosis, and stabilise respiratory and cardiac function.[23,28] Early rehabilitation with physiotherapy and occupational therapy is necessary to prevent or delay contractures and foot deformity and preserve function in children with CMT. An accurate genetic diagnosis is also becoming increasingly important for counselling about risks with future pregnancies, for screening pregnancies, and for enrolment in clinical trials.

OTHER CAUSES OF MOTOR COORDINATION PROBLEMS

Difficulties with motor coordination may be identified in children who have other diagnoses. These include:

- **Autism spectrum disorder and Asperger syndrome** – In addition to their social and language difficulties, children with autism may also have a delay with their gross and fine motor skills and awkwardness with their coordination and gait.[29]
- **Down syndrome** – Children with Down syndrome are often hypotonic and show a delay and persisting difficulties with their gross and fine motor skills.[30]
- **Other inherited disorders** – Difficulties with motor coordination may also be seen with Klinefelter syndrome, Spondyloepiphyseal dysplasia, storage disorders (Hurler and Hunter syndromes), etc.

MANAGEMENT

The first step is to exclude medical/neurological causes of coordination problems, in particular cerebral palsy and neuromuscular disorders, through a detailed history and physical examination. The paediatrician needs to ensure that the neurological examination is normal, and consider referral to a paediatric neurologist if there are abnormalities. Continued follow-up is essential to ensure that there is no progression or worsening of the motor or cognitive difficulties.

Improved outcomes following early intervention for children with DCD is supported by research.[31,32] For the motor coordination difficulties, referral to an occupational therapist (OT) and a physiotherapist is recommended. The therapist will assess the child and develop a program to facilitate the child's fine and gross motor skill development. Ideally the therapist works closely with the parent or carer in a family-centered manner to ensure that the family can continue the techniques used during therapy sessions at home.

The OT assists with training in functional daily living skills like dressing, doing buttons and shoelaces, feeding and personal hygiene. The OT also assesses the child's handwriting and other fine motor difficulties that the child might experience in the school environment and suggests interventions. Physiotherapy intervention for improving gross motor skills is important, particularly in targeted areas relevant to the particular child's interests, e.g. goal scoring in netball and ball skills in soccer. Some schools have therapists either on staff or visiting the school on a regular basis.

Psychological support and counselling may be necessary where poor self-esteem resulting from poor motor skills, e.g. the child who is bullied by their classmates because of poor performance in sporting activities or general awkwardness.

It also helps to find a skill that the child is good at and focus therapy and intervention to develop that skill in order to improve self-esteem and to encourage a sense of achievement, e.g. music and art in the child who is clumsy due to poor gross motor skills.

Comorbid difficulties must also be addressed as a part of effective intervention. The child who has expressive speech difficulty (verbal dyspraxia) needs early referral to a speech and language therapist for targeted intervention. Where attention difficulties hinder learning progress, the child might need medication and special educational intervention. See Chapters 6 and 8.

Approaches to intervention

Modern intervention for DCD fits into one of two approaches.[14]

Process or deficit approach

- Aims to remedy a process deficit with intervention targeted at a neural structure, e.g. the cerebellum or sensory systems (balance/proprioception).
- Intervention involves **Sensory Integration Therapy (SIT)** based on the work of Ayres[33] who suggested that motor difficulties are not related to motor execution problems but are likely to be related to difficulty with processing sensory information.
- SIT involves proprioceptive, tactile/kinaesthetic and vestibular stimulation, which is believed to remedy the underlying sensory deficit.
- A fairly recent review has challenged this approach and concluded that it had little empirical support and does not follow current understanding on motor control.[34]

Functional skill approach

- Aims to teach activities of daily living, but is not directed at remediation of a neural or structural deficit.
- Early work involved a cognitive motor approach, which emphasised planning and execution of movement and the use of cognitive skills. This approach was updated and renamed **Ecological Intervention (EI)**. EI places emphasis on actual control of movement and aims to provide intervention in a family and community setting.[14]
- **Cognitive Orientation to Daily Occupational Performance program (CO-OP)**, developed in Canada, targets skill development, cognitive strategy use, generalisation and transfer of learning.[35] Cognitive strategies are used to facilitate task acquisition where the child is engaged in choosing therapy goals and is guided in the learning process so that specific difficulties for the child are addressed. Hence the approach is goal orientated and child centred.

> **Practice Point**
>
> While there is a lack of consensus on the most effective intervention for DCD and no comprehensive guide available,[14] there are a number of strategies that are useful irrespective of the type and degree of motor and coordination difficulty:
> - The goals for therapy should be directed towards activities that are functionally relevant to the child.
> - Focus therapy on functional activities necessary for daily living, like feeding, writing and dressing.
> - Therapy should be evidence based and supported by scientific knowledge of motor control and learning.
> - Family life and routines must be taken into account.
> - Involve important individuals in the child's life as far as possible, e.g. parents, teachers, community support persons, health professionals.

CONCLUSION

The child with motor coordination difficulty or DCD requires careful assessment to avoid undue emphasis on the inability to perform physical tasks that are not essential for daily living and are not of interest or relevance to the child. Children of different ages have varied skills and ability, and there is a broad range of ability in typically developing, healthy children.

The clinician plays an important role in assessing whether motor problems are significantly delayed and whether these problems negatively impact on the child's life. In the absence of such findings, reassurance for parents and encouraging activities that are consistent with the child's interests are important to help protect the child's sense of self worth. The aim of management and intervention is to improve the child's ability to function at home and at school without 'medicalising' a perceived difficulty, which could be within the broad range of normal development.

REFERENCES

1. American Psychiatric Association. Developmental Coordination Disorder. 2010. Online. Available: http://www.dsm5.org/ProposedRevision/Pages/proposedrevision.aspx?rid=88#; 5 May 2011
2. Kirby A, Sugden DA. Children with developmental coordination disorders. Journal of the Royal Society of Medicine 2007;100(4):182–6
3. Blondis TA. Developmental Coordination Disorder and ADHD. In: Accardo PJ, editor. Attention deficits in children and adults. New York: Marcel Decker; 2000. p. 344–5
4. American Psychiatry Association. Diagnostic and statistical manual of mental disorders (DSM IV–TR). 4th ed. Washington DC: American Psychiatric Association; 2000
5. Roberts G, Anderson PJ, Davis N, et al. Developmental coordination disorder in geographic cohorts of 8-year-old children born extremely preterm or extremely low birth weight in the 1990s. Dev Med Child Neurol 2011;53(1):55–60
6. Pitcher TM, Piek JP, Hay DA. Fine and gross motor ability in males with ADHD. Developmental Medicine and Child Neurology 2003;45:525–35

7. Sergeant JA, Piek JP, Oosterlaan J. ADHD and DCD: A relationship in need of research. Human Movement Science 2006;25:76–89
8. Fliers E, Vermeulen S, Rijsdijk F, et al. ADHD and poor motor performance from a family genetic perspective. Journal Am Acad Child Adolesc Psychiatry 2009;48(1):25–34
9. Kopp S, Beckung E, Gillberg C. Developmental coordination disorder and other motor control problems in girls with autism spectrum disorder and/or attention deficit hyperactivity disorder. Research in Developmental Disabilities 2010;31:350–61
10. Kadesjo B, Gillberg C. Developmental coordination disorder in Swedish 7-year-old children. J Am Acad Child Adolesc Psychiatry 1999;38(7):820–8
11. Cummins A, Piek JP, Dyck M. Motor coordination, empathy and social behaviour in school-aged children. Develop Med Child Neurol 2005;47(7):437–42
12. Cairney J, Veldhuizen S, Szatmari P. Motor coordination and emotional–behavioral problems in children. Current Opinion in Psychiatry 2010;23(4):324–9
13. Cairney J. Gross motor problems and psychiatry disorders in children. Develop Med Child Neurol 2010;53(2):104
14. Sugden D. Current approaches to intervention with developmental coordination disorder. Develop Med Child Neurol 2007;49:467–71
15. Piek JP, Barrett NC, Allen LS, et al. The relationship between bullying and self-worth in children with movement coordination problems. British Journal of Educational Psychology 2005;75(13):453–63
16. Losse A, Henderson SE, Elliman D, et al. Clumsiness in children – do they grow out of it? A 10-year follow-up study. Developmental Medicine & Child Neurology 1991;33:55–68
17. Sigurdsson E, Van Os J, Fombonne E. Are impaired childhood motor skills a risk factor for adolescent anxiety? Results from the 1958 UK Birth Cohort and the National Child Development Study. Am J Psychiatry 2002;159:1044–5
18. Sewry C. Muscular dystrophies: an update on pathology and diagnosis. Acta Neuropathol 2010;120(3):343–58
19. Sewry CA, Jimenez-Mallebrera C, Muntoni F. Congenital myopathies. Curr Opin Neurol 2008;21(5):569–75
20. Mercuri E, Pichiecchio A, Allsop J, et al. Muscle MRI in inherited neuromuscular disorders: past, present, and future. J Magn Reson Imaging 2007;25(2):433–40
21. Johnsen B, Fuglsang-Frederiksen A. Electrodiagnosis of polyneuropathy. Neurophysiologie Clinique/Clinical Neurophysiology 2000;30(6):339–51
22. Tesi-Rocha C, Hoffman E. Limb–girdle and congenital muscular dystrophies: current diagnostics, management, and emerging technologies. Current Neurology and Neuroscience Reports 2010;10(4):267–76
23. Bushby KM, Hill A, Steele JG. Failure of early diagnosis in symptomatic Duchenne muscular dystrophy. Lancet 1999;353(9152):557–8
24. Fenton-May J, Bradley DM, Sibert JR, et al. Screening for Duchenne muscular dystrophy. Archives of Disease in Childhood 1994;70:551–2
25. Bushby K, Finkel R, Birnkrant DJ, et al. Diagnosis and management of Duchenne muscular dystrophy, Part 1: diagnosis, and pharmacological and psychosocial management. Lancet Neurology 2010;9(1):77–93
26. Pareyson D, Marchesi C. Diagnosis, natural history, and management of Charcot-Marie-Tooth disease. Lancet Neurology 2009;8(7):654–67
27. Dyck PJ, Chance P, Lebo R, et al. Hereditary motor and sensory neuropathies. In: Dyck PJ, Thomas PK, Griffin JW, et al, editors. Peripheral Neuropathy. Philadelphia: WB Saunders; 1993. p. 1094–136
28. Moxley RT, Ashwal S, Pandya S, et al. Practice parameter: corticosteroid treatment of Duchenne dystrophy: report of the Quality Standards Subcommittee of the American Academy of Neurology and the Practice Committee of the Child Neurology Society. Neurology 2005;64(1):13–20
29. Jeste SS. The neurology of autism spectrum disorders. Curr Opin Neurol 2011;24(2):132–9
30. Spano M, Mercuri E, Rando T, et al. Motor and perceptual–motor competence in children with Down syndrome: variation in performance with age. Europ J Paediatr Neurol 1999;3:7–13

31 Mandich AD, Polatajko HJ, Missiuna CP, et al. Cognitive strategies and motor performance in children with developmental coordination disorder. Phys Occup Ther Pediatr 2001;20:125–43
32 Sugden DA, Chambers ME. Intervention approaches and children with developmental coordination disorder. Pediatric Rehabilitation 1998;2:139–47
33 Ayres AJ. Sensory Integration and the Child. Los Angeles: Western Psychological Services; 1979
34 Wilson PH. Approaches to assessment and treatment of children with DCD: an evaluative review. Journal Child Psychology Psychiatry 2005;46:806–23
35 Polatajko HJ, Mandich A. Enabling occupation in children. The Cognitive Orientation to Daily Occupational Performance (CO-OP) approach. Ottawa, ON: CAOT Publications ACE; 2004

FURTHER READING

Hall DMB. Clumsy children. British Medical J 1988;296:375–6
Developmental coordination disorder. Online. Available: http://www.dcd-uk.org/; 15 Feb 2012
Dyspraxia. Online. Available: http://www.dyspraxiafoundation.org.uk/; 15 Feb 2012
Chun RW, Shapiro SM. Movement disorders, ch 9. In: David RB, editor. Pediatric Neurology for the Clinician. Norwalk, Connecticut: Appleton & Lange; 1992
Lock T. Neurophysiologic Basis for the Treatment of Movement Disorders, ch 23. In: Capute AJ, Accardo PJ, editors. Developmental Disabilities in Infancy and Childhood. Baltimore, Maryland: Paul H Brookes Publishing; 1991
Jones HR, De Vivo DC, Darras BT, editors. Neuromuscular disorders of infancy, childhood, and adolescence: a clinician's approach. Philadelphia: Butterworth Heinemann; 2003

4 Hearing and vision loss

Shirley Russ

HEARING LOSS

DEFINITIONS

While there is no universally agreed definition of hearing loss in children, practically this refers to the loss of some or all hearing in one or both ears that may be temporary or permanent. The term 'deafness' is imprecise, and is generally reserved for those children who have no useable residual hearing. The United States *Individuals with Disabilities Education Act (IDEA)(2004)* defines deafness as 'a hearing impairment that is so severe that the child is impaired in processing linguistic information through hearing, with or without amplification'. IDEA further defines hearing impairment as 'an impairment in hearing whether permanent or fluctuating, that adversely affects a child's educational performance'.[1] In general, families prefer the terms 'hearing loss' and 'deaf' or 'hard of hearing', often abbreviated to DHH over 'hearing impairment'.

TYPES OF HEARING LOSS

There are three major types of hearing loss:
1. **Sensorineural hearing loss (SNHL):** caused by a defect in the cochlea, auditory nerve or central connections
2. **Conductive hearing loss:** resulting from disorders in the external or middle ear
3. **Mixed hearing loss:** in which there are features of both sensorineural and conductive losses.

A fourth type of loss, auditory neuropathy, has emerged as a distinct entity over the past decade. **Auditory neuropathy spectrum disorder (ANSD)** is a disorder of hearing in which cochlear function is essentially spared while auditory nerve activation is impaired. Children with ANSD may have speech perception and word discrimination problems that are disproportionate to their hearing thresholds.

> **Practice Point**
>
> Although the term 'impairment' is widely used in medical practice, it comes from a disability model and can carry negative connotations. Many deaf people do not regard their condition as a handicap, but rather as a part of their identity. Consequently, terms such as 'impairment' or 'loss' can be troubling to them. Paediatricians should be aware of families' preferences for terminology. Many prefer the terms 'deaf' or 'hard of hearing'.

PREVALENCE

Reported prevalence of hearing loss varies significantly depending on definitions used and methods of ascertainment of hearing ability, but multiple studies from the United States, United Kingdom, Australia and Europe suggest that approximately 1–2 per thousand children are born with a hearing loss of sufficient degree to adversely affect speech and language development.[2–4] If milder degrees of loss and unilateral losses are included, the prevalence at birth rises to 2–3 per thousand.[5,6] The prevalence of hearing loss in the childhood population rises with age, with one United Kingdom study of moderate or greater losses showing 0.9–1.07 per 1000 at age 3 years, to 1.65–2.05 per 1000 for children aged 9–16 years.[7] A Danish study found the prevalence of all degrees of hearing loss to reach about 5.32 per 1000 by age 10–14 years.[8]

Studies based on parent report have produced higher estimates of prevalence, with one study showing 1.98 per cent reported hearing loss of any degree among United States children under the age of 17 years. The National Health and Nutritional Examination Survey (NHANES) that used formal audiologic evaluation and included even very mild measured degrees of hearing loss, including isolated low and high frequency losses, gave an estimated prevalence of 14.9 per cent.[9] The clinical relevance of these very mild losses is presently uncertain, and research is underway to determine whether there could be clinical associations with milder forms of language disorder, or with specific learning disorders.

AETIOLOGY AND RISK FACTORS

Hearing loss is a heterogeneous condition with multiple causes. Aetiology of hearing loss remains unknown in 35–55 per cent of most reported case series.[10,11] Over the past two decades, however, there has been an explosion in understanding of the genetic basis of deafness, and over half of sensorineural hearing losses (SNHLs) in newborns are now believed to have a genetic cause.

Sensorineural hearing loss

Genetics

About 70 per cent of genetically determined hearing loss occurs without other clinical abnormalities, i.e. is non-syndromic, while in 30 per cent the hearing loss is part of a syndrome.[12] More than 400 genetic syndromes are now known to be associated with hearing loss, and researchers have identified over 140 genetic loci associated with non-syndromic hearing loss, and over 60 specific genes.[13] Hereditary hearing loss can be inherited as an autosomal dominant, autosomal recessive, X-linked or mitochondrial (maternally inherited) condition. Most newborns with inherited forms of hearing loss are born to hearing parents and have recessive, non-syndromic losses. Some genes have been identified that are associated with both dominant and recessive non-syndromic deafness, and also with both syndromic and non-syndromic deafness, emphasising the complexity of this fast-growing field and the difficulties inherent in providing accurate genetic counselling.[14]

Autosomal dominant
The presence of a clinically affected parent will point to this mode of inheritance. Autosomal dominant (AD) hearing loss may present as an isolated anomaly (non-syndromic) or be associated with other clinical signs such as pigmentary changes (Waardenburg's syndrome) and facial anomalies (Brachio-Oto-Renal Syndrome

or BOR), the latter resulting from mutations in the EYA1 gene. The gene responsible for Waardenburg's syndrome has been mapped to the long arm of chromosome 2.[15] Waardenburg's syndrome Type 2 is caused by mutations in the human microphthalmia-associated transcription factor (MITF) gene. A number of deafness-associated pigmentary disorders are caused by mutations in genes that in some way regulate MITF expression or activity.[16] Unusual AD phenotypes include DFNA1 (HDIA1), which results in low-frequency hearing loss, DFNA8/12 (TECTA), which results in mid-frequency hearing loss, and DFNA9 (COCH) in which there are vestibular symptoms and signs.[12]

Autosomal recessive

Autosomal recessive (AR) forms of deafness that occur as part of syndromes include Pendred's syndrome (associated with goitre), Usher syndrome (associated with retinitis pigmentosa and progressive visual impairment)[17] and Jervell-Lange-Nielson syndrome (associated with ECG abnormalities where cardiac arrhythmias secondary to prolonged QT interval may result in syncopal episodes or loss of consciousness).

Recessive mutations in the PDS gene are the common cause of Pendred syndrome. Mutations in the same gene can cause non-syndromic hearing loss associated with temporal bone abnormalities, which cross the spectrum from isolated enlargement of the vestibular aqueduct (EVA) to Mondini dysplasia. These temporal bone abnormalities may be caused by a side-splice mutation in the PDS gene.[18] For Usher syndrome, three clinical types (USH1, USH2 and USH3) and 11 mutated genes or loci have been described. Mutations in MYO7A and USH2A are responsible for about 40 and 60 per cent of Usher syndromes type 1 and 2 respectively.[19]

In some cases, AR hearing impairment occurs without any additional phenotypic abnormalities. Consanguinity of the parents or an affected sibling might suggest an AR aetiology. In the absence of any other apparent aetiology, some authors estimate that the likelihood for an AR aetiology of hearing loss may be as high as 80 per cent. Recessive mutations at a single locus, GJB2 or Connexin 26, are now thought to account for more than half of all genetic cases of deafness in some, but not all, populations.[12] The single base deletion mutation 35delG in the GJB2/DFNB1 gene is believed to be the most important single cause of genetic hearing loss in European and American populations,[20] with a carrier rate of 3 per cent – similar to that for cystic fibrosis.[21] Another deletion mutation 167delT, which has a carrier rate of about 4 per cent in the Ashkenazi Jewish population, has also been described.

Hearing loss due to Connexin 26 mutations can vary from mild to profound, even within the same sibship, and is non-syndromic, accompanied by normal vision, vestibular responses, and no malformations of the inner ear detectable by CT scanning. Progressive and asymmetrical hearing loss has been noted, but accounts for less than one-third of cases.[21] In general, phenotypes caused by truncating GJB2 mutations are more severe than those caused by missense mutations.[22]

Most cases of genetic deafness arise from mutations at a single locus, but an increasing number of examples are being recognised in which recessive mutations at two loci are involved. Digenic interactions are an important cause of deafness in individuals who carry a single mutation of the Connexin 26 locus together with a deletion involving the functionally related Connexin 30 locus. This mechanism complicates genetic counselling, but provides an explanation for why some Connexin 26 heterozygotes are deaf.[12] Molecular screening of the GJB2 (Connexin 26) gene should be considered in all cases of non-syndromic deafness, if desired by parents, where the cause cannot be identified. Connexins are the building blocks of gap junctions with six connexins oligomerising to form a hexameric torus called a connexon.[23] Gap junctions play a critical role in cell–cell communication.

Most forms of AR non-syndromic hearing impairment cause a prelingual hearing loss, generally severe–profound, and not associated with any radiological abnormality. However exceptions exist such as DFNB2 (MYO7A) where age of onset may be later in childhood; DFNB 4 (SLC26A4) where there may be dilated vestibular aqueducts and endolymphatic sacs, and DFNB 9 (OTOF) where there may be auditory neuropathy.[24]

X-linked
X-linked inheritance accounts for only 3 per cent of cases of non-syndromal deafness, where deafness is the only anomaly or may be associated with other anomalies such as in Hunter's and most types of Alport syndromes. X-linked Alport's syndrome (XLAS) results from mutations in the X-linked collagen gene COL4A5.[25] The syndrome includes sensor neural hearing loss, eye abnormalities and progressive kidney dysfunction leading to end-stage renal disease (ESRD) in almost all cases. Affected males usually eventually require kidney transplantation. Heterozygous females have widely varying outcomes, with some having normal urinalysis and kidney function, while others develop deafness and ESRD. The variation in females may be due in part to skewing of X-chromosome inactivation.[26]

Mitochondrial
Several mitochondrial DNA mutations associated with hearing loss have been identified over the last decade. Some are associated with systemic neuromuscular disorders, such as Kearns–Sayer syndrome, while others are associated with non-syndromic hearing loss.[27] Mitochondrial mutations are maternally inherited. One specific mutation, A1555G, is associated with predisposition to aminoglycoside toxicity and hearing loss. Although mutation screening in this gene has been recommended prior to aminoglycoside use as a preventive strategy, in practice the mutation does not occur with sufficiently high frequency in the population to justify this approach. Presence of the mutation alone, even in the absence of aminoglycoside exposure, may result in sensorineural hearing loss.[28]

Non-Mendelian malformation syndromes
This type includes syndromes such as cervocio-oculo-acusticus (Wildervanck's) syndrome, which may be a clinical variant of Klippel-Feil sequence. Both conditions are sporadic, with a female preponderance. Wildervanck's may have a genetic cause of uncertain inheritance, or an environmental aetiology such as a vascular disruption sequence during embryonic development.[29]

Environmental causes of sensorineural hearing loss
A variety of environmental factors have been associated with childhood hearing loss. These are generally categorised as prenatal, perinatal and postnatal causes.

Prenatal
Maternal infections including rubella, toxoplasmosis, cytomegalovirus (CMV), syphilis, herpes and AIDS are all associated with development of hearing loss in the fetus. Although prenatal ototoxic drug exposures, e.g. due to maternal

> **Practice Point**
>
> The aetiology of hereditary hearing loss is very complex. The audiologic phenotypes associated with many genes overlap, while some syndromes have variable penetrance of phenotypic features, making the distinction between syndromic and non-syndromic hearing loss challenging, especially in infancy and early childhood. Testing for individual genes associated with non-syndromic hearing loss, with the exception of Connexin 26, is generally expensive and of relatively low yield, but advances in DNA sequencing are changing this picture. It is likely that in the next decade it will become possible to identify aetiology in almost all cases of genetic deafness. The complexities of interpretation of genetic test results and appropriate counselling mean that referral to a medical geneticist should be offered to families in all cases of hearing loss.

ingestion of aminoglycosides and other toxins, are frequently cited as causes of congenital hearing loss, the epidemiologic evidence for these associations is weak. Consequently caution is advised in ascribing maternal drug ingestion as a cause of childhood hearing loss.

Rubella
The fetus is most susceptible to the effects of the virus during the first trimester, when maternal infection is thought to result in damage to the fetus in over 20 per cent of cases. Although congenital rubella syndrome (CRS) is now rare in developed countries that have efficient vaccination programs, it remains common in developing countries where such programs are lacking. Recently experts have expressed concern that congenital rubella may undergo a resurgence due to refusal of the MMR vaccine among some population subgroups.[30] Diagnosis is relatively easy in cases of confirmed maternal infection where infants have classic features of CRS, such as cataracts, congenital heart defects and mental retardation, but is very challenging in the absence of a history of maternal infection, and in cases where SNHL is the only manifestation of the disease, as is common when infection occurred later in pregnancy. Although retrospective diagnosis of congenital rubella has been attempted using lymphocyte responsiveness in combination with serological testing, these techniques remain controversial and are not widely used.

Toxoplasmosis
Maternal infection with toxoplasmosis is frequently mild and unnoticed. Pregnant women who have cats as house pets are at increased risk of infection and should avoid cleaning cat litter boxes. Raw meat is another potential source of infection. Up to half of affected infants are born prematurely. Signs of infection include hepatosplenomegaly, eye damage, cerebral calcifications, macrocephaly and petechiae. Although congenital toxoplasmosis has been associated with hearing loss, prevalence of SNHL varies from 0–28 per cent in reported studies, at least in part related to treatment. Children receiving limited or no treatment have a 28 per cent prevalence of hearing loss, those in whom treatment started after age 2.5 months and with uncertain compliance have an SNHL prevalence of 12 per cent, while children receiving 12 months of anti-parasitic therapy initiated prior to 2.5 months of age with serologically-confirmed compliance have a reported 0 per cent prevalence of SNHL.[31]

Cytomegalovirus

Cytomegalovirus (CMV) is a herpes virus with the ability to lay dormant in the body after initial infection. Up to 90 per cent congenital CMV infections remain undetected in the newborn period. SNHL occurs in about 35 per cent of symptomatic newborns, who may present with retinitis, hepatosplenomagealy, petechiae and microcephaly, and in about 10 per cent of asymptomatic infected newborns. CMV-associated hearing loss is often progressive, so any child with proven CMV requires close audiologic follow-up, even if initial hearing tests are normal.

Both primary and secondary maternal infections are reported to be associated with CNS disturbances, including deafness. Symptomatic newborns shed the virus, and a diagnosis of congenital CMV infection can be made if the virus is detected in the infant's urine, blood, saliva or other body tissues within 2–3 weeks of birth. Recently, real-time polymerase chain reaction (PCR) assays of saliva specimens have been shown to be highly sensitive and specific for detection of CMV infection, offering a potential screening tool for CMV in newborns.[32] The proportion of cases of childhood hearing loss attributable to CMV is presently unknown, but recent studies based on retrospective diagnosis using PCR assays of Guthrie card bloodspots suggest that it could account for up to 40 per cent of severe–profound losses.[33]

Perinatal

Babies born prematurely that receive care in a neonatal intensive care unit (NICU) are known to be at increased risk of hearing loss, with the prevalence of SNHL in babies spending more than 5 days in the NICU approaching ten times that of infants in the general population (1 per 100 versus 1 per 1000). Although the precise factors accounting for this increased risk have not been well delineated, the following are recognised associations with SNHL.

Hyperbilirubinemia

Historical evidence suggests an association between very high bilirubin levels and hearing loss.[34] Risks for moderately high bilirubin levels are less clear, though their effects may be more profound on premature babies where the blood–brain barrier is less well formed and offers less resistance to the passage of toxins. There is considerable debate, which remains unresolved, about the need for aggressive treatment of neonatal jaundice in term babies without hemolysis. Some experts regard the risks of bilirubin toxicity in this group as low and aggressive treatment unwarranted, while others argue that sequelae such as hearing loss are presently low due to the aggressive management – phototherapy together with exchange transfusion if required – currently employed, and that there is little justification for a change in approach.

Hyperbilirubinemia has recently been associated with the clinical picture of auditory neuropathy spectrum disorder (ANSD). Some newborns with high bilirubin levels have transient auditory brainstem evoked response (ABR) abnormalities that normalise as bilirubin levels fall, suggesting that in some cases 'recovery' from the effects of bilirubin toxicity is possible. The relationship between jaundice in the newborn period and milder degrees of hearing loss has not been well studied.

Prematurity

Premature infants are a vulnerable group who are exposed to a number of potential ototoxins including aminoglycosides, hypoxia and hyperbilirubinemia. Consequently it is difficult to estimate the effect of 'prematurity' alone on an infant's risk of developing SNHL, and for this reason prematurity should be regarded as a 'risk factor' for infant hearing loss rather than an etiologic factor per se. Reported rates of SNHL in premature infants have varied from 1–10 per cent. Extremely premature infants (<28 weeks) appear to be at highest risk, with one large longitudinal study showing a 3 per cent risk of permanent hearing loss.[35] It is also important to note that premature babies have a high incidence of transient conductive hearing problems that can make assessment of definitive hearing status difficult.[36]

Birth asphyxia
Practically defined as an Apgar of less than 4 at 5 minutes of age, birth asphyxia has been associated with the development of hearing loss in newborns, but the association is not strong where asphyxia is the only risk. Like prematurity, asphyxia may be a 'marker' for a group of related insults that can impact on an infant's hearing ability, and should be regarded as a risk factor for both SNHL and ANSD.

Hypoxia
Chronic hypoxia is associated with hearing loss in newborns. In Robertson's recent study of extremely premature infants, prolonged oxygen therapy was the most significant predictor of severe–profound hearing loss.[35] Infants who have received extacorporeal membrane oxygenation therapy (ECMO), prolonged (>5 days) mechanical ventilation or have a diagnosis of hypoxic ischaemic encephalopathy (HIE) are at increased risk of hearing loss. ECMO particularly is associated with delayed onset and progressive losses.

Postnatal
Meningitis
Meningitis is thought to account for about 6 per cent of all childhood hearing loss. A meta-analysis of the better studies gives a 9.5 per cent incidence of hearing loss among children surviving meningitis.[37] The mechanism is probably suppurative labyrinthitis, although direct nerve fibre damage may also be involved. There are reports of hearing loss improving after meningitis, so the ideal time for definitive audiologic evaluation is about 4–6 weeks after the illness. Widespread use of the haemophilus influenzae B (Hib) vaccine, streptococcus pneumoniae (Prevnar) vaccine, and the newer neisseria meningitides (Menactra) vaccine is expected to result in a significant reduction in cases.

Some children with congenital SNHL are at increased risk of developing meningitis. Presence of the Mondini malformation, characterised by a short, flat cochlea, large vestibule, wide, small or missing semicircular canals, and an immature sensorineural structure, is often accompanied by anomalies of the footplate of the stapes.[38] This can lead to spontaneous perilymphatic fistula and meningitis. Sometimes cases are detected only after onset of meningitis. Some experts advocate CT scanning of the inner ear in all cases of SNHL to detect these malformations.

Ototoxins
Drugs such as aminoglycosides, loop diuretics, cisplatin and salicylates have been associated with SNHL. Use of these drugs should be avoided wherever possible, especially in vulnerable populations such as premature babies. When these drugs must be used, drug levels should be monitored closely to avoid toxicity. As noted above, children with the mitochondrial mutation A1555G are at particular risk of aminoglycoside toxicity.[27]

Tumour
Acoustic neuroma is the commonest primary tumour causing deafness. Prevalence is 15–800 per 100,000 in the general population and is even rarer in children. This may occur as part of neurofibromatosis. Metastatic lesions causing deafness are virtually unknown in childhood.

Injury
Skull fractures or penetrating injuries of the middle ear may result in SNHL or permanent conductive losses. Radiation-induced injury may result in nerve deafness. These are rare in childhood.

Noise
Noise exposure, especially prolonged industrial exposure, is associated with acquired hearing loss in adults. The importance of noise as an aetiologic factor in childhood hearing loss is uncertain. It may play a role, along with acoustic trauma, in the hearing loss observed in association with prolonged mechanical ventilation, but this mechanism is uncertain. There are case reports of children who have had a sudden onset of SNHL, sometimes unilateral, after exposure to a very loud noise such as a gunshot.

Widespread use of iPods and other portable entertainment devices among adolescents and increasingly among pre-teens has raised questions regarding risks for hearing ability. One recent study indicated that widespread exposure to recreational noise and minimal use of hearing protection may have led to an increase in noise-induced threshold shift (NITS) prevalence among female youths in the US,[39] but there is no definitive evidence of increasing rates of permanent clinical hearing loss. Nonetheless, it is prudent to encourage use of ear protection and limits on device volume in an effort to prevent future hearing problems.

Practice Point
Experts advise caution when ascribing hearing loss to environmental causes that are not well defined. For example, it is not unusual to find cases of hearing loss that were initially thought to have an environmental cause, such as exposure to aminoglycoside therapy, subsequently prove to be genetic in origin when a second sibling is born with the same condition. Even when an environmental cause is suspected, offer genetic referral to the family to avoid these types of error.

Conductive hearing loss
Conductive losses result from disorders of the external or middle ear. Aetiology is best considered as hereditary or acquired.

Hereditary
Autosomal dominant
Autosomal dominant (AD) forms of conductive loss include mandibulofacial dysostosis (Treacher-Collins) and otosclerosis.

Treacher-Collins syndrome results from an embryonic aberration involving first and second brachial arch derivatives. The external auditory canal is usually absent, and malformations of the external and middle ear are common. Clinical features include hypoplasia of the zygomatic bones and mandible, coloboma, absence of the lower eyelid cilia and preauricular hair displacement. This disorder of facial development results from mutations in TCF01. There is wide variation in clinical presentation, and up to 60 per cent of cases arise de novo, resulting in challenges for diagnosis of milder cases. Conductive hearing loss occurs in 40–50 per cent of cases of Treacher-Collins. Direct sequencing of the coding and flanking intronic regions of TCOF1 detects mutations in 90–95 per cent of affected individuals, facilitating diagnosis.[40]

Otosclerosis affects about 0.4 per cent of the population and is usually bilateral. Fixation of the stapes footplate results in conductive hearing loss, and involvement of the endosteum of the inner ear may cause a concomitant SNHL. Otosclerosis is usually slowly progressive, and hearing loss does not usually present until adulthood. Both genetic and environmental factors appear to be involved in the development of this complex condition.[41]

X-linked dominant (XD)
Otopalatodigital syndrome (OPD) Type 1 is a rare disorder resulting from mutations in the FLNA gene that codes for filamin A, a protein that helps build the cytoskeleton. Affected individuals have wide-set eyes and chest deformities. Hearing loss results from malformations in the ossicles of the middle ear, resulting in conductive hearing loss. There is considerable overlap with OPD Type II and with Larsen syndrome.[42]

Non-Mendelian malformation syndromes
Goldenhar's syndrome is a congenital ipsilateral deformity of the ear and face with coloboma and vertebral anomalies. It is associated with predominantly conductive, and occasional sensorineural, congenital hearing loss. The aetiology is poorly understood and may represent an early developmental field defect.

Acquired conductive hearing loss
Otitis media with effusion
By far the most common cause of conductive hearing loss in children is otitis media with effusion (OME) or 'glue ear'. Hearing loss is usually mild, temporary and reversible, although the long-term effects of this condition are unclear and its management, which may include insertion of typanostomy tubes, remains the subject of controversy.[43] Fluid in the middle ear, one of the chief markers of the condition, has a high point prevalence in childhood of 15–25 per cent, with a cumulative prevalence in the childhood years of close to 80 per cent. There has been considerable debate as to whether mild transient hearing loss associated with OME, if occurring at critical periods in language development such as early infancy and persisting for sufficient time, will interfere with language acquisition and learning, but extensive meta-analyses and longitudinal studies have failed to show such a link in children who have no other medical conditions or cognitive disabilities.

In a small proportion of cases, the condition becomes chronic with tympanic membrane retraction, erosion of portions of the ossicular chain and cholesteatoma. Tympanic membrane disruption may also occur. These changes may result in permanent hearing loss. Chronic otitis media is particularly common in Australian Aboriginal children, in whom it is a significant cause of hearing loss.

TYPES OR CLASSIFICATION

Hearing loss in childhood is heterogeneous, and a variety of classification approaches have been used including degree, type, and time of onset.

Degree of hearing loss

The degree of a child's hearing loss will greatly influence their ability to acquire language by the oral route, and is best understood by comparing the child's hearing ability with that of a normally hearing child. Sounds consist of complex combinations of pure tones that vary in frequency (pitch) and intensity (loudness). Sound intensity is measured on a logarithmic decibel (dB) scale. Conversational voice intensity is 50–60 dB, a shout may be 100–105 dB. Children with hearing loss have perceptual thresholds that exceed 15–20 dBHL. The human ear can detect sounds between 16 and 20,000 Hz, but it is the speech frequencies, usually 250–8,000 Hz, that are functionally the most important, and most tests used in clinical practice are confined to these frequencies. Vowel sounds tend to be low frequency (250–1000 Hz) and consonants high frequency.

For children with hearing loss, classification systems have been developed based on an average level of hearing loss in decibels dBHL (where 0 dBHL represents audiometric '0', the average threshold for pure tone in normal hearing adults) for pure tones presented at 500, 1000 and 2000 Hz (usually termed three-frequency average hearing loss in the better ear). In some countries, including the United Kingdom, four-frequency average hearing loss in the better ear across 500, 1000, 2000 and 4000 Hz is used. Degrees of hearing loss are functionally classified as mild, moderate, severe and profound, and details are shown in Table 4.1.

Type of hearing loss

Sensorineural hearing loss

Sensorineural hearing loss (SNHL) is the commonest type of permanent hearing loss. SNHL may be of any degree, slight to profound, and higher frequencies are usually most affected. Comparison of air and bone conduction thresholds is used to differentiate SNHL from conductive deafness. In SNHL air and bone conduction thresholds are identical, whereas in conductive losses air thresholds are higher than bone thresholds, i.e. there is an 'air-bone gap'. Most SNHL is permanent. Most congenital losses are sensorineural in type, reflecting pathology in the cochlea, auditory nerve or central connections.

Conductive hearing loss

Most conductive losses are transient in nature and secondary to OME. Permanent conductive losses are encountered in cases of external auditory atresia, and in syndromes such as Treacher-Collins and Goldenhar's. Conductive losses tend to affect hearing more at low frequency ranges. Children with transient conductive losses do not receive amplification with hearing aids, and rarely receive any special educational approaches. Children with permanent conductive losses tend to have more severe losses than those encountered with OME and may be offered bone-anchored hearing aids (see below).

Children with conductive losses can discriminate speech if it is loud enough, and tend to be softly spoken as they hear their own speech more loudly. The maximum amount of hearing loss accountable for by a conductive problem is 50 dBHL approximately. At louder sound intensities, bone conduction occurs.

TABLE 4.1 Degrees of hearing loss[44]

Degree of hearing loss	Hearing threshold	Clinical characteristics
Slight	16–20 dBnHL	Uncertain significance. May be difficulty hearing soft-spoken speech.
Mild	21–40 dBnHL	Difficulty with soft-spoken speech. May result in articulation and perception errors with high frequency consonant word endings such as 's', 'z' and 'sh'.
Moderate	41–70 dBnHL	Difficulty understanding speech at a distance and in groups. Speech production difficulties – speech may be unintelligible to some listeners due to articulation errors and poor voice quality.
Severe	71–95 dBnHL	May understand close loud speech. May distinguish vowels but have problems even with hearing aids in distinguishing consonants. Poor voice quality and articulation errors.
Profound	>95 dBnHL	Little residual hearing – aware of only the loudest noises. Auditory channel cannot serve as primary mode of communication. Reliant on visual perception for communication.

Consequently, if a child has a hearing threshold >50 dBHL it is very unlikely that conductive hearing loss is the sole cause.

Mixed hearing loss
Some conditions, such as Down syndrome, are associated with an increased prevalence of both SNHL and conductive hearing loss, and mixed types of loss containing features of both are often seen in this condition. It is not unusual to have a permanent underlying SNHL co-occurring with a transient conductive loss secondary to fluid in the middle ear. This combination can present challenges clinically in determining the true type and degree of loss, and is typically encountered in children that have failed newborn hearing screens.

Auditory neuropathy spectrum disorder
The term 'auditory neuropathy' was first coined to describe a series of patients that had evidence of normal cochlear outer hair cell function, as evidenced by normal oto-acoustic emissions (OAEs) and cochlear microphonics (CMs), and abnormal auditory pathway function characterised by absent or severely abnormal auditory brainstem potential. These patients were different from those with 'typical' SNHL who were assumed to have hair cell dysfunction with or without accompanying loss of auditory neuron function and hence demonstrated absence

of OAEs and CMs. This problem was originally regarded as a type of 'neuropathy' of the auditory nerve, but it has become clear that the auditory nerve is not always the site of the lesion. Disruption of the inner hair cell–cochlear nerve synapse from a mutation in the Otoferlin (OTOF) gene has also been shown to be associated with the audiologic symptoms of auditory neuropathy spectrum disorder (ANSD).[45] Given the possibility of non-neural sites for the lesion, the term 'auditory neuropathy spectrum disorder' is now used.

Recent reports suggest that ANSD accounts for 8–40 per cent of cases of severe–profound hearing loss, and 10 per cent all infants in the United Kingdom identified with permanent hearing loss have a pattern of ANSD.[46] ANSD appears to have multiple aetiologies, including associations with premature birth, hyperbilirubinemia, asphyxia and sepsis, and to affect all age groups. In some children, ANSD occurs together with peripheral neuropathies, e.g. Charcot-Marie-Tooth, or as a component of other genetic disorders, e.g. Wolfram and Mohr syndromes. Much research is currently underway on this condition that has only recently emerged as a distinct clinical entity whose pathophysiology is poorly understood. Some, but not all, children with ANSD are helped by hearing aid use and by cochlear implantation.

Time of onset

Although classifications by degree and type of loss are most important clinically, losses are also classified by time of onset (congenital versus perinatally or postnatally acquired); pre-lingual (onset before the acquisition of speech and language) versus postlingual; duration (temporary versus permanent); aetiology (genetic versus environmental, hereditary versus sporadic) and extent (unilateral versus bilateral). Each of these factors is important in gaining a full picture of the child's hearing loss. An additional important clinical distinction is between those children who have hearing loss as their sole condition, compared with those children with additional developmental challenges, or in whom hearing loss occurs as part of a defined syndrome.

CLINICAL PRESENTATION

Prior to the mid-1990s, late diagnosis of congenital hearing loss was the norm with most cases presenting with delayed speech and language acquisition that usually became apparent around the age of 12–18 months. Most deaf babies develop double-syllable babble at about the expected time, suggesting that this developmental milestone may not be dependent on auditory input. Emergence of first words is delayed however. Technological advances have resulted in the ability to screen all newborns for hearing loss at birth. Over 95 per cent of newborns in the United States and United Kingdom are now screened, and Australia is implementing similar programs across states. Consequently most cases of congenital hearing loss are now detected through newborn screening, rather than presenting with delayed speech and language or through parental concerns about hearing ability. Common clinical signs of childhood hearing loss are listed in Text Box 4.1.

Despite widespread implementation of newborn hearing screening, paediatricians need to remain vigilant to the possible diagnosis of hearing loss in their patients. Some children, e.g. some babies born at home or migrating from

> **TEXT BOX 4.1** Signs of childhood hearing loss[47]
>
> **Infants and toddlers**
> *Birth to 4 months*
> - Does not waken or stir to loud noises
> - Does not startle to loud noises
> - Does not calm at the sound of a familiar voice
> - Does not respond to mother's voice by smiling or cooing.
>
> *4–9 months*
> - Does not turn towards source of familiar sounds
> - Does not smile when spoken to
> - Appears not to notice rattles or other sound-making toys
> - No variation in cry for different needs.
>
> *9–15 months*
> - Little variation in babbled sounds
> - Does not respond to their own name
> - Does not respond to changes in tone of caregiver's voice
> - No single words
> - Does not use their voice to attract attention.
>
> *15–24 months*
> - Does not point to familiar objects when named
> - Does not listen to stories, songs or rhymes
> - Does not follow simple commands
> - Does not use several different words
> - Does not point to body parts when asked
> - Does not name common objects
> - Does not put two or more words together.
>
> **Preschool and older children**
> - Turns up volume of television excessively high
> - Responds inappropriately to questions
> - Does not reply when called by name
> - Watches others to imitate what they are doing
> - Has articulation problems or speech/language delays
> - Has problems academically
> - Complains of earache, ear pain or head noises
> - Has difficulty understanding what people are saying
> - Speaks differently from other children their own age.

countries without established screening programs, may miss their initial screen. A small number of families decline newborn screening. The screen may miss some mild and progressive losses, and in other children the loss will develop after screening. It is very important for paediatricians to take a proactive role in continued hearing surveillance after the newborn period and to refer promptly

CHAPTER 4 Hearing and vision loss 63

> **TEXT BOX 4.2** Risk indicators associated with permanent congenital, delayed-onset or progressive hearing loss in childhood.[48]
>
> 1. Caregiver concerns* regarding hearing, speech, language or developmental delay.
> 2. Family history* of permanent childhood hearing loss.
> 3. NICU stay of more than 5 days or any of the following regardless of length of stay: ECMO*, assisted ventilation, exposure to ototoxic medications (gentamycin and tobramycin) or loop diuretics (e.g. furosemide/lasix) and hyperbilurubinemia that requires exchange transfusion.
> 4. In utero infections such as CMV*, herpes, rubella, syphilis and toxoplasmosis.
> 5. Craniofacial anomalies, including those that involve the pinna, ear canal, ear tags, ear pits, and temporal bone anomalies.
> 6. Physical findings such as white forelock, associated with a syndrome known to include a sensorineural or permanent conducive hearing loss.
> 7. Syndromes associated with hearing loss or progressive or late-onset hearing loss*, such as neurofibromatosis, osteopetrosis, and Usher syndrome; other frequently identified syndromes including Waardenburg, Alport, Pendred, and Jervell and Lange-Nielson.
> 8. Neurodegenerative disorders*, such as Hunter syndrome, or sensory motor neuropathies, such as Friedreich ataxia and Charcot-Marie-Tooth syndrome.
> 9. Culture-positive postnatal infections associated with sensorineural hearing loss*, including confirmed bacterial and viral (especially herpes viruses and varicella) meningitis.
> 10. Head trauma, especially basal skull/temporal bone fractures* that required hospitalisation.
> 11. Chemotherapy*
>
> Risk indicators marked* are of greater concern for late-onset loss.

for audiologic evaluation any child in whom there is concern about hearing ability, or who has significant speech and language delay, even if the newborn screen was passed.

Children who have known risk factors for hearing loss need particularly close audiologic supervision, even if a newborn hearing screen was passed. In areas where universal newborn hearing screening is not yet available, children with known risk factors for early hearing loss should be referred directly to an audiologist for full audiologic evaluation. A list of relevant risk factors is given in Text Box 4.2. It is also recommended that any child with recurrent or persistent otitis media with effusion for at least 3 months be referred for audiologic evaluation.

In some areas, additional hearing screens are performed during the preschool years, and most children in the United States, Australia and United Kingdom receive a further hearing screen at school entry, followed by additional screenings throughout the school-age years.

> **Practice Point**
>
> Expressed parental concern about a child's hearing ability should result in referral for a full audiologic evaluation, even if a newborn or other previous screen was passed. Prior to the introduction of formal screening programs, parents frequently reported being falsely reassured by medical professionals that their concerns about their child's hearing were unfounded. Ignoring parental concerns can lead to delayed diagnosis of permanent hearing loss.

HEARING SCREENING

Oto-acoustic emissions and auditory brainstem evoked responses

Physiologic measures used to screen newborns and infants for hearing loss include oto-acoustic emissions (OAEs) and auditory brainstem evoked responses (ABRs). OAE measures are obtained from the ear canal using a sensitive microphone with a probe assembly that records cochlear responses to acoustic stimuli. OAEs reflect the status of the peripheral auditory system extending to the cochlear outer hair cells. ABRs are obtained from surface electrodes that record neural activity generated in the cochlea, auditory nerve and brainstem in response to acoustic stimuli delivered via an earphone. Automated ABRs (AABRs) reflect the status of the peripheral auditory system, VIIIth nerve and brainstem auditory pathway.

OAEs and AABRs can both be used to detect sensory (cochlear) hearing loss,[49] but both may be affected by outer or middle ear dysfunction. Temporary conductive losses may result in a failed OAE or AABR even in the presence of normal cochlear and/or neural function. Conversely, an OAE may be passed even in the presence of a neural conduction disorder in the absence of accompanying sensory dysfunction, as in auditory neuropathy. As infants in the NICU are at increased risk of ANSD, the Joint Committee on Infant Hearing recommends that AABR technology be used to screen this group of infants. For infants in the well baby nursery, either OAE or AABR may be used.[48]

Screen results should be communicated to families promptly and in a culturally sensitive manner, preferably in both verbal and written forms, and to the child's paediatrician or other primary care provider. Some protocols call for a rescreen to be performed on all babies that fail their initial screen, either as an inpatient or an outpatient, no later than one month of age in order to decrease the number of referrals for audiologic evaluation. However no more than two screens should be performed in total.

Ease of use of OAEs, together with their non-invasive nature, have lead to suggestions that intermittent OAE screening could be used throughout infancy and early childhood to detect developing hearing losses. However fluid in the middle ear, which results in loss of OAEs in many cases, is such a prevalent condition in this age group that there are concerns that this form of screening would lead to numerous false positives. More studies are needed on the utility of this type of screening before it can be implemented.

Pure tone audiometry

After the newborn period, there are no widely used population-based screens of hearing until the child enters the preschool age years. Pure tone audiometry (PTA) may be used to screen (or test) hearing from about the age of 3 years. A number of pure tones are presented to the child via headphones at varying frequencies and intensities, and the child is asked to indicate to the tester whether they have heard the tone. Cooperation and a certain level of understanding are necessary for accurate completion of the test. An audiogram can be plotted giving precise information about the child's hearing ability in each ear at different frequencies and intensities. PTA can be used as a diagnostic test, or as a screening tool when sounds at only a few frequencies and intensities are presented. Children failing the screen are referred to an audiologist for a full audiogram. PTA testing also forms the basis of school entry hearing screening and ongoing screening throughout the school years.

ASSESSMENT

A variety of assessment approaches are employed by audiologists to make a definitive determination of children's hearing ability. Diagnostic testing in infants and young children should be performed by experienced paediatric audiologists. For infants referred after hearing screening, diagnostic evaluation should be completed no later than age 3 months.[48]

Diagnostic ABR

When used as an automated screen, the ABR uses a limited series of clicks at defined intensities, and screen outcome is determined as pass or fail by a computerised algorithm set to a pre-determined threshold. The ABR can be used as a diagnostic test as well as a screen when click stimuli at multiple intensities are presented, allowing for accurate determination of the infant's individual hearing threshold. Both air and bone conductor ABRs may be used to distinguish SNHL from conductive losses. The ABR is particularly useful for those infants who are too young for behavioural assessment methods. Infants undergoing a diagnostic ABR must be either asleep or drowsy. Most infants less than three months old have little difficulty in falling asleep naturally for the test, but as infants become older it may prove necessary to use sedation. As use of sedation is not without risk, it is strongly recommended that it be avoided wherever possible. Parents should be advised to bring their infant tired and hungry at the time of testing, with the aim of feeding the infant then testing during natural sleep.

Steady state evoked potential testing

Steady state evoked potential (SSEP) testing offers a means to obtain accurate, frequency-specific estimates of the hearing threshold in subjects with hearing loss. The frequency-specific information adds to the evaluation obtained through conventional diagnostic ABR, and is particularly important in evaluating children with severe and profound losses in the preoperative evaluation of cochlear implant candidates.[50,51] This specialised testing should be conducted in a unit experienced in test interpretation.

Visual reinforcement audiometry

Auditory stimuli of varying intensities are presented to the child in free field conditions. The child responds by turning to the source of the noise, and these responses are reinforced and conditioned by a visual stimulus such as the appearance of a puppet. Visual reinforcement audiometry (VRA) can be completed with ear-specific techniques using insert phones or headphones, and is most widely used to assess the hearing threshold children aged 6–30 months. The test must be performed in a soundproof booth requiring attendance at an audiological testing facility, and can be difficult to interpret in some groups, e.g. developmentally delayed children.

Other assessment techniques employed include **infant toy tests**, where children aged 18 months – 3 years are conditioned to carry out simple repetitive actions, such as putting a peg in a board in response to a sound stimulus; **speech discrimination tests**; and **acoustic reflex** thresholds. **Pure tone audiometry**, as described above, is widely used as a diagnostic test in children over 3 years of age.

Tympanometry

Tympanometry is widely used during diagnostic assessment of hearing ability in young children. A hand-held device or tympanometer is placed in the ear canal and a seal made adjacent to the ear drum. A tympanogram trace is obtained providing a measure of the acoustic energy that is passed through the middle ear system (admittance), or the energy reflected back by the middle ear system (impedance). Tympanograms are interpreted in terms of peak pressure point, peak amplitude and shape. When a serous effusion is present in the middle ear, a 'flat' tympanogram is obtained. A flat tympanogram in the presence of a mild hearing loss may mean that the loss is transient and conductive, but it is not possible to exclude a sensorineural loss due to the presence of a flat tympanogram as SNHL may co-exist with fluid in the middle ear. For this reason, tympanometry does not have a place in hearing screening protocols.

Communicating test results

Results of diagnostic audiometric evaluation should be given to families both verbally and in writing, and a copy together with the audiologist's interpretation of the findings sent to the child's paediatrician. If a diagnosis of permanent hearing loss has been made, the child and family should be referred to early intervention services.

MANAGEMENT

As well as close ongoing audiologic supervision with regular hearing evaluations by a trained paediatric audiologist, all children diagnosed with permanent hearing loss need additional evaluations to guide management. The paediatrician should coordinate the medical evaluation, including clinical history, family history, physical examination, identification of any syndromes and need for further radiologic and lab study. This evaluation should inform aetiology investigations and recommendations for management. The paediatrician should ensure that appropriate referrals are made, and that results are obtained and acted upon.[48] These include:

- ENT consultation is often required prior to fitting of hearing aids. ENT may help guide aetiology investigations and determine optimal management of any middle ear effusions, including placement of tympanostomy tubes.
- Ophthalmology evaluation at diagnosis and annually thereafter as children with hearing loss have a higher prevalence of vision problems.
- Developmental paediatrician if the child's hearing loss is part of a syndrome that has developmental implications or if there is concern about global development on developmental surveillance.
- Neurology, cardiology and nephrology referrals as needed if associated conditions.
- Genetics referral should be offered to determine whether the hearing loss has a genetic cause, whether there is a genetic diagnosis with additional management implications, e.g. Usher's syndrome, and recurrence rate.
- Offer referral for hearing aid fitting and monitoring. Hearing aids are available for all children in Australia though Australian Hearing. In contrast, in the United States some health insurers do not cover aids, presenting a financial challenge to families. For families that elect amplification, aids should be fitted within one month of referral. Digital programmable aids can be customised to provide maximum amplification where most needed. Infancy is a period of rapid growth, and frequent changes of ear moulds will be required to ensure appropriate fit.
- Consider referral for cochlear implantation. Implantation should be considered for any child receiving limited benefit from a trial of appropriately fitted hearing aids. Implantation is now being performed as young as 12 months. Additional developmental conditions, such as autism, causing developmental delays do not preclude consideration of implantation. Recent studies suggest that implants provide substantial language, academic and social benefit. The auditory cortex may have sensitive periods for development, and the balance of current evidence suggests that the best language outcomes occur in recipients that were implanted at a younger age, and are in an environment rich in oral communication.[48] Bilateral implantation offers some acoustic advantages but some providers prefer to perform unilateral implantation, delaying the second implant to allow for potential advances in implant technology.

EARLY INTERVENTION

Ideally, all families of children with any degree of bilateral or unilateral permanent hearing loss should be considered eligible for early intervention services. Referral for intervention should be initiated within two days of a diagnosis of permanent loss, and intervention commenced no later than 6 months of age. Intervention should be provided by professionals with expertise in hearing loss, including educators of the deaf and specialised speech–language pathologists. Both home- and centre-based interventions should be offered. A range of communication approaches is available for families of children with hearing loss, including Australian Sign Language, aural/oral, and signed English. Families should be given information about all communication options and available hearing technologies. It is important that this information be provided in an unbiased manner. Informed family choice and desired outcome should guide the family's decision-making process.[46]

Families frequently seek the advice of their paediatrician about decisions related to intervention approaches. Paediatricians should become knowledgeable about the available options, and know how to direct families to appropriate resources to obtain more detailed information. There is good evidence that intervention commenced early, prior to the age of 6 months, results in improved language development,[48] however age at diagnosis is not the only factor influencing outcomes. Research suggests that family engagement in intervention is at least as, if not more, important while other factors such as the presence of additional conditions also play a role.

Based on the limited evidence currently available, no one intervention approach or communication modality has been proven to be superior to any other in terms of outcome, however this is a rapidly evolving field in need of much research. Some experts suggest that children should initially be exposed to all the communication modalities, rather than having families make the difficult decision of which approach to adopt. Where sign language is used, it is very important that training in sign language acquisition be provided to all family members and to extended family, in addition to the child themself. Families of children with hearing loss should be informed of family-to-family support services that can be invaluable sources of information, and offered access to deaf mentors.

As children with hearing loss enter school, many benefit from the use of FM systems in which a microphone is worn by the teacher and a receiver by the student to amplify the teacher's voice. Children with mild losses could also potentially benefit from these devices but their use for this group has not been well studied. Many deaf students are now integrated into mainstream education with use of aides and teachers of the deaf. Students may need individual supports on transitioning to higher education where FM systems are rarely used.

> **Practice Point**
>
> It is very important that children who do not pass a newborn hearing screen receive appropriate follow-up. Australia and the United Kingdom have well-developed public health infrastructures with limited loss-to-follow-up after screening, but in the United States almost half of the babies that do not pass their screens are not documented to receive audiologic evaluation by the age of 3 months and close to one-third of children with hearing loss are not documented to receive early intervention. Paediatricians can play a pivotal role in ensuring infants are not 'lost' to the system, but obtain and follow-through with all appropriate referrals. At the same time families have the right to refuse interventions if they so wish, but providers must ensure that families have all relevant information on which to base an informed decision.

PROGNOSIS

Prior to the introduction of newborn hearing screening, children with severe–profound bilateral hearing loss on average were reported to leave high school with a 4th grade reading level.[52] However, these data have been criticised as most studies did not adequately evaluate sign language skills, or report the successes of some student groups. Infants with mild–profound losses that are diagnosed early and commence intervention in the first 6 months of life have been demonstrated to have better outcomes than later diagnosed children in vocabulary development, receptive and expressive language, speech production and social–emotional development. However many questions remain about the relative importance of various aspects of intervention, e.g. intensity of services, degree of family engagement, method of communication and curricula.[48]

Some studies have shown that even children with mild and unilateral losses have worse outcomes in terms of educational attainment than normally hearing children,[53] but not all studies have shown these deficits.[54] Consequently there is debate as to how much, and what type of intervention is warranted for these types of loss. Most programs now offer services to all children with any degree of hearing loss. Some parents, such as those of infants with unilateral losses, choose only developmental monitoring supplemented with intermittent consultation, while children with more severe bilateral losses receive much more intense services from a variety of providers.[48] More research is needed on the long-term educational and social outcomes of different intervention approaches, and on quality of life among children that are deaf or hard of hearing. Studies are also needed that separate the impact of hearing loss per se from that of associated conditions on developmental outcomes.

Intervention programs should assess the language, cognitive skills, auditory skills, speech, vocabulary and social–emotional development of all children with hearing loss at six-monthly intervals during the first three years of life, preferably using norm-referenced assessment tools. Children using sign language should have their language development assessed in that modality.

Practice Point

Families report that there is frequently little communication between healthcare and intervention providers. Families should be encouraged to provide written permission for health and educational professionals to collaborate when forming an individualised educational plan for each child. Interventions must focus on the whole child. Over half of children with hearing loss have additional conditions that will impact the intervention approach.

KEY POINTS

- The introduction of universal newborn hearing screening has made early diagnosis of permanent hearing loss the norm.
- Prompt diagnostic testing for infants that fail screens, and entry to intervention for children with hearing loss are vital to the success of these screening programs.
- Early diagnosis is associated with improved language outcomes, but other factors such as family engagement are very important.
- Much of the hearing loss previously classed as having unknown aetiology is now understood to have a genetic basis, and genetics consultation is recommended for all children with permanent hearing loss.
- Children with profound losses can now receive cochlear implantation as early as 12 months of age.

VISION LOSS

DEFINITIONS

Although the term 'vision impairment' may refer to any type of defect, disease or dysfunction of any part of the optical system, in the educational context it is defined as 'an impairment in vision that, even with correction, adversely affects a child's educational performance'.[55] Four terms describe levels of visual impairment:[56]

- **Partially sighted:** some type of vision problem that has resulted in the need for special education.
- **Low vision:** a severe visual impairment, not necessarily limited to distance vision. Children have some vision, but would be unable to read newspaper-size print at a normal viewing distance, even with the aid of eyeglasses or contact lenses. Children with low vision use a combination of vision and other senses to learn, and may require adaptations in lighting, the size of print, and sometimes Braille.
- **Legally blind:** child has less than 20/200 (6/60 metric) vision in the better eye or a very limited field of vision (20 degrees at its widest point).
- **Totally blind:** students learn via Braille or non-visual media.

PREVALENCE

As with hearing loss, prevalence estimates for vision loss vary widely based on definitions used and methods of case ascertainment. Vision losses of any degree are reported to occur at the rate of about 12.2 per 1000 in individuals in the United States under the age of 18 years. Severe visual impairment (legally or totally blind) occurs in 0.06 per 1000.[56] One United States study estimated the prevalence of vision impairment using a more restrictive definition of best corrected visual acuity in the better eye of 20/70 or worse and found a prevalence of 10.7 per 10,000 among 6–10-year-old children in Atlanta, Georgia.[57] Of these, 59 per cent had low vision, and almost two-thirds had coexisting disabilities. A systematic review of the literature on the prevalence of any type of vision loss among children under the age of 5 years conducted for the United States Preventive Services Task Force estimated the prevalence to be as high as 7–8 per cent. The same review found that about 3 per cent of children under the age of five years had amblyopia.[58]

AETIOLOGY AND RISK FACTORS

Vision impairment is a term used to describe the consequence of a functional loss of vision, rather than the eye disorder itself. Eye disorders that can lead to vision impairments have a range of aetiologies including the following.

Infections

Congenital

Important causes of congenital blindness include congenital infections, such as the protozoal infection toxoplasmosis and the viral infection rubella. If the mother becomes infected with toxoplasmosis during pregnancy, the infection may be passed to the fetus during pregnancy, labor or delivery. Infection earlier in gestation causes more severe problems. The classic eye condition associated with toxoplasmosis is chorioretinitis. Diagnosis can be made based on antibody studies on cord blood, while a computed tomography (CT) scan of the brain may reveal cerebral calcifications. Pregnant women who have cats as house pets may be at increased risk so they should avoid contact with potentially infected cat faeces, or with flies and cockroaches that could have had contact with infected faeces. Pregnant women are also at risk of contracting toxoplasmosis from undercooked meat.[59]

Congenital rubella is now rare in the developed world due to immunisation, but is still seen in developing countries that lack such immunisation programs. Congenital rubella can cause cataracts, glaucoma or retinitis.[60] Children born with congenital cytomegalovirus (CMV) experience eye disorders but these are not as common as hearing loss and developmental delays. Vision loss may result from retinitis with macular scars, cortical vision loss and optic atrophy. Congenital CMV has also been associated with strabismus and, rarely, with incomplete formation of the eyes. Although rarely seen in developed countries, congenital syphilis is associated with particular eye pathology, namely interstitial keratitis. Congenital herpes is also associated with retinitis and keratitis.

Acquired
Trachoma is rare in developed countries. It is caused by *Chlamydia trachomatis*, the organism being transmitted from person to person by direct contact and by flies. Children act as a reservoir of infection, while blindness that occurs after repeated infection and is caused by corneal scarring principally affects adults. Trachoma is endemic in 55 countries, and is prevalent in Australian Aboriginal populations.

In developing countries, **measles**-related corneal ulceration and scarring remain a significant cause of blindness, though this is very rare in developed countries with effective measles immunisation programs.

Genetics
In the developed world, it is estimated that up to half of all cases of congenital blindness have a genetic origin.[61] Molecular genetics has allowed characterisation of mutations that cause congenital eye disorders, and for comparison with mutations in model organisms. A common genetic network appears to underlie eye development in flies, mice and humans, including several master control genes that direct distinct pathways of development and differentiation. Mutations that lead to clinically relevant phenotypes highlight important steps in eye development – some affect the genes that function at the top of the regulatory hierarchy and therefore affect the initial stages of eye development. Mutations in these genes such as PAX6 and SOX2 lead to anophthalmia, microphthalmia and aniridia. Other genes function downstream or later in development and cause anterior segment malformations, iris anomaly and glaucoma (FOXC1) and Peter's anomaly (FOXE3). Some mutations define genes that are important for only one tissue, e.g. the crystalline-encoding genes in development of the lens and PAX2 in the optic nerve.[61] Some genes appear to be frequently affected by mutations, others rarely.

Albinism occurs when one of several genetic defects results in the body being unable to produce melanin resulting in little or no color in the skin, hair and iris of the eye. Type I is caused by defects that affect production of the pigment melanin, while Type 2 is due to a defect in the 'P' gene. Oculocutaneous albinism is a severe form, while ocular albinism type 1 affects only the eyes, with no coloring in the retina. Albinism is associated with strabismus, photophobia, nystagmus (rapid eye movements) and functional blindness.[62] Mutations in several genes have been associated with albinism including the tyrosinase gene (TYRP1) and OCA1, 2 and 3.[63]

Leber's optic atrophy (LHON) and **autosomal dominant optic atrophy (DOA)** are the two most common inherited optic neuropathies. Three mitochondrial DNA point mutations account for over 90 per cent of LHON cases, while most cases of DOA result from mutations in OPA1, which codes for a mitochondrial inner membrane protein. Patients can exhibit a broad phenotypic spectrum suggesting that environmental factors may also play a role in the selective loss of retinal ganglion cells.[64]

Similar to the genetics of deafness, the genetics of vision loss is complex. Some clinical eye phenotypes can be caused by different mutations in different genes, yet conversely, mutations in the same gene do not necessarily cause the same phenotype.

Retinopathy of prematurity

Retinopathy of prematurity (ROP) refers to abnormal blood vessel development in the retina of the eye in a premature infant. Fragile vessels may grow abnormally from the retina into the normally clear gel that fills the back of the eye. The vessels can leak, causing bleeding in the eye. Scar tissue may develop, and the retina can detach from the eye's inner surface. Severe cases can result in vision loss.[65] Despite current treatment, ROP remains a major cause of blindness in premature infants and its incidence is rising worldwide as more infants born at a very early age survive.[66] Historically, use of excess levels of oxygen in the treatment of premature infants stimulated abnormal vessel growth, but close monitoring of oxygen therapy has made this cause of ROP rare.[65] Nonetheless, it is still uncertain which oxygen saturation target should be adopted.[67] Today, the smallest and sickest premature babies have the highest risk.

Risk factors for ROP[63] include:
- Prematurity, especially ≤25, and 26–28 weeks' gestation
- Sepsis
- Apnoea
- Bradycardias
- Acidosis (low blood pH)
- Heart disease
- Respiratory distress.

Early low and late high oxygen saturations are associated with decreased risk of ROP in infants <30 weeks' gestation,[68] and antenatal steroids may also offer protection, though late postnatal use of steroids, starting after 3 weeks' of life, especially if continued for 2 weeks or more, is associated with greater risk.[69]

There are five stages of ROP:
Stage I: Mildly abnormal blood vessel growth
Stage II: Moderately abnormal blood vessel growth
Stage III: Severely abnormal blood vessel growth
Stage IV: Severely abnormal blood vessel growth and retinal detachment
Stage V: Total retinal detachment.

Specialised eye examination is needed to reveal the blood vessel changes. An infant is classed as having 'plus disease' if dilation and twisting of blood vessels matches or exceeds a standard photograph. Symptoms of severe ROP include abnormal eye movements, crossed eyes, severe nearsightedness, and white-looking pupils (leukocoria).

Cataracts

A congenital cataract is clouding of the lens of the eye that is present at birth. If the cataract is mild and does not affect vision, no treatment is required. In many patients with cataract, no specific cause can be found. In addition to the causes of cataract already listed, i.e. congenital infections or genetic causes, cataracts may also be seen as a component of a number of syndromes including **Down, Pierre-Robin** and **Lowe**. Cataracts are also seen in **galactosemia**, a recessively inherited disorder in which deficiency of an enzyme, most commonly galactose-1 phosphate uridyl transferase deficiency, results in an inability to break down the simple sugar galactose.

Vitamin A deficiency

Vitamin A deficiency is rarely seen in developed countries but persists in the developing world. The ocular disease is known as xerophthalmia, with ocular changes including conjunctival and corneal drying (xerosis), corneal ulceration and melting (kerotomalacia), night blindness (nyctalopia) and retinopathy. The condition is most likely to occur when there is a combination of vitamin A and protein deficiency. The most severe blinding complications occur in children aged 6 months to 3 years born to vitamin-A deficient mothers, who then consequently get little vitamin A from breastfeeding.[70]

Retinal degeneration

Retinal degeneration may occur as a component of a range of eye pathologies. Retinitis pigmentosa (RP) refers to damage to the retinal rods or cones, resulting in the presence of dark deposits visible in the retina. It is usually inherited and affects only about 1 in 4,000 people in developed countries. Symptoms first appear in childhood, but severe problems do not usually develop until early adulthood. Patients with RP develop cataracts at an early age, and macular oedema. A combination of hearing loss and RP is seen in Usher's syndrome (autosomal recessive), and similar eye pathology to RP is seen in Friederich's ataxia and myotonic dystrophy.[71]

Glaucoma

Primary congenital glaucoma (PCG) is characterised by elevated intraocular pressure (IOP), enlargement of the globe, oedema and opacification of the cornea. Visual acuity may be reduced and visual fields restricted. Untreated, the condition leads to blindness. CYP1B1, the gene encoding cytochrome P450 1B1, is the only gene known to be associated with PCG. Mutations are inherited in an autosomal recessive manner. Infantile and juvenile types of glaucoma are also seen clinically.

Corneal disorders

The cornea is the outermost layer of the eye that helps shield the eye from germs and dust. Abnormalities include **corneal dystrophies**, in which parts of the cornea lose clarity due to a build-up of cloudy material. Development of genotyping analyses has revolutionised knowledge of the corneal dystrophies, revealing many inaccuracies in the dystrophy nomenclature. It has been proposed that these conditions now be classified as 'inherited corneal diseases' with four categories based on evidence for the condition as a distinct entity. Dystrophies are further now classified anatomically according to the layer chiefly affected: epithelial and subepithelial; Bowman layer; stromal; and those affecting Descement's membrane and the endothelium.[72]

Refractive errors result from irregularities in the shape of the cornea. There are four common types of refractive error:[73]

- **Myopia or nearsightedness:** clear vision close up, but blurry in the distance. The cornea is curved too much or the eye is longer than normal. Myopia is often diagnosed in children aged between 8 and 12 years and may worsen during the teen years. People whose parents have myopia are more likely to get the condition but its aetiology is poorly understood. About 20 per cent of the population of the United States is affected.
- **Hyperopia or farsightedness:** clear vision in the distance, but blurry close up. The cornea is curved too little or the eye is shorter than normal. Hyperopia affects about 5–10 per cent of the population of the United States, and is commoner in children whose parents have the condition.
- **Presbyopia:** an inability to focus as a result of ageing.
- **Astigmatism:** focus problems caused by variations in curvature of the cornea, blurring vision at all distances. In corneal astigmatism, the cornea is curved more steeply in one direction than another. In lenticular astigmatism it is the lens that is unevenly curved. Astigmatism may be present at birth or may develop after an eye injury, disease or surgery.

Amblyopia

Amblyopia or 'lazy eye,' with the loss of one eye's ability to see details, is the most common cause of vision problems in children. It occurs when the nerve pathway from one eye to the brain does not develop, usually because the abnormal eye sends a blurred image to the brain which then 'ignores' the abnormal image. The most common cause of amblyopia is strabismus (or squint) in which the eye turns in or out; however amblyopia can occur even in the absence of strabismus. Amblyopia may also occur secondary to cataracts, farsightedness, nearsightedness or astigmatism, especially if it is greater in one eye.[74]

Practice Point

Children with amblyopia are at risk of blindness if they lose vision in their 'good' eye. These children need to be counselled about the importance of eye protection, especially during participation in sports such as ball games. Wearing glasses may provide protection to the 'good eye' in children with amblyopia.

Strabismus

Strabismus results from imbalance of the muscles that control positioning of the eye. The eye may turn inward (**esotropia**), outward (**exotropia**), upward (**hypertropia**) or downward (**hypotropia**), and the defect may be constant or intermittent. '**Phoria**' is a mild tendency for misalignment of the eyes, whereas '**tropia**' is a constant visible deviation of the eyes. Strabismus may cause diplopia (double vision) in an older child and amblyopia in a younger child.

Infantile esotropia develops before 6 months' of age, tends to run in families and can be severe. Accommodative esotropia is inward turning of the eyes that develops between ages 6 months and 7 years, and is usually corrected with treatment. Paralytic strabismus may result from a nerve disorder, brain injuries, certain viral illnesses or a brain tumour that increases pressure within the skull and compresses the nerves. Temporary paralysis may be seen in Guillan-Barré syndrome. Strabismus may also be associated with the presence of a large haemangioma involving the eyelid.[75]

Eye injury

Although rare, partial or total loss of vision in an eye may result from injuries; including direct injury and penetrating trauma. Most eye injuries are preventable. Common mechanisms include a direct blow to the eye by a ball, or puck, traveling at high speed e.g. squash, hockey, and pellet gun injuries. In children with amblyopia, traumatic injury to the non-amblyopic eye may result in blindness in both eyes.

Uveitis

Childhood uveitis can lead to vision-threatening complications, and is best understood as a significant risk factor for vision loss. Uveitis refers to inflammation of the uvea, a component of the eye that is made up of three parts: the iris, the ciliary body and the choroid.

Uveitis may be infectious, as occurs in toxoplasmosis, chickenpox, and in toxocariasis in which a parasitic worm is transmitted to people from dogs and cats. Children may come into contact with the parasite when they play in sandboxes and on playgrounds contaminated with the parasite's eggs. The worm's larva can invade the eye, causing uveitis.

Uveitis can also be endogenous. The leading cause of uveitis in children is juvenile rheumatoid arthritis. Uveitis may also result from other inflammatory diseases including sarcoidosis, lupus, and Bechet's disease. Longitudinal studies have shown the prevalence of visual acuity of 20/200 or worse in at least one eye after diagnosis of paediatric uveitis is close to 70 per cent after 5 years,[76] while about 7.6 per cent are legally blind after ten years.[77] Uveitis therefore poses a serious risk to long-term vision.

Cortical or cerebral visual impairment

Cortical or cerebral visual impairment (CVI) is a neurological disorder resulting in bilateral impairment in visual acuity caused by damage to the central nervous system, meaning that visual acuity is decreased as a result of non-ocular disease.

CVI may occur in the absence of any pathology in the eye itself but, in practice, patients with CVI frequently have associated ophthalmologic abnormalities.

There is evidence that with increasing survival of children with severe medical problems the prevalence of CVI is increasing such that it is now the leading cause of bilateral vision impairment in children in Western countries. The most common cause of CVI is hypoxic-ischaemic injury. At least 60 per cent of children with neonatal hypoxic-ischaemic encephalopathy (HIE) are reported to have CVI. Head injuries, shunt failure, infections, and complications of cardiac treatment can all lead to CVI, and it frequently coexists with other serious neurologic impairment.[78] Most patients with CVI will not regain normal vision, but improvement is often seen over time.

Tumour

Rarely, vision impairment is caused by a tumour such as retinoblastoma. Retinoblastomas are bilateral in up to one-third of cases, and occur in about 1 in 15,000 births. Inherited forms are associated with a mutation on chromosome 13, the RB1 gene. About 50 per cent of cases have this mutation.

TYPES OR CLASSIFICATION

There is no single universally agreed classification system for vision loss. In addition to the four-category classification of partially sighted, low vision, legally blind and totally blind, there are alternate classification systems, e.g. based on the ICD-9 classification of Visual Acuity Impairment designating medical necessity for rehabilitation.[79] In this system, vision impairment is classified as follows:
- Moderate impairment: Best corrected acuity <20/60
- Severe impairment (legal blindness): Best corrected acuity <20/160 or visual field ≤20 degrees
- Profound impairment: Best corrected acuity <20/400 or visual field ≤10 degrees
- Near-total impairment: Best corrected acuity ≤20/1000 or visual field ≤5 degrees
- Total impairment: No light perception.

A third system, the WHO Classification of Visual Acuity Loss, avoids use of the term 'legally blind' and is designed to give a better description of the vision loss:
- Normal acuity: 20/25 or better
- Mild vision loss: 20/32 to 20/63
- Moderate vision loss: 20/80 to 20/160
- Severe vision loss: 20/200 to 20/400
- Profound vision loss: 20/500 to 20/1000
- Near blindness: <20/1000
- Blindness: no light perception.

This latter system allows for classification of mild vision loss, which is much more prevalent in the childhood population than the more severe vision impairments. In 2006 the United States Social Security Administration revised its guidelines on measurement of visual acuity so that a person would be considered legally blind if they are unable to read any letters on the 20/100 line on the alternate ETDRS chart.[80]

Existing classification systems are regarded as imperfect, leading to recommendations that a newer system based on functional loss of the patient rather than visual acuity or field loss be adopted. The ICD 10-ICIDH has been developed for this purpose but it is not yet widely adopted.[80]

Vision impairment has also been classified by aetiology, where known, divided into genetic, prenatal, perinatal and childhood categories,[81] however some aetiologies could fall into more than one of these categories making classification challenging. In addition, as more vision impairments are understood to have an underlying genetic aetiology, continual revision of categories is essential.

CLINICAL PRESENTATION

Severe vision impairments usually present early but can sometimes be missed, especially when there are other conditions present. Signs of vision loss in the child may include:
- Unable to fix their eyes on even a close object
- Random or roving eye movements
- Does not smile by age of 6 weeks
- Eyes may be abnormally large and cloudy if glaucoma present
- Baby may lie quietly to maximise use of their hearing
- May be less responsive than other babies.

Signs of vision loss in older children may include:
- Squinting to see
- Difficulty in recognising people
- Poor school performance
- Deteriorating school performance
- Finding light too bright or too dim
- Bumping into objects
- Moving about cautiously
- May be delay in other areas of development, e.g. gross and fine motor skills.

Any signs of vision loss or parental concern about a child's vision at any stage should lead to a full ophthalmologic evaluation conducted by a trained paediatric ophthalmologist or optometrist (see below).

Although there is no universally agreed list of risk factor for vision loss, children diagnosed with conditions known to be associated with vision impairment need regular ophthalmologic evaluation, even if vision appears normal at first examination, e.g. infants with congenital toxoplasmosis, CMV, paediatric uveitis.

For children with mild vision loss, or with more severe loss affecting only one eye, there may be few outward signs of a problem with vision in the early preschool years. These children are unlikely to be diagnosed in the absence of either routine vision assessment or vision screening. The United States Preventive Services Task Force (USPSTF) conducted an extensive evidence review and determined that there is insufficient evidence to assess the balance of benefits and harms of vision screening for children under the age of 3 years.[82] An Australian literature review conducted just prior to the USPSTF's work reached the same conclusion.[83] The USPSTF did, however, recommend vision screening for all children at least once between the ages of 3 and 5 years (Australian recommendation is between 3.5 and 5 years).[83]

It is important for providers to understand that the main target condition for screening is amblyopia and its risk factors, not refractive error. While there is good evidence to suggest that early detection of amblyopia between the ages of 3 and 5 years, followed by appropriate management with use of cycloplegic agents, patching and eyeglasses (see management) leads to improved vision outcomes, there is no existing evidence that shows unequivocally that there are benefits to the early detection and correction of relatively mild refractive errors in young children. In fact, there are concerns that such screening could lead to over-referral and inappropriate treatment. This is an area in need of much further research. Vision screening is also recommended at school entry, and bi-annually thereafter.

> **Practice Point**
>
> In contrast to the auditory system, which is relatively fully developed at birth, the visual system is believed to continue to mature throughout the first year of life and beyond. GIven our existing state of knowledge and technology, vision screening in the newborn period is not currently recommended. Efforts to develop age-related visual acuity norms in preschool children are underway.[84]

SCREENING TESTS

Typical components of vision screening include evaluations of visual acuity, strabismus and stereoacuity. Younger children, below the age of three years, are unable to cooperate with some of the screening tests performed in clinical practice, such as visual acuity testing. Stereoacuity testing is often omitted in this age group or performed incorrectly when attempted. False positives may result from young children being unable to cooperate with screening. Whenever there are positive findings on a screen, the child must be referred for a full ophthalmologic examination to confirm the presence of vision problems and to guide further treatment.[82] Vision screening tests that could feasibly be used in paediatric primary care are listed in Table 4.2.

There are few Australian data on patterns of vision screening in preschool-aged children, but in the United States evidence suggests that many paediatricians do not follow recommendations for screening and referral. Two-thirds do not begin visual acuity testing at age three, and about one-fifth do not test until age five years. One-quarter do not perform cover tests or stereopsis testing at any age.[85] National United States data based on parent report suggest that only 36 per cent of children aged five and under had ever had their vision screened. Widespread efforts are underway to increase vision screening rates among 3–5-year-old children, and to ensure that all children are screened at school entry and biannually thereafter.

ASSESSMENT

Any child who is referred after vision screening or who has risk factors for vision loss requires a full ophthalmologic evaluation. This may be carried out by an

TABLE 4.2 Vision screening tests

Visual screening test	Description	Comments
Visual acuity		
Snellen chart	Black letters on a white background. 6.10 m (20 ft) represents optical infinity. Numerator refers to distance in feet between subject and chart. Denominator indicates size of letters, specifically separation at which lines making up the letters would be separated by a visual angle of 1 arc minute, which for lowest line read with no refractive error would be 6.10 m (20 ft).	20/20 normal vision; 20/40 would be half normal acuity for distance vision. Snellen cannot be used with children who do not know letters. Widely used for school-age children.
Lea symbols	Uses common picture optotypes, e.g. house, heart in an effort to improve testability among young children and eliminate cultural biases.	Use of both single and surrounded Lea symbols have yielded modest sensitivities in children aged 2–6 years. May be useful in developmentally delayed children.[86]
HOTV	Uses surround bars combined with four single letters.	High testability in ages 4–7 years, reliable completion in only 50% of children aged 2–4 years.[86]
Glasgow acuity cards	Test performed at 3 m instead of 6 m. Linear progression of letters using a log scale. Letters of equal legibility and equal number of letters per line.	Some evidence of improved test reliability in young children.
Teller acuity cards preferential looking	Technician presents cards from behind a window in wall to check if child is more visually attentive to random vertical or horizontal bars on one side versus blank page on other side. Bars become progressively closer together.	Reliant on behavioural response so some subjectivity.
Visual evoked potentials	Brain waves created by presentation of black and white stripes or checkerboard patterns are recorded.	VEPs are mature by 1 year of age. Behavioural responses typically lag behind VEP responses.

TABLE 4.2 Continued

Visual screening test	Description	Comments
Visual acuity		
Monocular autorefractor e.g. SureSight, Retinomax	Automatically determines refractive state of each eye. Cannot directly detect amblyopia or strabismus.	Sensitive screen for ages 3–5 years but some false positives. Low testability for children <3 years.[87]
Photorefraction	Simultaneous recording of corneal and fundus reflexes by flash or video photography may allow detection of conditions that can give rise to amblyopia, including strabismus, ametropia, anisometropia and cataracts.	Limited testing in primary care settings. Reliability uncertain with inexperienced operators.
Strabismus		
Cover–uncover test	Child focuses on a near object and cover is placed over eye for a brief moment, then removed while observing eye for movement. A 'lazy eye' will wander in or out. Process is repeated on both eyes, and with focus on a distant object.	Subjective interpretation may be less reliable in inexperienced screeners.
Hirschberg test	Light shone into both eyes while observe where light reflects off the corneas. Light lands on centre of both corneas if normal ocular alignment.	In exotropia light lands on medial aspect of cornea; in esotropia light lands on lateral aspect of the cornea.
Stereoacuity		
Stereo fly, stereo butterfly, randot and preschool and random dot E tests	Tests depth perception and functioning of both eyes together. Fly and butterfly used with children as young as 4 years. Randot requires identification of 6 geometric shapes from random dot backgrounds. Preschool version is a matching test used in children as young as 2 years. Random Dot E used with children 3 years and up to distinguish a raised E from a non-stereo target.	For children aged 30–72 months, 80% can be tested using randot preschool stereoacuity test, and 97% children over age of 4.[88]

ophthalmologist, a medical doctor who specialises in eye and vision disorders, or an optometrist, a licensed provider trained to diagnose common visual acuity problems. Evidence from outside of Australia suggests that follow-up after vision screening is very variable. Barriers to effective follow-up include lack of parental knowledge or understanding about referral on a vision screen, and lack of access to diagnostic testing.

Many of the same techniques used in screening are used in diagnostic evaluations of visual ability. Assessment should include a comprehensive history including family and general health history, together with a comprehensive ocular examination. This includes comprehensive age-appropriate testing of visual acuity, ocular motility and binocular vision, visual field assessment, tonometry (eye pressure measurement), and central and peripheral fundi examination. Supplemental testing may include colour vision testing that may affect educational and vocational decisions in older children, visual evoked potentials, electro-retinograms (ERGs) and electro-oculograms. Electrodiagnostic tests may be important in certain conditions, e.g. Usher's syndrome, or when the patient is very young or has multiple handicaps.

Vision loss often occurs in the context of conditions that result in additional developmental challenges. In a British study of children with severe vision impairment or blindness, over two-thirds had associated non-ophthalmic impairment.[89] In addition, significant vision loss may result in delayed development in other areas, e.g. gross and fine motor function. Vision and hearing difficulties may coexist, so a full audiologic evaluation is also recommended. In most cases, especially where aetiology is unclear, referral for genetics evaluation and counselling is recommended. Any child with vision impairment should have an annual eye evaluation and review of treatment.

MANAGEMENT

Some vision loss is preventable. Prevention strategies focus on aetiology, e.g. rubella immunisation for prevention of congenital rubella syndrome, prevention of premature births, meningitis prevention through immunisations. Some eye conditions require specialised management, e.g. laser therapy for retinopathy of prematurity (ROP), anti-viral therapy for congenital CMV, vitamin A replacement therapy in vitamin A deficiency.

For children with established vision loss, correction of refractive errors with glasses or contact lenses is a mainstay of management. Glasses are used to treat nearsightedness, farsightedness and astigmatism. The place of laser eye surgery in children is not yet established, and most providers regard the long-term consequences as too uncertain to recommend this procedure prior to adulthood; however this recommendation may change. For amblyopia, patch therapy is advised. The 'healthy' eye is 'disabled' by putting a patch over it or by using eye drops such as atropine to blur vision, forcing the 'lazy' eye to work, strengthening its vision and stimulating the formation of new neural connections between the brain and the eye. As vision in the 'worse' eye improves, the brain becomes able to integrate the images it is receiving from both eyes, achieving binocular vision.

Corrective lenses may also be used to correct strabismus, together with surgery to alter the pull of the eye muscles where needed. Surgery is also needed to remove cataracts, following which children must either wear contact lenses or glasses to replace the eye's natural lens, or receive an intra-ocular lens (IOL) implant. Rarely, surgery is required to remove retinoblastoma, sometimes requiring enucleation of the eye and insertion of a prosthesis. In recent years, there have been attempts to avoid eye removal with greater use of chemotherapy and cryotherapy aimed at eye preservation.

Children with serious visual impairment face mobility challenges, and can benefit from tools such as a white cane with a red tip that can be used to sweep across the path ahead. Some older children use guide dogs to assist mobility, and may supplement these tools with technology such as a GPS for the visually impaired. These children will benefit from occupational therapy to help with adaptations to the tasks of daily living.

Reading may be assisted through use of large print or magnification devices. Use of Braille (raised print reliant on a dot system), talking books and reading machines offer further access to the written word. Specialised computers can also magnify text or offer screen reading.

The management of mild refractive error problems in young children remains controversial, and the optimal 'cut-off' visual acuity for the prescription of corrective lenses remains uncertain. Visual acuity of 20/40 (6/12) or worse is generally managed with corrective lenses. National United States data show that about 25 per cent of children aged 6–18 years have corrective lenses.[90] A number of studies have suggested that there may be an association between myopia and higher IQ levels. It is speculative whether this reflects a preference for children with myopia to engage in near-work, such as reading, which increases IQ, or whether extensive reading leads to myopia, although the latter is thought unlikely. Lack of exposure to sunlight has also been implicated as predisposing to myopia.

Several studies have addressed vision problems in children with learning difficulties and reading problems. The place of correction of very minor refractive errors, and of techniques such as vision exercises in the management of reading difficulties, remain controversial and there is currently no evidence that these interventions are warranted. However, given the high prevalence both of learning problems and vision problems in childhood much further research is needed in this area.

PROGNOSIS

Prognosis depends on that of the underlying condition, the nature and extent of the vision loss, the patient's physical and mental abilities, and on comorbidities outside of the ocular system. Once established, refractive errors generally do not improve. Similarly, improvement of blindness is rare with management focusing on uses of assistive and adaptive technology. Amblyopia, however, can be treated effectively, although further research is needed on optimal age at treatment and treatment intensity.

Children with vision impairment require careful monitoring throughout the school years, and may require additional support during the transition to adulthood and to further education. Relatively little is known about the long-term effects of childhood amblyopia and low vision in terms of quality of life and health through the course of life. Successful outcomes depend on a collaborative effort between the child, family, health and vision care providers, together with optimal use of technology.

KEY POINTS

- Immaturity of the vision system prior to the age of 3 years makes very early screening for vision loss challenging at population level.
- Severe vision impairment is usually diagnosed early, but milder forms of vision loss and amblyopia are often missed in the absence of screening.
- Early treatment for amblyopia is associated with improved vision outcomes.
- A significant amount of vision loss is now understood to have a genetic aetiology, and referral for genetic evaluation is recommended for all children with significant visual impairment.
- Over two-thirds of children with severe vision loss or blindness have additional conditions that may impact their developmental progress.

REFERENCES

1. National Dissemination Center for Children with Disabilities (NICHCY). Deafness and Hearing Loss. NICHCY Disability Fact Sheet, June 2010. Online. Available: http://nichcy.org/disability/specific/hearingloss; 20 Feb 2012
2. Russ SA, Poulakis Z, Barker M, et al. Epidemiology of congenital hearing loss in Victoria, Australia. Int J Audiol 2003;42:385–90
3. Davis A, Wood S. The epidemiology of childhood hearing impairment: factors relevant to planning of services. Br J Audiol 1992;26:77–90
4. Mehl A, Thomson V. The Colorado Newborn Hearing Screening Project, 1992–1999: On the threshold of effective population-based universal newborn hearing screening. Pediatrics 2002;109(1):e7
5. Finitzo T, Albright K, O'Neal J. The newborn with hearing loss: detection in the nursery. Pediatrics 1998;102:1452–60
6. Barsky-Firsker L, Sun S. Universal Newborn Hearing Screenings: A three-year experience. Pediatrics 1997;99(6):E4
7. Fortnum HM, Summerfield AQ, Marshall DH, et al. Prevalence of permanent childhood hearing impairment in the United Kingdom and implications for universal neonatal hearing screening: questionnaire based ascertainment study. BMJ 2001 Sept 8;323(7312): 536–40
8. Parving A, Christensen B. Epidemiology of permanent hearing impairment in children in relation to costs of a hearing health surveillance program. Int J Pediatr Otorhinolaryngol 1996;34:9–23
9. Niskar AS, Kieszak SM, Holmes A, et al. Prevalence of hearing loss among children 6 to 19 years of age: the Third National Health and Nutrition Examination Survey. JAMA 1998;279(14):1071–5
10. Smith RJ, Bale JF, White KR. Sensorineural hearing loss in children. Lancet 2005;365: 879–90
11. Das VK. Aetiology of bilateral sensorineural hearing impairment in children: a 10-year study. Arch Dis Child 1996 Jan;74(1):8–12
12. Bitner-Glindzicz M. Hereditary deafness and phenotyping in humans. Br Med Bull 2002;63:73–94
13. Alford RL. Nonsyndromic hereditary hearing loss. Adv Otorhinolaryngol 2011;70:37–42
14. Peterson MB. Non-syndromic autosomal-dominant deafness. Clin Genet 2002 Jul;62(1):1–13
15. Farrer LA, Arnos KS, Asher JH, et al. Locus heterogeneity for Waardenburg syndrome is predictive of clinical subtypes. Am J Hum Genet 1994;55(4):728–37

16 Hershey CL, Fisher DE. Genomic analysis of the microphthalmia locus and identification of the MITF-J/mitf-J isoform. Gene 2005;347(1):73–82
17 McLeod AC, McConnell FE, Sweeney A, et al. Clinical variation in Usher's syndrome. Arch Otolaryng 1971;94:321
18 Yang JJ, Tsai CC, Hsu HM, et al. Hearing loss associated with enlarged vestibular aqueduct and Mondini dysplasia is caused by splice-side mutation in the PDS gene. Hear Res 2005 Jan;199(1–2):22–30
19 Maubaret C, Griffoin JM, Arnaud B, et al. Novel mutations in MYO7A and USH2A in Usher syndrome. Ophthalmic Genet 2005 Mar;26(1):25–9
20 Kelley PM, Cohn E, Kimberling WJ. Connexin 26: required for normal auditory function. Brain Res Brain Res Rev 2000 Apr;32(1):184–8
21 Cohn ES, Kelley PM. Clinical phenotype and mutations in connexin 26 (DFNB1/GJB2), the most common cause of childhood hearing loss. Am J Med Genet 1999 Sep 24;89(3):130–6
22 Oguchi T, Ohtsuka A, Hashimoto S, et al. Clinical features of patients with GJB2 (connexin 26) mutations: severity of hearing loss is correlated with genotypes and protein expression patterns. J Hum Genet 2005;50(2):76–83
23 Chang EH, Van Camp G, Smith RJ. The role of connexins in human disease. Ear Hear 2003;24(4):314–23
24 Varga R, Kelley PM, Keats BJ, et al. Non-syndromic recessive auditory neuropathy is the result of mutations in the otoferlin (OTOF) gene. J Med Genet 2003;40(1): 45–50
25 Hanson H, Storey H, Pagan J, et al. The value of clinical criteria in identifying patients with X-linked Alport syndrome. Clin J Am Soc Nephrol 2011;6(1): 198–203
26 Rheault MN. Women and Alport Syndrome. Pediatr Nephrol 2012 Jan;27(1):41–6
27 Fischel-Ghodsian N. Mitochondrial deafness. Ear Hear 2003 Aug;24(4):303–13
28 Matsunaga T, Kumanomido H, Shiroma M, et al. Audiologic features and mitochondrial DNA sequence in a large family carrying mitochondrial A1555G mutation without use of aminoglycoside. Am Otol Rhino Laryngol 2005 Feb;114(2):153–60
29 Corsello G, Carcione A, Castro L, et al. Cervico-oculo-acusticus (Wildervanck's) syndrome: a clinical variant of Klippel-Feil sequence? Klin Padiatr 1990 May–Jun;202(3):176–9
30 Berger BE, Omer SB. Could the United States experience rubella outbreaks as a result of vaccine refusal and disease importation? Hum Vaccin 2010;6(12):1016–20
31 Brown ED, Chau JK, Atashband S, et al. A systemic review of neonatal toxoplasmosis exposure and sensorineural hearing loss. Int J Pediatr Otorhinolaryngol 2009;73(5): 707–11
32 Boppana SB, Ross SA, Shimamura M, et al. Saliva polymerase chain reaction assay for cytomegalovirus screening in newborns. N Engl J Med 2011;364(22):2111–18
33 Barbi M, Binda S, Caroppo S, et al. A wider role for congenital cytomegalovirus infection in sensorineural hearing loss. Pediatr Infect Dis J 2003;22(1):39–42
34 Valaes T. Bilirubin toxicity: the problem was solved a generation ago. Pediatrics 1992;89:819–21
35 Robertson CM, Howarth TM, Bork DL, et al. Permanent bilateral sensory and neural hearing loss of children after neonatal intensive care because of extreme prematurity: a thirty-year study. Pediatrics 2009;123(5):e797–807
36 Tudehope D, Smyth V, Scott J, et al. Audiological evaluation of very low birthweight infants. J Pediatr Child Health 1992;28:172–5
37 Fortnum HM. Hearing impairment after bacterial meningitis: a review. Arch Dis Child 1992;67:1128–33
38 Schuknecht HF. Mondini dysplasia. Ann Otol Rhinol Laryngol 1980;89:3–21
39 Henderson E, Testa MA, Hartnick C. Prevalence of noise-induced hearing-threshold shifts and hearing loss among US youths. Pediatrics 2011;127(1):e39–46
40 Huston Katsanis S, Cutting GR. In: Pagon RA, Bird TD, Dolan CR, et al, editors. Gene reviews. Seattle, WA: University of Washington; 1993–2004. Updated Oct 2006
41 Schrauwen I, Van Camp G. The etiology of otosclerosis: a combination of genes and environment. Laryngoscope 2010;120(6):1195–202

42 Robertson SP, Twigg SR, Sutherland-Smith AJ, et al. Localized mutations in the gene encoding the cytoskeleton protein filamin A cause diverse malformations in humans. Nat genet 2003;33(4):487–91
43 Browning GG, Rovers MM, Williamson I, et al. Grommets (ventilation tubes) for hearing loss associated with otitis media with effusion in children. Cochrane Database Syst Rev 2010;10:CD001801
44 British Society of Audiology, Descriptors for Pure Tone audiograms. British Journal of Audiology 1988;22:123
45 Rodriguez-Ballesteros M, del Castillo FJ, Martin Y, et al. Auditory neuropathy in patients carrying mutations in the otoferlin gene (OTOF). Hum Mutat 2003;22(6):451–6
46 Uus K, Bamford J. Effectiveness of population-based newborn hearing screening in England: ages of interventions and profile of cases. Pediatrics 2006;117(5):e887–893
47 Palo Alto Medical Foundation. Hearing Loss in Children. 2011 Online. Available: http://www.pamf.org/hearinghealth/facts/children.html; 20 Feb 2012
48 Joint Committee on Infant Hearing. Year 2007 Position Statement: principles and guidelines for early hearing detection and intervention programs. Pediatrics 2007;120(4):898–921
49 Norton SJ, Gorga MP, Widen JE, et al. Identification of neonatal hearing impairment: evaluation of transient evoked otoacoustic emission, distortion product otoacoustic emission and auditory brainstem evoked response test performance. Ear Hear 2000;21:508–28
50 Yoon PJ. Pediatric cochlear implantation. Curr Opin Pediatr 2011;23(3):346–50
51 Swanepoel D, Hugo R. Estimations of auditory sensitivity for young cochlear implant candidates using the ASSR: preliminary results. Int J Audiol 2004;43(7):377–82
52 Traxler CB. The Stanford Achievement test, 9th edn: national norming and performance standards for deaf and hard of hearing students. J Deaf Stud Deaf Educ 2000;5:337–48
53 Brookhouser PE, Worthington DW, Kelly WJ. Unilateral hearing loss in children. Laryngoscope 1991;101:1264–72
54 Wake M, Tobin S, Cone-Wesson B, et al. Slight/mild sensorineural hearing loss in children. Pediatrics 2006;118(5):1842–51
55 Pierangelo R, Guliani G. The educator's manual of disabilities and disorders. San Francisco: John Wiley & Sons; 2007
56 National Dissemination Center for Children with Disabilities (NICHCY) Fact Sheet 13: Vision Impairment. 2004 Online. Available: http://www.nichcy.org; 20 Feb 2012
57 Mervis CA, Boyle CA, Yeargin-Allsopp M. Prevalence and selected characteristics of childhood vision impairment. Dev Med Child Neurol 2002;44:538–41
58 Kemper A, Harris R, Lieu T, et al. Screening for visual impairment in children younger than age 5 years: A systematic evidence review no 27 (Prepared by the Research Triangle Institute–University of North Carolina Evidence-based Practice Center). Rockville, MD: Agency for Healthcare Research and Quality; May 2004. Online. Available: http://www.ncbi.nlm.nih.gov/books/bv.fcgi?rid=hstat3.chapter.33443; 20 Feb 2012
59 Remington JS, McLeod R, Thulliez P, et al. Toxoplasmosis (ch 31). In: Remington JS, editor. Infectious Diseases of the Fetus and Newborn Infant, 6th ed. Philadelphia: Saunders Elsevier; 2006
60 Edlich RF, Winters KL, Long 3rd WB, et al. Rubella and congenital rubella (German measles). J Long Term Eff Med Implants 2005;15(3):319–28
61 Graw J. The genetic and molecular basis of congenital eye defects. Nat Rev Genet 2003;4:876–88
62 Summer GS. Albinism: classification, clinical characteristics, and recent findings. Optom Vis Sci 2009;86:659–62
63 Oetting WS, King RA. Molecular basis of albinism: mutations and polymorphisms of pigmentation genes associated with albinism. Hum Mut 1999;13(2):99–115
64 Yu Wai-Man P, Griffiths PG, Chinnery PF. Mitochondrial optic neuropathies: disease mechanisms and therapeutic strategies. Prog Retin Eye Res 2011;30(2):81–114
65 US National Library of Medicine, National Institutes of Health. Retinopathy of Prematurity. 2009 Online. Available: http://www.nlm.nih.gov/medlineplus/ency/article/001618.htm; 20 Feb 2012

66 Chen J, Stahl A, Hellstrom A, et al. Current update on retinopathy of prematurity: screening and treatment. Curr Opin Pediatr 2011;23(2):173–8
67 Quinn GE, Gilbert C, Darlow BA, et al. Retinopathy of prematurity: an epidemic in the making. Clin Med J (Engl) 2010;123(20):2929–37
68 Chen ML, Guo L, Smith LE, et al. High and low oxygen saturation and severe retinopathy of prematurity: a meta-analysis. Pediatrics 2010;125(6):e1483–92
69 Karna P, Muttineni J, Angell L, et al. Retinopathy of prematurity and risk factors: a prospective cohort study. BMC Pediatr 2005;5(1):18
70 Smith J, Steinemann TL. Vitamin A deficiency and the eye. Int Ophthalmol 2000;40(4):83–91
71 Berson EL. Retinitis pigmentosa and allied retinal diseases (ch 24). In: Tasman W, Jaeger EA, editors. Duane's Ophthalmology, 15th ed. Philadelphia: Lippincott Williams & Wilkins; 2009
72 Weiss JS, Moller HU, Lisch W, et al. The ICD3 classification of the corneal dystrophies. Cornea 2008;27(Suppl 2):S1–S42
73 Facts about refractive error. National Eye Institute, National Institutes of Health. 2009 Online. Available: http://www.nei.nih.gov/CanWeSee/qa_refractive; 20 Feb 2012
74 Olitsky SE, Coats DK. Amblyopia and its management (ch 10). In: Tasman W, Jaeger EA, editors. Duane's Ophthalmology, 15th ed. Philadelphia: Lippincott Williams & Wilkins; 2009
75 Olitsky SE, Hug D, Smith LP. Disorders of eye movement and alignment (ch 622). In: Kliegman RM, Behrman RE, Jenson HB, et al, editors. Nelson Textbook of Pediatrics, 18th ed. Philadelphia: Saunders Elsevier; 2007
76 Rosenberg KD, Feuer WJ, Davis JL. Ocular complications of pediatric uveitis. Ophthalmology 2004;111(12):2299–306
77 Smith JA, Mackensen F, Sen HN, et al. Epidemiology and course of disease in childhood uveitis. Ophthalmology 2009;116(8):1544–51
78 Good WV, Jan JE, Burden SK, et al. Recent advances in cortical visual impairment. Developmental medicine and child neurology 2001;43:56–60
79 The International Classification of Disease, 9th rev., Clinical Modification (ICD-9-CM). 2001 Online. Available: http://www.cdc.gov/nchs/about/otheract/icd9/abticd9.htm; 20 Feb 2012
80 Freeman KF, Cole RG, Faye EE, et al. American Optometric Association Consensus Panel on the care of the patient with low vision. Optometric clinical practice guideline care of the patient with visual impairment (low vision rehabilitation). St Louis, MO: American Optometric Association; 2007
81 Khan RI, O'Keefe M, Kenny D, et al. Changing pattern of childhood blindness. Ir Med J 2007;100(5):458–61
82 US Preventive Services Task Force. Vision screening for children 1 to 5 years of age: US Preventive Services Task Force Recommendation Statement. Pediatrics 2011;127:340–6
83 Mathers M, Keyes M, Wright M. A review of the evidence on the effectiveness of children's vision screening. Child Care Health Dev 2010;36(6):756–80
84 Pan Y, Tarczy-Hornoch K, Cotter SA, et al. Visual acuity norms in pre-school children: the Multi-Ethnic Pediatric Eye Disease Study. Optom Vis Sci 2009;86(6):607–12
85 Wall TC, Marsh-Tootle W, Evans HH, et al. Compliance with vision-screening guidelines among a national sample of pediatricians. Ambul Pediatr 2002;2(6):449–55
86 Repka MX. Use of Lea symbols in young children. Br J Ophthalmol 2002;86(5):489–90
87 Kemper AR, Keating LM, Jackson JL, et al. Comparison of monocular autorefraction to comprehensive eye examinations in preschool-aged and younger children. Arch Pediatr Adolesc Med 2005;159(5):435–9
88 Tarczy-Hornoch K, Lin J, Deneen J, et al. Stereoacuity testability in African-American and Hispanic pre-school children. Optom Vis Sci 2008;85(3):158–63
89 Rahi JS, Cumberland PM, Peckham CS for the British Childhood Visual Impairment Interest Group. Improving detection of blindness in childhood: the British Childhood Vision Impairment Study. Pediatrics 2010 Oct;126(4):e895–903
90 Kemper AR, Bruckman D, Freed G. Prevalence and distribution of corrective lenses among school-age children. Optom Vis Sci 2004;81(1):7–10

FURTHER READING

Hearing Loss
Joint Committee on Infant Hearing. Year 2007 Position Statement: principles and guidelines for early hearing detection and intervention programs. Pediatrics 2007;120(4):898–921

Vision Loss
US Preventive Services Task Force. Vision screening for children 1 to 5 years of age: US Preventive Services Task Force Recommendation Statement. Pediatrics 2011;127:340–6

RESOURCES

These sites available 20 February 2012.

Hearing Loss
Aussie Deaf Kids. http://www.aussiedeafkids.org.au/
Australian Hearing. http://www.hearing.com.au/
Centers for Disease Control and Prevention Hearing Loss in Children. http://www.cdc.gov/ncbddd/hearingloss/index.html
Hands and Voices. http://www.handsandvoices.org/
US National Center for Hearing Assessment and Management. http://www.infanthearing.org/
Victorian Infant Hearing Screening Program. http://www.rch.org.au/vihsp/index.cfm?doc_id=7461

Vision Loss
Vision Australia. Blindness and Low Vision Services. http://www.visionaustralia.org.au/
Australian Blindness Forum. http://www.australianblindnessforum.org.au/
Prevent Blindness America. http://www.preventblindness.org/hcp/
Vision 2020. The Right to Sight. http://www.vision2020.org/main.cfm?type=WIBCHILDHOOD

5 Autism spectrum disorders

Natalie Silove

HISTORY

With the increase in awareness and recognition of autism spectrum disorders there has been concern that the incidence has increased in recent years. However, autistic behaviour has been described in early folklore long before it was described by Leo Kanner.

> Folklore includes stories about changelings. They describe a child who exhibits remarkable and sudden changes in behaviour and/or appearance, explaining that supernatural folk steal normal children and replace them with one of their own, or some other substitute. The new child – the changeling – is characterised by unresponsiveness, resistance to physical affection, obstreperousness, inability to express emotion, and unexplained crying and physical changes such as rigidity and deformity. Some are unable to speak.[1]

These folklore stories are a reminder that perhaps autism is not a new disorder. They are particularly reminiscent of parental reports of children who appear to be developing well and then regress in their second year of life.

The word 'autism' comes from the Greek word 'autos', meaning 'self.' The term describes conditions in which a person is removed from social interaction – hence, an 'isolated self'. Eugen Bleuler, a Swiss psychiatrist, in around 1911 was the first to use the term in relation to symptoms seen in adult schizophrenia.

In 1943 Leo Kanner, a child psychiatrist at Johns Hopkins University in the United States, described a small group of children who demonstrated extreme aloofness and total indifference to others, failure to use language for the purpose of communication, and an 'anxiously obsessive desire for the maintenance of sameness, resulting in marked limitation in the variety of spontaneous play'. In 1944 Hans Asperger published an article in which he described a group of children demonstrating similar symptoms but with better verbal and cognitive skills. His work was unknown because it was published in German and little translated into English until Lorna Wing, a British psychiatrist, wrote a paper in 1981 describing 34 cases similar to Asperger's and referred to his original publication.

Descriptive terms and diagnostic criteria for autism have varied over time as there is increasing epidemiologic and biological evidence that contributes towards the understanding of aetiology and clinical manifestations.

'Infantile autism' first appeared as a separate category in the DSM-III in 1980.[2] The Autistic Disorder (AD) criteria were broadened and the new subthreshold category, Pervasive Developmental Disorder-Not Otherwise Specified (PDD-NOS) was included in the DSM-III in 1987. Asperger syndrome (AS) was included in the DSM-IV in 1994.[3] The DSM-IV-TR in 2000 refined the text description of PDD-NOS, but Autistic Disorder and AS remained largely unchanged.[4] This correlates better with the International Statistical Classification of Diseases and Related Health Problems (10th edn).[5]

The DSM-IV-TR[6] refers to the term 'Pervasive Developmental Disorders' which includes: autistic disorder, Asperger's disorder, pervasive developmental disorder not otherwise specified, Rett's disorder and childhood disintegrative disorder.

The explosion of information and better understanding of the continuum of the spectrum over the last decade has led to the recently favoured term 'autism spectrum disorders' which includes autistic disorder, Asperger's disorder and pervasive developmental disorder not otherwise specified.[6]

The proposed DSM-V will most likely result again in a change in the nosology, as well as recommend changing the classic 'triad' to two domains: social communication and interaction, and restricted repetitive patterns of behaviours, interest and activities.[7]

DEFINITIONS
DSM-IV-TR classification[4]
Autistic disorder
This has previously been described as early infantile autism, childhood autism or Kanner's autism.

Autism is a **pervasive, developmental neurobiological** disorder characterised by core deficits in three main developmental domains, i.e. the classic 'triad' of impairment:
- Reciprocal social interaction skills
- Communication
- Restricted, repetitive and stereotyped patterns of behaviour, interests and activities.

Autism is **pervasive** as it affects all aspects of an individual's life (home, school and community); **developmental** as the clinical presentation may change with age; and **neurobiological** because it involves biological changes affecting the developing brain.

The 12 DSM-IV-TR criteria for autistic disorder[4] are listed in Text Box 5.1. Diagnosis of autistic disorder is dependent on six criteria with at least two relating to qualitative impairment of social development, and at least one each relating to qualitative impairment of communication and restricted repetitive and stereotyped patterns of behaviour, interests and activities. Manifestations should be evident prior to the age of three years, and vary markedly depending on developmental level and chronological age of the individual.

It is essential to have an in-depth understanding of the developmental trajectories of the clinical manifestations described in each component of the triad, as without that knowledge it is not possible to know whether the acquired skill is appropriate for the individual's developmental/mental age.

Asperger's disorder (also known as Asperger's syndrome)
The essential features of Asperger's disorder are the severe and sustained impairment in social interaction and the development of markedly restricted, repetitive patterns of behaviour and interests (see Text Box 5.2). The disturbance must cause

> **TEXT BOX 5.1** DSM-IV-TR diagnostic criteria for 299.00 Autistic Disorder
>
> A A total of six (or more) items from (1), (2) and (3) with at least two from (1) and one each from (2) and (3).
>   1 Qualitative impairment in social interaction as manifested by at least two of the following:
>   a Marked impairment in the use of multiple nonverbal behaviours, such as eye-to-eye gaze, facial expression, body postures, and gestures to regulate social interaction
>   b Failure to develop peer relationships appropriate to developmental level
>   c A lack of spontaneous seeking to share enjoyment, interests, or achievements with other people (e.g. by a lack of showing, bringing, or pointing out objects of interest)
>   d Lack of social or emotional reciprocity.
>   2 Qualitative impairments in communication as manifested by at least one of the following:
>   a Delay in, or total lack of, the development of spoken language (not accompanied by an attempt to compensate through alternative modes of communication such as gesture or mime)
>   b In individuals with adequate speech, marked impairment in the ability to initiate or sustain a conversation with others
>   c Stereotyped and repetitive use of language or idiosyncratic language
>   d Lack of varied, spontaneous make-believe play or social imitative play appropriate to developmental level.
>   3 Restricted repetitive and stereotyped patterns of behaviour, interests, and activities, as manifested by at least one of the following:
>   a Encompassing preoccupation with one or more stereotyped and restricted patterns of interest that is abnormal either in intensity or focus
>   b Apparently inflexible adherence to specific, nonfunctional routines or rituals
>   c Stereotyped and repetitive motor mannerisms (e.g. hand or finger flapping or twisting, or complex whole-body movements)
>   d Persistent preoccupation with parts of objects.
> B Delays or abnormal functioning in at least one of the following areas, with onset prior to age three years; (1) social interaction, (2) language as used in social communication, or (3) symbolic or imaginative play.
> C The disturbance is not better accounted for by Rett's disorder or childhood disintegrative disorder.

clinically significant impairment in social, occupational or other areas of functioning. By definition, intellectual ability and early formal language development (single words by two years and two-word spontaneous phrases by three years) must be within the average range. As a result, parents or caregivers often only become concerned at a later age as the social relationships fail to develop as

TEXT BOX 5.2 DSM-IV-TR diagnostic criteria for 299.80 Asperger's disorder

A Qualitative impairment in social interaction, as manifested by at least two of the following:
   1 Marked impairment in the use of multiple nonverbal behaviours, such as eye-to-eye gaze, facial expression, body postures, and gestures to regulate social interaction
   2 Failure to develop peer relationships appropriate to developmental level
   3 A lack of spontaneous seeking to share enjoyment, interests or achievements with other people (e.g. by a lack of showing, bringing, or pointing out objects of interest to other people)
   4 Lack of social or emotional reciprocity.
B Restricted repetitive and stereotyped patterns of behaviour, interests and activities as manifested by at least one of the following:
   1 Encompassing preoccupation with one or more stereotyped and restricted patterns of interest that is abnormal either in intensity or focus
   2 Apparently inflexible adherence to specific, nonfunctional routines or rituals
   3 Stereotyped and repetitive motor mannerism (e.g. hand or finger flapping or twisting, or complex whole-body movements)
   4 Persistent preoccupation with parts of objects.
C The disturbance causes clinically significant impairment in social, occupational, or other important areas of functioning.
D There is no clinically significant general delay in language (e.g. single words used by age two years, communicative phrases used by age three years).
E There is no clinically significant delay in cognitive development or in the development of age-appropriate self-help skills, adaptive behaviour (other than in social interaction) and curiosity about the environment in childhood.
F Criteria are not met for another specific pervasive developmental disorder or schizophrenia.

expected or the restricted, repetitive patterns of behaviour and interests emerge. While the definition requires that early language be present, it does not mean that the communication skills in Asperger's disorder are 'normal'. Affected individuals may have qualitatively impaired reciprocal communication, and unusual language. Semantic (understanding) pragmatic (social use of) language impairment is the language impairment most commonly described.

Asperger's disorder is not mild autism, as commonly thought. The functional impact of Asperger's disorder or autistic disorder for an individual varies from mild to severe at different ages, depending on the demands of the environment and the acquired skills of the individual.

Pervasive developmental disorder – not otherwise specified

The category pervasive developmental disorder – not otherwise specified (including atypical autism) (PPD) should be used when there is a severe and pervasive

> **TEXT BOX 5.3** Pervasive developmental disorder not otherwise specified (including atypical autism)
>
> This category should be used when there is a severe and pervasive impairment in the development of reciprocal social interaction or verbal and nonverbal communication skills, or when stereotyped behaviour, interests, and activities are present, but the criteria are not met for a specific pervasive developmental disorder, schizophrenia, schizotypal personality disorder, or avoidant personality disorder. For example, this category includes 'atypical autism' – presentations that do not meet the criteria for autistic disorder because of late age at onset, atypical symptomatology, or subthreshold symptomatology, or all of these.

impairment in development of reciprocal social interaction associated with impairment in either verbal or nonverbal communication skills or with the presence of stereotypic behaviour, interests, and activities. It includes 'atypical autism'; presentations which do not meet criteria for a diagnosis of autistic disorder because of late age of onset, atypical or sub-threshold symptomatology, or all of these (see Text Box 5.3).

Rett's disorder is included as a pervasive developmental disorder because behaviours observed in persons with Rett's are similar to characteristic of autism – particularly in the preschool years. However the course and onset of Rett's is very distinctive; very early development is normal, head growth then decelerates, usually in the first months of life and a loss of purposeful hand movements occurs. Motor involvement is quite striking and profound, intellectual disability is typical. Characteristic hand-wringing stereotypic behaviours develop. Historically, Rett's was thought to only affect girls. Since the discovery of the MECP2 gene responsible for Rett's, variants of the syndrome have been reported in males who have mutations of MECP2 with some overlap in the symptomatology observed in girls.[8]

Childhood disintegrative disorder is characterised by a marked regression (loss of established skills) in multiple areas of functioning following a period of at least two years of apparently normal development (previously called Heller's syndrome or dementia infantilis).

Accepted current terms for **autism spectrum disorders** (ASD) include autistic disorder, Asperger's disorder and pervasive developmental disorder not otherwise specified (or atypical autism).

Broader autism phenotype
Broader autism phenotype (BAP) refers to siblings and family members who have some autism features.[9]

PREVALENCE

Autism was once considered a rare condition affecting only 3–4 per 10,000 children. Recent Australian figures estimate the prevalence of ASD in Australia to be on average 1 in 160 children.[10] This is consistent with other international studies where prevalence varies from 22 per 10,000 (1 in 455) for autistic disorder and 59 per 10,000 (1 in 169) for all PDD's under six years old.[11] Explanations for this increased prevalence include: changing diagnostic criteria and broadening of the spectrum, differences in methodology, referral patterns, diagnostic substitution (e.g. students who may have been identified with an intellectual disability only, as the autism did not receive special compensation), availability of services, migration, and public and professional awareness[6,8]. However, it is not possible at this stage to exclude the possibility of environmental factor(s) interacting with a genetic predisposition.

AETIOLOGY

The exact cause of ASDs remains unknown, but they are clearly biologically-based, highly heritable developmental disorders. The sex ratio of male to female is 4:1, similar to other developmental disorders. The concordance rate between monozygotic twins is 90 per cent. Currently a genetic cause can be identified in 20–25 per cent of children with autism. A small number can be traced to specific teratogen exposure. The cause in the remaining 75–80 per cent remains unknown.[12]

Genetics

- **Cytogenetically visible chromosomal abnormalities (high resolution chromosome analysis and FISH ~5–8 per cent):** Maternally derived duplication of the Prader-Willi or Angleman syndrome critical region (15q11-q13), trisomy 21, 45X, Turner syndrome, and a number of other deletions and sex chromosome aneuploidies have been reported in individuals with ASD.
- **Copy number variants (CNVs)** or submicroscopic deletions and duplications (10–20 per cent). Array comparative genomic hybridisation (aCGH) is increasingly recommended as a first tier test.[13] Several pathogenic genomic changes in genes encoding for neuronal cell adhesion molecules and in genes involved in the ubiquitin pathways have been idenitified.[12]
- **Single gene disorders** in which neurologic findings are associated with ASD (~5 per cent). These include Fragile X syndrome (1–3 per cent of ASD), PTEN (phosphatase and tensin homolog) macrocephaly syndrome, Sotos syndrome, Rett's syndrome, tuberous sclerosis complex (TSC), neurofibromatosis (NF-1), Timothy syndrome, and Joubert syndrome, metabolic conditions, Duchenne muscular dystrophy.[14]

Environmental risks

Infectious diseases (e.g. congenital rubella, postnatal encephalitis), inborn errors of metabolism (e.g. phenylketonuria or metabolic error in cholesterol biosynthesis in Smith-Lemli-Opitz syndrome) and toxins (e.g. fetal alcohol syndrome, thalidomide, valproic acid),[14] and more recently terbutaline in pregnancy, severe fetal hypoxia[15] and assisted reproductive technologies have been implicated.[16] It is highly recommended that women taking valproate in pregnancy be informed of the risks.[14]

A number of rigorous studies show no epidemiological evidence to support the theory of a link between measles–mumps–rubella vaccination, or between thimerosol-containing vaccines and autism. (The MMR vaccine has never contained thimerosol.) There is also no rationale for giving separate vaccinations as opposed to the combination vaccine.[17] Consensus is to continue with the recommended immunisation schedules.

Neuropathology and neuroimaging

The head circumference at birth is within the typically normal range. However, there is evidence that the brains of autistic infants at 2–4 months of age are on average 10 per cent larger than those of normal infants, and that there is a spurt of brain growth in the first years of life (which is not as marked in typically developing infants). However after the spurt of growth there is a plateau, so that the adolescent and adult autistic brain is no larger than the normal brain[18,19] It is suggested that during this time of excessive growth in infancy, mini columns (anatomical and physiological units of the neocortex) are laid down and generated in excess in autistic brains.[20] It is suggested that the reduction in the size of neuronal bodies and of the nucleoli in the neurons in the smaller mini columns could reflect a bias towards shorter connecting fibres in the autistic cortex, since the distances between adjacent neurons are shorter. It is possible that this bias would favour local computation between neurones at the expense of the formation of connections between cortical areas and connectivity across the corpus callosum.[20]

Post mortem neuropathological studies of brain tissue have revealed several abnormalities, not the least of which includes reduced numbers of Purkinje cells in the cerebellum, reduced neuronal cell size, stunted dendritic arbors, increased cell-packing density in limbic structures, shortening of the brainstem associated with anatomic deficits in the region of the facial and superior olivary nuclei and neocortical malformation (e.g. heterotopias).[6] None of these findings are pathognomonic.

Functional neuro-imaging (using SPECT and PET) scans show differences in the active processing of information with the autistic brain responding differently to both visual and auditory information. Neurochemical differences have been demonstrated with regards to serotonin and specific neurotransmitters.[6] None of these finding are pathognomonic or sufficiently consistent to be helpful in the diagnosis or management of ASD, and therefore are not indicated routinely.

Cognitive theories underlying the core deficits in ASD

- **Theory of mind** (ToM)[21] refers to a human's ability to infer mental state in others. It is the ability to explain observable events based on desires or emotions, knowing that other people think differently from you, being able to take another person's perspective, put other people's feelings before your own, and thinking about the consequences of your actions before engaging in them.
- **Central coherence theory** describes an inability to bring together various details to make a meaningful whole.[22,23] A lack of cognitive central coherence or gestalt processing can easily cause a person to miss the importance of the subtle cues that create meaning in a social context, including the difficulty of intuitively understanding the main idea of a conversation or a passage in literature. In other words, they miss the 'big picture'.
- **Executive dysfunction** reflects impairment in the higher-order processes that enable a person to plan, sequence, initiate, and sustain their behaviour towards a particular goal, incorporating feedback and making adjustments along the way.[24]
- **Cortical under connectivity theory** of autism proposes that autism is a cognitive and neurobiological disorder associated with under-functioning of integrative brain circuitry, resulting in a deficit in integration of information

at the neural and cognitive levels. There is therefore reduced functional connectivity between parts of the brain.[25]

CLINICAL PRESENTATION

Understanding and knowing age-appropriate milestones and 'typical development' is imperative in being able to identify atypical development. It is only obvious that a child is unable to do something when they have reached the age at which they are expected to have achieved a particular skill.

The clinical presentation varies significantly between individuals with ASD depending on level of intellectual ability, communication skills, and presence of comorbidity. Severe social skills deficits, and restrictive, repetitive and stereotyped patterns of behaviour, interests and activities are core features of all ASDs. Significant language delays are characteristic of autistic disorder and PDD-NOS, and not Asperger's disorder. The qualitative impairments in all three developmental areas in the triad do not necessarily parallel each other in severity or timing of presentation. Many individuals may be more impaired in communication than socialisation, or vice versa, and the restricted repetitive behaviours and interests may be present to varying degrees at different developmental ages. Many children do not present with stereotypic and ritualistic behaviours until much later, and when they are present in infancy it appears to be a poorer prognostic sign.

Parents may become concerned during the second and third year of life when it becomes clear that their child's development appears to have plateaued or, in 25–30 per cent of children, regressed.[6]

Speech delay is a common presenting feature. Often it is thought that the child is 'deaf' as they do not respond to their name, and a hearing assessment is requested.

In a child who is making what appears to be developing 'typical' language, motor and cognitive skills, it may only become clear at a much later stage that they are having difficulty with social relationships, understanding social cues and the emotional states of others, and that their interests are not developing and expanding as one would expect. This is often when the diagnosis of Asperger's disorder is considered.

Social

Failure to make eye contact, respond to a social smile or settle with a cuddle, are often early subtle features of ASD. These can be masked by other issues at the time, such as feeding or sleeping difficulties, and so may be missed. While there is no pathognomonic feature of ASD, delayed or absent **joint attention** seems to be a fairly reliable 'red flag' for ASD. Joint attention (JA) is a spontaneously occurring behaviour whereby the infant shows enjoyment in sharing an object or event with another person by looking back and forth between the two. Later, gestures and/or speech can also be used to engage others' attention with regard to the object and event simply for the enjoyment of sharing the experience.

At approximately 12 to 14 months of age a typically developing child will begin to point to request an object (imperative pointing), and by 15 months of age pointing to share or show an object or activity in the distance (protodeclarative pointing). As the child points, they will look alternatively between the object of interest and the parents (cross-referencing).[6] *These very early social engagement and reciprocal skills may be absent or delayed in children with autism.*

At a later age they may have little or no interest in their peers and be content to play on their own. Higher functioning children may be aware of their peers, initiate interaction, but be unable to sustain any relationships or activities. Often their relationships evolve around their own special interests. They may have difficulty in understanding another's point of view (theory of mind skills), unable to understand a behaviour or verbal response in context, have difficulty seeing the 'big picture' (lack of central coherence) and tend to focus on detail. On the other hand, many have the ability to form strong attachments to particular individuals, usually parents and caregivers initially, and subsequently with other individuals who may share similar interests.

Communication

The communication deficits in autism include both verbal and nonverbal forms of communication.

Verbal communication consists of a number of components: expressive (spoken), receptive (understanding/semantics), pragmatic (social use of language), motor (articulation) and expression (prosody). Many have very delayed onset of language. In others, early expressive language may develop which consists predominantly of 'naming words'. However further development is impaired as children are expected to use language to initiate, share and communicate needs and interests. Echolalia (parroting words or phrases) may be a prominent feature, or they may have the ability to recite large chunks of dialogue from their favourite movies or nursery rhymes, but be unable to put a simple spontaneous sentence together. Higher functioning individuals may have very good expressive speech, but speech tends to be pedantic, idiosyncratic, and at times socially inappropriate or focused on their own agenda and not reciprocal. Some will have unusual prosody (sing song, monotone or staccato quality), or take on unusual accents, e.g. from the BBC or American movies.

There is often an associated limited or awkward use of gestures, e.g. pointing, waving or descriptive gestures.

Play skills

Play is often repetitive, and the ability to imitate and engage in spontaneous make-believe imaginative play is lacking or delayed. They may enjoy lining up, grouping or stacking toys rather than playing appropriately. Symbolic (i.e. using an object or something other than what it was intended for, e.g. using a pencil as a wand or a sword) play may be delayed. Many persist at the sensory-motor stage of play where they explore objects by mouthing/smelling, swirling, banging and manipulating the object in an unusual way. They often tend to play with parts of the object and not with the object as a whole, e.g. become obsessed with the wheels rather than play with the car in a creative way. Many children enjoy the sensory aspects of play, e.g. being swung or thrown high up in the air, or bounced up and down on someone's knee. As further skills are developed, play tends to be more 'object' focused (puzzles, computer games), rather than 'person' focused.

Stereotypic behaviours

This includes restricted, repetitive and stereotyped patterns of behaviour, interests and activities.

Stereotypic behaviours are repetitive, non-functional, atypical behaviours, such as hand-flapping, rocking, twirling, unusual hand and finger movements. Although most are harmless, they can get in the way of learning new skills and making progress. At times they can draw attention to the child, which may lead to further isolation or bullying. Stereotypes may not appear until after the age of three.

Unusual and persistent attachment to objects can occur long past the age when these may be developmentally appropriate. In higher functioning individuals, interests may be more related to topics and facts rather than actual objects. While the interest or topic of interest may be age-appropriate, it is the degree, persistence and pervasiveness of the interest that is abnormal, e.g. they may persist in talking about dinosaurs or space long after the other children have moved on to a different activity.

Self-injurious behaviours, e.g. head banging or skin picking, may also be stereotypic and can become problematic, particularly in children with severe developmental disabilities. Self-injurious behaviours may be precipitated by frustration due to unsuccessful communication, significant anxiety, a change in the routine, transition from one activity to another, boredom, depression, sleep deprivation or pain.

Rigidities around mealtimes and food can be very problematic. The reasons for this may be varied, including differences in smell, texture, colour or taste perception. Reduced flexibility of thought or ideas is often problematic.

Sleep disturbance of all types are more common in ASD and require specific attention.

Savant skills

Savant skills occur in 1–10 per cent of people with autism. It refers to an extraordinary splinter skill, which is out of keeping with the other developmental and mental abilities of that particular individual. Savant skills are found usually in the fields of numerical calculation, music and art.

Common strengths described in ASD

It is important to identify absolute or relative strengths in individuals with ASD as this will often provide a platform to allow for engagement and success. Clinical experience reveals that strengths may include (but are not limited to) the ability to memorise rote material, understand concrete concepts, think and learn visually, focus on detail, have unusual long-term memory, learn chunks of information quickly, have good sense of direction, be perfectionist, understand and follow rules and sequences, reliability, honesty and a strong sense of integrity.

DIFFERENTIAL DIAGNOSES OF THE AUTISM SPECTRUM DISORDERS

1. **Sensory impairment:** vision and hearing.
2. **Global developmental delay (DD) and intellectual disability (ID):** Global DD and ID may occur together with an ASD, however increasingly more students are being identified who have an ASD with average and above average intellectual ability.

3. **Specific language impairment (SLI):** Labels and definitions of language disorders vary. However the fundamental concept is that a SLI is a developmental language disorder that can affect both expressive and receptive language, is significantly behind that expected for the intellectual ability of the individual, and is not related to or caused by other developmental disorders, hearing loss or acquired brain injury.
4. **Anxiety disorders:** These include selective mutism, generalised anxiety disorder, social phobia and obsessive–compulsive disorder.
5. **Reactive attachment disorder of infancy and early childhood:** This presents with markedly disturbed and developmentally inappropriate social relatedness. In most contexts it begins before age five years and is associated with grossly pathological care.[4] Developmental learning allowances are made for up to two years after a child has been in a caring, stimulating and nurturing environment, after which the standard diagnostic testing and assessments can be applied (with regards to learning and developmental milestones), while emotional and other supportive care is ongoing.
6. **Attention deficit hyperactivity disorder (ADHD):** ADHD presents with a persistent pattern of inattention, sustained attention with goal-directed activities, distractibility, hyperactivity–impulsivity, that is more frequent and severe than observed in an age-related peer of comparable development. It is often associated with difficulty in planning and organising of thoughts, activities and environment, and may have a significant impact on socialisation and learning. Up to 60 per cent of child with ASD may have ADHD.

EARLY IDENTIFICATION IN PRESCHOOL CHILDREN

The earlier the identification and intervention, the better the life outcomes.

There are several 'red flags' in the preschool age child, which alert the clinician to the possibility of ASD.[26]

1. Impairment in social interaction:
    - Lack of appropriate eye gaze
    - Lack of warm, joyful expressions
    - Lack of sharing interest or enjoyment
    - Lack of response to name.
2. Impairment in communication:
    - Lack of showing gestures
    - Lack of coordination of nonverbal communication
    - Unusual prosody (little variation in pitch, odd intonation, irregular rhythm, unusual voice quality).
3. Repetitive behaviours and restricted interests:
    - Repetitive movements with objects
    - Repetitive movements or posturing of body, arms, hands or fingers.
4. Absolute indications for urgent referral for an autism-specific assessment of a preschool-aged child include:
    - No babbling, pointing or other gestures by 12 months
    - No sharing of interest in objects with another person
    - No single words by 16 months
    - No two-word spontaneous phrases by 24 months
    - Any loss of any language or social skills at any age.

EARLY IDENTIFICATION AND SCREENING

The identification of children with autism requires **developmental surveillance** (see Table 5.1). Opportunities arise for this at all routine health checks or visits to the general practitioner (GP) for acute illness (see Chapter 2 Developmental assessment in the young child).

Following or concurrent with developmental surveillance, consideration should be given to screening for ASD. A number of autism-specific screening tools are available, and include the Autism Detection in Early Childhood (ADEC)[27] for children age 12 months to 3 years, Checklist for Autism in Toddlers-23 (CHAT 23)[28] for children age 18–24 months, Autism Behaviour checklist[29] and the Modified Checklist for Autism in Toddlers (M-CHAT)[30] validated for screening toddlers between 16 and 30 months of age. A follow-up interview for use in conjunction with the M-CHAT is available. A significant number of the children who fail the M-CHAT will not be diagnosed with an ASD; however these children are at risk for other developmental disorders or delays and, therefore, evaluation is warranted for any child who fails the screening.

Most Asperger syndrome/high functioning autism (HFA) screening tools concentrate on social and behavioural impairment in children four years of age and older (up to adulthood), who usually develop without significant language delay. Qualitatively these tools are quite different from the early childhood screening tools, highlighting more social–conversational and perseverative–behavioural concerns. These include Autism Spectrum Screening Questionnaire (ASSQ),[31] Social Communication Questionnaire (SCQ)[32] or Australian Scale for Asperger Syndrome (ASAS).[33]

While these screening tools provide helpful information, there remains a high rate of false positives and false negatives. The screening tools are age-specific (to allow for the developmental changes) and care is required to use the correct screener for the chronological age of the child or adolescent. Clinical experience is the most important factor in identifying children who require further evaluation.

DIAGNOSTIC TOOLS

These diagnostic tools are included in Table 5.2.
- **The Childhood Autism Rating Scale, 2nd edn (CARS2)**[34] consists of two fifteen-item rating scales completed by qualified professionals and a parent or caregiver questionnaire. The standard version rating booklet (CARS2-ST) is used for <6 years age for children with communication difficulties and below average intellectual ability. The high functioning version rating booklet (CARS2-HF) is used for >6 years, verbally fluent children with average or above average intellectual ability. The CARS2 is to be used by qualified professionals *as part of* a comprehensive assessment and should not be used as a screening tool in the school-aged population. The CARS2 may be best considered a diagnostic aid.
- **The Autism Diagnostic Interview-Revised (ADI-R)**[35] is a structured interview used for diagnosing autism, planning treatment, and distinguishing autism from other developmental disorders. The ADI-R has proven highly useful for formal diagnosis as well as treatment and educational planning. To administer the ADI-R, an experienced clinical interviewer questions a parent or caretaker who is familiar with the developmental history and current

TABLE 5.1 ASD screening measures

Screening tool	Age	Format (no. of items)	Time to complete (min)	Availability
Checklist for Autism in Toddler-23 (CHAT-23)[28]	16–86 mo (all had mental ages of 18–24 mo)	Parent interview or questionnaire and interactive (parent: 23, clinician: 5)	10	Combination of M-CHAT and CHAT items; protocol available in Wong et al[28]
M-CHAT[30]	16–30 mo	Questionnaire completed by parent (23)	5–10	Download http://www.firstsigns.org/downloads/m-chat_scoring; 23 Feb 2012 Purchase: PsychCorp/Harcourt Assessment http://www.harcourtassessment.com; 23 Feb 2012
The Australian Scale for Asperger's syndrome (ASAS)[33]	Primary school years	Check list	5–10	Downloads and links can be found on the http://www.firstsigns.org; 23 Feb 2012
Autism Detection in Early Childhood (ADEC)[27]	12 mo–3 yr	Observational	10–15	http://www.acer.edu.au/autism; 23 Feb 2012
Autism Behavior Checklist (ABC)[29]	≥18 mo	Behaviour checklist completed by interviewer (57)	10–20	Purchase: Pro-Ed http://www.proedinc.com; 23 Feb 2012 as part of the Autism Screening Instrument for Educational Planning (ASIEP-2)
Autism Spectrum Screening Questionnaire (ASSQ)[31]	6–17 yr	Questionnaire completed by parent (27)	10	Questions are included as an appendix in Ehlers et al[31]
Social Communication Questionnaire (SCQ) (formerly Autism Screening Questionnaire (ASQ))[32]	≥4 yr	Questionnaire completed by parent (40)	5–10	Purchase: Western Psychological Services http://www.wpspublish.com; 23 Feb 2012
Childhood Autism Rating Scale, 2nd edn (CARS2)[34]	CARS-ST <6 yr + CARS-HF >6 yr	Two behavioural checklists completed by trained interviewer or observer (15) One parent questionnaire, not meant to use as a screener but as part of a diagnostic assessment	Variable	Purchase: Western Psychological Services http://www.wpspublish.com; 23 Feb 2012

CHAPTER 5 Autism spectrum disorders 101

TABLE 5.2 Diagnostic assessment tools

Screening tool	Age	Format (no. of items)	Time to complete	Availability
Autism Diagnostic Observation Schedule (ADOS)[36]	2+ yr	Four modules available. Module delivered is determined by expressive language and chronological age. Differentiates between autism ASD and other	30–45 min	Purchase: Western Psychological Services http://www.wpspublish.com; 23 Feb 2012
The Autism Diagnostic Interview-Revised (ADI-R)[35]	Mental age above 2.0 years	Structured interview for diagnosing autism, planning treatment, distinguishing autism from other developmental disorders	1½–2½ h	Purchase: Western Psychological Services http://www.wpspublish.com; 23 Feb 2012
Diagnostic Interview for Social and Communication Disorders (DISCO)[37]	Children and adults	Detailed semi-structured interview. In clinical work its purpose is to facilitate understanding of the pattern over time of the skills and impairments underlying the overt behaviour. Identifies comorbidity	2–3 h	http://www.autism.org.uk; 23 Feb 2012

behaviour of the individual being evaluated. The interview can be used to assess both children and adults, as long as their mental age is above 2.0 years. Typically, administration and scoring requires about 1½ to 2½ hours.

- **Autism Diagnostic Observation Schedule (ADOS)**[36] is a semi-structured assessment used to evaluate someone suspected of having autism – from toddlers to adults, from children with no speech to adults who are verbally fluent. The ADOS includes four modules, each requiring just 35–40 minutes to administer. The individual being evaluated is given just one module, depending on their expressive language level and chronological age. The activities provide a 30–45 minute observation period and scoring takes a further 15 minutes approximately. Algorithm scores differentiate between the broader diagnosis of PDD–atypical autism–autism spectrum and autism.
- **Diagnostic Interview for Social and Communication Disorders (DISCO)**[37] is a detailed semi-structured interview used with an informant who has known the person concerned well, preferably since infancy, and is designed to collect information in a systematic way so that the impairments associated with autistic spectrum disorders can be recognised and identified. In clinical work, its purpose is to facilitate understanding of the pattern over time of the skills and impairments that underlie the overt behaviour. Recommendations for helping the person follow from the information gained. The findings from the DISCO are relevant for children and adults of any age, and for any level of ability from profound learning disability to the superior range. It can assist in identifying conditions associated with the spectrum such as ADHD, tics, dyspraxia etc.

MULTIDISCIPLINARY DIAGNOSIS AND ASSESSMENT OF AUTISM SPECTRUM DISORDERS[38]

Stages of assessment

Stage 1 Identification of concerns
Concern is usually raised by parents, carers, teachers or healthcare professionals. Once concern has been raised, parents should consult with their GP or paediatrician. Consideration is given to the use of an ASD screening questionnaire.

Stage 2 General developmental and medical assessment
Information is collected from all those involved in the care of the child, including carers, teachers and therapists. This provides an insight that is not always possible in the office situation. It is most helpful when observations and concerns are outlined under the headings of learning, communication, socialisation, play, behaviour and attention. It is important to note the challenging behaviours, strategies trialled (what worked and what did not work), as well as to identify the child's personal strengths.
- A thorough medical, developmental and psychosocial history is taken.
- A medical and neurological examination is carried out with specific consideration given to growth parameters, neurocutaneous stigmata and dysmorphism. Formal testing of hearing and vision is essential.

Formal developmental assessments often require referral to particular allied health disciplines. These include:
- Communication (speech pathologist)
- Motor, sensory, play (occupational therapist)

- Development, cognitive, attention, adaptive functioning, mental health (psychologist)
- Education and academic progress (psychologist and teacher).

It may be possible to then make a diagnosis of an ASD at this point. If the diagnosis is not clear, then further autism specific assessment is required.

Stage 3 Autism-specific assessment

There are a number of autism-specific diagnostic tools that can be used in the more challenging diagnostic presentations. These include parental questionnaires, e.g. Autism Diagnostic Interview – Revised (ADI-R), and Diagnostic Interview for Social and Communication Disorders (DISCO). The Autism Diagnostic Observation Schedule (ADOS) is a semi-structured standardised assessment of communication, social interaction, and play for individuals who have been referred due to concern about a pervasive development disorder (PDD). These autism-specific diagnostic tools require specialist training (usually a few days), are expensive to undertake and can take 2–5 hours to administer and score. Training and use of these tools can be undertaken by any professional member of the multidisciplinary diagnostic team.

None of these tools are to be used in isolation. They form part of the comprehensive assessment using all the information gathered in the previous stages of the assessment process. A specialist clinician using the DSM-IV classification for the diagnosis of autism remains the gold standard.

Stage 4 Discussion and intervention planning

The family return to discuss the outcome of the assessment and recommendations, and are provided with a report. This may occur on the same day or at a review visit on another day. Once the diagnosis is made, the challenge of accessing early intervention and incorporating this into the daily and functional needs of the individual and family begins. This requires constant review and change as would be expected for any developmental disorder. Available financial and local government support should be discussed. This will vary according to country and region. (See Text Box 5.4.)

Stage 5 Ongoing multidisciplinary management and review

This stage requires ongoing collaborations between parents, teachers, allied health and doctors. Handover of relevant information from year to year, ongoing monitoring of educational progress and review of strategies to ensure they remain developmentally appropriate is essential. The doctor monitors general health and development, and emergence of comorbid medical and mental health issues for the student within the context of the family.

> **Practice Point**
>
> The diagnosis and assessment is multidisciplinary, and usually occurs over a number of visits.
>
> **Specific medical management in relation to diagnosis and assessment**
> *History*
> - **Developmental history:** speech and language, motor, cognitive, personal social, play, behaviour

- **Pregnancy and perinatal history:** method of conception, medications (anti-epileptics, thalidomide, tocolytics), delivery, perinatal history, feeding
- **Family history:** family composition, social circumstances, ASD, ADHD, language disorders, obsessive–compulsive disorder, depression, bipolar disorder, schizophrenia, addiction, genetic disorders
- **Neurological:** seizures, regression, coordination, vision
- **ENT:** middle ear infections, hearing
- **Gastrointestinal:** diet, vomiting, constipation, diarrhoea, reflux
- **Sleep:** sleep onset, frequent wakenings, parasomnias, nocturnal snoring.

Physical examination
- **Growth:** height, weight, head circumference (macrocephaly in 35 per cent, microcephaly 5–15 per cent)
- **Cardiovascular system:** heart rate, blood pressure (especially if on medication), murmurs
- **Skin:** depigmented and hyperpigmented lesions (including a Wood's lamp examination, tuberous sclerosis complex, NF-1)
- **Dysmorphology:** palate and voice (velo-cardio-facial syndrome)
- **Connective tissue:** hernias, ligamentous laxity
- **Genital examination:** testicular size large in fragile X and penile freckles in PTEN disorders (hamartomas, mucocutaneous lesions, macrocephaly predisposition to tumours and malignancies)
- **Neurological examination:** e.g. Moebius syndrome (facial muscle weakness, incomplete abduction of eyes), and mitochondrial disorders (failure to thrive, hypotonia, recurrent vomiting, episodes of regression), cerebral palsy.

Investigations
Recommended for all children with ASD:[12]
- Array comparative genomic hybridisation (aCGH)
- FMR1 molecular genetic testing
- Other investigations will need to be considered on a case by case basis, including standard cytogenetic examination to exclude an apparently balanced rearrangement not detectable with a CGH.

Investigations considered on an individual basis:
- Specific molecular genetic testing (e.g. MECP2 to exclude Rett's syndrome); serum lead level if there is a history of pica (eating sand or non-edibles) or living in an old house; a full blood count, iron and folate levels, and vitamin B12 levels (if dietary habits are limited); and, if clinically indicated, thyroid function tests, creatine kinase level, coeliac antibody levels, and urine metabolic screen (see Chapter 2 for investigations if there is associated global developmental delay).
- In the context of suspicion of seizures and language regression, a sleep deprived electroencephalography (EEG) is indicated to exclude aphasic epileptic syndromes, e.g. Landau Kleffner syndrome.
- Brain imaging is *not* routine and is only indicated if there is a neurological indication.

> **TEXT BOX 5.4** Support for families living in Australia
>
> **Autism specific**
> - Helping Children with Autism Package
>   http://www.fahcsia.gov.au/autism or contact the enquiry line on 1800 289 177
> - Autism Advisor Program
>   This program is part of the Helping Children With Autism federal initiative.
>   http://www.fahcsia.gov.au/autism or 1300 978 611
>   autismadvisor@autismspectrum.org.au
>   For a language interpreter call 13 14 50
>
> **For all children with developmental delays**
> - Enhanced Primary Care Program
>   http://www.medicareaustralia.gov.au
>   http://www.health.gov.au/mbsonline
> - Better access to mental health
>   http://www.medicareaustralia.gov.au
>   http://www.health.gov.au/mbsonline
> - Medicare Safety Net
>   http://www.medicareaustralia.gov.au
>
> **Carer allowance (caring for a child under 16 years)**
>   http://www.centrelink.gov.au

Genetic counselling

It is advisable to refer to a geneticist (if one is available) if there is any concern regarding dysmorphology or positive family history. In the presence of a *known* cause of autism, the genetic counselling is specific to that identified condition. In the case of autism with *no known* cause, the risk to siblings ranges from 5–10 per cent for autism and 10–15 per cent for milder symptoms including language, social and psychiatric conditions.[13] For families with two or more affected children the risk for autism approaches 35 per cent.

INTERVENTION

There is no one 'magic cure' for ASD. This is partly because there is no 'one cause' for ASD. In addition the clinical presentation, while having impairments within the triad, varies significantly depending on the cognitive, sensory, communication skills, and the medical and mental health comorbidity. All intervention therefore needs to be tailored to the individual and take account of family circumstances.

Elements of a successful early intervention program include:[39]
- Autism-specific intervention for a minimum of 20 hours a week over a period of two years or more: 'The earlier, the better, the more, the better'
- Individualised to the child's and family's needs (individual educational plan)
- Family partnership and culturally sensitive

- Functional approach to problem behaviours
- Generalisation and naturalisation of learnt skills
- Specific support during transition periods.

MODELS OF INTERVENTION[39,40]

Behavioural interventions

Behavioural approaches are based upon the principle of the learning theory: the idea that human behaviour is learned and governed by its antecedents and its consequences. The theory assumes that children can learn new skills by modification of stimuli and presentation of reinforcement. Behavioural interventions include applied behaviour analysis (ABA).[39,40] There is universal agreement that behavioural interventions have produced positive outcomes for children with autism that are well supported by research. However there continues to be controversy about particular behavioural interventions and programs, concerns about methodological issues, and differences in the interpretation of research findings. This controversy revolves around claims that behavioural programs can lead to 'recovery' of children with autism, recommendations by some service providers that applied behaviour analysis and discrete trial training approaches should be used to the exclusion of all other methods, and concerns that the intensity of treatment may not be appropriate for all children and families.

Developmental interventions

Developmental or relationship-based interventions focus on the child's ability to form positive, meaningful relationships with other people. Generally the aims of these programs are to promote attention, relating to and interacting with others, experience of a range of feelings, and organised logical thought.

To date, there is little research evidence to support the effectiveness of developmental interventions for children with autism. Examples include:
- Developmental social–pragmatic model
- Developmental individual–difference relationship-based model (DIR)
- Responsive teaching (RT)
- Relationship development intervention (RDI).

Therapy-based interventions

Communication-focused interventions

A number of communication-focused interventions are commonly used with children with autism. These may be used in isolation or integrated into a more comprehensive program. Strategies include:
- visual strategies and visually cued instruction
- manual signing
- the picture exchange communication system (PECS)
- social stories
- speech generating devices.

Functional communication training is a behavioural strategy for teaching people with autism to use augmentative and alternative communication (AAC) as substitutes for the 'messages' underlying their challenging behaviour. Functional communication training is currently considered to be a 'treatment of choice' in the management of challenging behaviours in children with autism.

Combined interventions
Treatment and Education of Autistic and Related Communication Handicapped Children (TEACCH) is a 'whole life' approach aimed at supporting children, adolescents and adults with autism through the provision of visual information, structure and predictability. The results of a small number of studies have indicated positive outcomes for children who access the TEACCH program. However there is a need for larger, systematic and controlled studies to be conducted by independent researchers in order to evaluate immediate and long-term outcomes of the program.

Other combined intervention models include Social Communication Emotion Regulation Transaction Support (SCERTS) model and Learning Experiences – An Alternative Program for Preschoolers and Parents (LEAP).

Family-based interventions
In family support programs, therapists and professionals work with parents, siblings and significant others rather than directly with the child with autism. Family support and education programs include:
- The Help! Program
- The Early Bird Program
- Family-Centred Positive Behaviour Support (PBS) Programs
- The Hanen Program (More Than Words).

Biological intervention
The role of medication[41]
The mainstay of intervention in individuals with autism remains individualised education, communication and behavioural strategies. No biological treatment has yet been rigorously shown to change the core social and communication impairment in autism. The only TGA (in Australia) and FDA (in the United States) approved medication for autism is risperidone, specifically indicated for severe irritability and aggression.[42]

However medication has a discrete but important role in the treatment of targeted symptoms impairing the quality of life and progress of an individual with autism.

In broad terms, the behaviours that may show some response with medication are divided into four main categories:
- attention deficit–hyperactivity disorder (ADHD)
- ritualistic–compulsive behaviours and anxiety
- sleep disorders
- challenging behaviour (e.g. aggression, self-injury).

With regards to challenging behaviour:
- Attempt to understand the function of the behaviour before simply trying to suppress it.
- Review the communication system with the therapists involved.
- Exclude a medical cause, e.g. ear infections, dentition, gastro-oesophageal reflux, pain, abuse.
- Consider medication together with a comprehensive intervention plan. The medication used will depend on the driving factor for the behaviour, i.e. impulsive, anxiety-related, or due to a ritual being interrupted.

Basic principles that are adhered to when prescribing medication include:
- Baseline assessments and identification of targeted symptoms
- Close monitoring and review before, during and after medication trial

- Medications are commenced in the lowest dose possible and increased slowly (start low, go slow)
- Enquiring about the method (and ease) of administering the particular medication
- Ensuring that the child's living arrangements allow for safe medication use
- Adequate informed consent.

Prescribing medication is usually initiated by a specialist with knowledge of autism and pharmacology.

Stimulants are commonly used to address the ADHD symptoms, but they may increase the aggression and stereotypical behaviours. Clonidine is somewhat helpful in treating the hyperactivity, impulsive aggression and sleep difficulty. Specific serotonin reuptake inhibitors (SSRI) should be considered on an individual basis (for anxiety, depression and obsessive compulsive behaviours).[43] Lithium and anticonvulsants (carbamazepine, valproic acid) may be used as mood stabilisers in the presence of cyclical behaviour patterns and aggression. Blood monitoring is required and may be problematic. Atypical antipsychotics, e.g. risperidone, have been noted to improve social relatedness, aggression, irritability agitation and hyperactivity.[42] Side-effects include significant weight gain, galactorrhea and potential for extrapyramidal movements. Emerging evidence suggest that melatonin is helpful for the sleep disorders. The role of glutamatergic drugs and oxytocin is being explored.[44]

It is worthwhile monitoring the progress of the Autism Treatment Network (ATN) in the United States.[45] The ATN is a consortium of 15 autism treatment centres which was formed with the support of Autism Speaks and the National Institutes of Health to develop a medically-based approach to the diagnosis and treatment of individuals with autism. Algorithms for the initial assessment of children with autism as well as guidelines for continued medical care and surveillance are being developed and can be accessed through the website as well as through planned publications.[12]

Complementary and alternative therapies, interventions and diet[45,46]

An increasing number of families of children with autism spectrum disorders use complementary and alternative therapies. The range of these therapies available increases daily, as do the medico-legal, ethical, and research debates. Common complementary and alternative therapies include:
- biologically-based practices (e.g. vitamins, herbs, dietary supplements, diets and foods)
- manipulative and body-based practices (chiropractic, massage, osteopathic and reflexology)
- mind body medicine (prayer, spiritual healing, breathing, cognitive behaviour practices)
- bio-field techniques (acupuncture, therapeutic touch)
- whole or traditional medical systems (homeopathy, naturopathy and traditional cultural healing systems).

In general, medical practitioners are encouraged to:
- ask about the use of complementary and alternative therapies in a non-judgemental way
- provide information that allows families to weigh up the evidence, safety and potential effectiveness

- caution against alternative therapies that may have a detrimental effect on the child's health
- be supportive of the family's decision, unless clearly dangerous.

Dietary interventions
The most common alternative biomedical intervention used in children with ASD is the gluten- and casein-free diet (GFCF). It is based on the unproven theory of the 'brain–gut' connection where it is proposed that certain food sensitivities, especially to gluten and casein, cause gut inflammation and increase gastro-intestinal permeability, causing a 'leaky gut' allowing toxins to cross over into the blood and subsequently the brain, to cause the autism symptoms.

There is abundant *anecdotal* evidence supporting the GFCF diet. Research is lacking, especially as the methodology and practicalities of a randomised control trial are difficult. Factors to consider about the GFCF diet are:
- the cost of the diet
- applying a further restriction on a child who may already have self-induced dietary restrictions
- further unnecessarily identifying that child as different
- exclusion from important daily social and family activities around meals, outings and food.

Should parents decide to proceed with the diet, they should be supported and encouraged to do it under the supervision of a qualified dietician. Parents often need reassurance and advice on sensible healthy eating practices suitable for any child (e.g. avoiding caffeinated drinks and high intakes of fruit juices; encouraging adequate water intake and sufficient fibre and fresh foods in the diet).

The evidence for replacing essential omega-3, -6 fatty acids is preliminary but encouraging. There is insufficient evidence to support replacement of other vitamins and minerals above the daily recommended allowance, and some have the potential for toxicity when given in supra-physiological doses. Other practices, e.g. metal chelation, not only have no evidence base but should be strongly discouraged due to the potential side-effects.

TRANSITION TO ADULTHOOD

The key element to transition is *planning*, as would occur for all adolescents. Planning needs to begin at least 3–4 years before the event, so that what is taught at school, and home, can be specifically targeted towards achievable and realistic goals. Planning should be done in a methodical and detailed manner.

Areas that require consideration include: health (transfer to adult medical service providers), education (whether it be tertiary academic, trade, supported or supervised employment), financial (money matters, banking, future security, insurance, social security), mobility (independence, public transport), personal appearance, social skills, safety, and recreation.

This process is ongoing, fluid and occurs over a long period of time. Assistance and guidance is obtained from all those who know the individual well and are involved in their care.

PROGNOSIS

ASD is a very heterogeneous condition and prognosis is difficult to predict for each individual. ASD is a life-long condition, and the impact it has at various stages of life depends on the skills acquired, the demands made on those skills and the comorbidity present. Intellectual ability (IQ over 70) and useful speech by age five are good prognostic factors. Other important factors affecting prognosis include medical comorbidity (epilepsy, severe anxiety), the degree of social skills attained and the amount of social support available.

Research suggests that 20 per cent may go on to receive academic qualifications at school, 30 per cent are in employment and 25 per cent have friendships that involve common interests or activities. Therapeutic and educational provisions have improved significantly over the past 30 years, and as such a significant number of adults with ASD may find work, live independently and develop meaningful relationships with others.[47]

REFERENCES

1. Leask J, Leask A, Silove N. Evidence for autism in folklore? Archives of Disease in Childhood 2005;90:271
2. American Psychiatric Association. Diagnostic and statistical manual of mental disorders, 3rd edn (DSM-III). Washington, DC: APA; 1980
3. American Psychiatric Association. Diagnostic and statistical manual of mental disorders, Version 4. Washington, DC: APA; 1994
4. American Psychiatric Association. Diagnostic and statistical manual of mental disorders, 4th edn, text revision (DSM-IV-TR). Washington, DC: APA; 2000
5. World Health Organization. International classification of diseases and health related problems, 10th edn (ICD-10). Geneva: WHO; 1992
6. Johnson CP, Myers SM and the Council on Children with Disabilities. Identification and evaluation of children with autism spectrum disorders. Pediatrics 2007;120(5):1183–215. Online. Available: http://aappolicy.aappublications.org/cgi/content/full/pediatrics; 120/5/1183; 22 Feb 2012
7. American Psychiatric Association. DSM-5 Development A 09 Autism spectrum disorder. Online. Available: http://www.dsm5.org/ProposedRevisions/Pages/proposedrevision.aspx?rid=94; 22 Feb 2012
8. Yale Child Study Center. Online. Available: http://www.med.yale.edu/chldstdy/autism/retts.html; 22 Feb 2012
9. Piven J, Palmer P. Psychiatric disorder and the broader autism phenotype: evidence from a family study of multiple-incidence autism families. Am J Psychiatry 1999;156:557–63
10. Williams K, MacDermott S, Ridley G, et al. The prevalence of autism in Australia. Can it be established from existing data? J Paeds and Child Health 2008;44:504–10
11. Chakrabarti S, Fombonne E. Pervasive developmental disorders in preschool children: confirmation of high prevalence. Am J Psychiatry 2005;162:1133–41
12. Miles J, McCathren R, Stitchter J, et al. Autism Spectrum Disorders. NCBI bookshelf. National Institutes of Health 2003. Online. Available: http://www.ncbi.nlm.nih.gov/books/NBK1442/; 22 Feb 2012
13. Miller DT, Adam MP, et al. Consensus Statement: Chomosomal microarray is a first-tier clinical diagnostic test for individuals with developmental disabilities or congenital anomalies. American Journal of Human Genetics 2010;86:749–64
14. Bromley RL, Mawer G, Clayton-Smith J, et al. Autism spectrum disorders following in utero exposure to anti epileptic drugs. Neurology 2008;71:1923–4
15. Badawi N, Dixon G, Felix JF, et al. Autism following a history of newborn encephalopathy: more than a coincidence? Dev Med Child Neurol. 2006;48:85–9
16. Connors S, Levitt P, Matthews SG, et al. Fetal mechanisms in neurodevelopmental disorders. Pediatr Neurol 2008;38:163–76
17. Taylor B, Miller E, Farrington C, et al. Autism and measles, mumps, and rubella vaccine: no epidemiological evidence for a causal association. Lancet 1999;353:2026–9
18. Courchesne E. Brain development in autism: early overgrowth followed by premature arrest of growth. Ment Retard Dev Disabil Res Rev 2004;10:106–11

19 Courchesne E, Pierce K. Brain overgrowth in autism during a critical time in development: implications for frontal pyramidal neurone and inter neurone development and connectivity. Int J Devl Neurosci 2005;23:153–70
20 Blatt GJ. The neurochemical basis of autism: From molecules to mini columns. New York: Springer; 2010
21 Baron-Cohen S, Leslie AM, Frith U. Does the autistic child have a 'theory of mind'? Cognition 1985;21:37–46
22 Frith U. Autism: explaining the enigma. Oxford, UK: Blackwell; 1989
23 Happé FGE. Wechsler IQ profile and theory of mind in autism: A research note. Journal of Child Psychology & Psychiatry 1994;5:1451–71
24 Ozonoff S, Jensen J. Specific executive function profiles in three neurodevelopmental disorders. J Autism Dev Disord 1999;29:171–7
25 Just MA, Cherkassky VL, Keller TA, et al. Cortical activation and synchronization during sentence comprehension in high-functioning autism: evidence of underconnectivity. Brain 2004;127:1811–21
26 Wetherby A, Woods J, Allen L, et al. Early indicators of autism spectrum disorders in the second year of life. Journal of Autism and Developmental Disorders 2004;34:473–93
27 Young RL. Autism detection in early childhood (ADEC) manual. Camberwell, Australia: ACER; 2007
28 Wong V, Hui LH, Lee WC, et al. A modified screening tool for autism (Checklist for Autism in toddlers (CHAT-23) for Chinese children. Pediatrics 2004;114(2). Available at www.pediatrics.org/cgi/content/full/114/2/e166
29 Krug DA, Arick J, Almond P. Behavior checklist for identifying severely handicapped individuals with high levels of autistic behaviour. J Child Psychol Psychiatry 1980;21:221–9
30 Robins DL, Fein D, Barton ML, et al. The Modified Checklist for Autism in Toddlers: an initial study investigating the early detection of autism and pervasive developmental disorders. J Autism Dev Disord 2001;31:131–44
31 Ehlers S, Gillberg C, Wing L. A screening questionnaire for Asperger syndrome and other high-functioning autism spectrum disorders in school age children. J Autism Dev Disord 1999;29:129–41
32 Berument SK, Rutter M, Lord C, et al. Autism Screening Questionnaire: diagnostic validity. Br J Psychiatry 1999;175:444–51
33 Attwood T, Asperger's syndrome: A guide for parents and professionals. London: Jessica Kingsley Publishers; 1997
34 Schopler E, Reichler RJ, DeVellis RF, Daly K. Toward objective classification of childhood autism: Childhood Autism Rating Scale (CARS). J Autism Dev Disord 1980;10(1):91–103
35 Lord C, Rutter M, Le Couteur A. Autism Diagnostic Interview-Revised: A revised version of a diagnostic interview for caregivers of individuals with possible pervasive developmental disorders. J Autism Dev Disord 1994;24(5):659–85
36 Lord C, Risi S, Lambrecht L, et al. The autism diagnostic observation schedule – generic; a standard measure of social and communication deficits associated with the spectrum of autism. J Autism Dev Disord 2000;30(3):205–23
37 Wing L, Leekam SR, Libby SJ, et al. The Diagnostic Interview for Social and Communication Disorders: Background, inter-rater reliability and clinical use. J Child Psychol Psychiatry 2002;43(3):307–25
38 Silove N, Blackmore R, Warren A, et al. Consensus approach for the paediatrician's role in the diagnosis and assessment of autism spectrum disorders in Australia (PDF: 176 KB) 2008. Online. Available: http://www.racp.edu.au; 22 Feb 2012
39 Prior M, Roberts J. Early intervention for children with autism spectrum disorders. Australian Government Department of Health and Ageing, 2006. 22 Feb 2012
40 Roberts JM. A review of the research to identify the most effective models of best practice in the management of children with autism spectrum disorders. Sydney: Centre for Developmental Disability Studies; 2004
41 Gringas P. Practical paediatric pharmacological prescribing in autism: The potential and the pitfalls. Autism 2000;4(3):229–48

42 McDougle CH, Scahill L, Aman MG, et al. Risperidone for the core symptom domains of autism: results from the study by the autism network of the research units on pediatric psychopharmacology. Am J Psychiatry 2005;162:1142–8

43 Wheeler DM, Hazell P, Silove N, et al. Selective serotonin reuptake inhibitors for the treatment of autism spectrum disorders. Cochrane Database of Systematic Reviews 2010, Issue 1. Art. No. CD004677. DOI: 10.1002/14651858.CD004677

44 Posey DJ, Erickson CA, McDougle CJ. Developing drugs for core social and communication impairment in autism. Child Adolesc Psychiatr Clin N Am Oct 2008;17(4):787-ix.DOI.10.1016/j.chc.2008.06.010

45 Levy S, Hyman S. Alternative/complementary approaches to treatment of children with autistic spectrum disorders. Infants Young Child 2002;14:33–42

46 Levy S, Mandell D. Use of complementary and alternative medicine among children recently diagnosed with Autistic Spectrum Disorder. Journal of Developmental and Behavioural Paediatrics 2003;24(6):418–23

47 Howlin P, Goode S, Hutton J, et al. Adult outcome for children with autism. J Child Psych and Psychiatry 2004;45(2):212–29

6 Specific learning disorders

Sandra Johnson

DEFINITION

Specific learning disorder (SLD) is the term used to refer to significant learning problems in childhood. It is worth noting that other terms, such as specific learning disabilities (sometimes shortened to learning disabilities) and specific learning difficulties are often used interchangeably.

In American literature the term tends to imply significant learning problems specific to one or more areas, such as reading, spelling, writing and/or mathematics – irrespective of intellectual function. In some European literature the term 'learning disabilities' refers to individuals who have intellectual impairment. In Australia the term 'intellectual disability' would be used rather than learning disability in these circumstances.

When identifying or diagnosing SLD, the child's reading, spelling, mathematics and/or writing skill is found to be significantly weaker than their intellectual potential on formal psychometric tests. For example, the child's intellectual ability on psychometric testing can be in the average range for age (with full scale IQ scores between 90 to 110 depending on the test used), but their learning skills may be at least two years delayed compared to their IQ score. Neuropsychologists sometimes refer to a significant discrepancy (>15 points being more than one standard deviation from the mean) between verbal and performance scores on psychometric testing as being significant and in keeping with SLD. However, researchers have legitimately challenged this discrepancy model and the clinician needs to be aware that the debate continues.[1] Also, the discrepancy between verbal and performance scores has a wide distribution even in the 'normal' population. (See Chapter 7 Language disorders and Chapter 8 Attention deficit hyperactivity disorder for more on discrepancy.)

Many clinicians prefer the term 'learning disorder' to learning disability, because children who have these disorders may have intellectual and functional skills that are in the average and even above average range for their age.[2] This means that they do not strictly have a 'disability' with respect to their daily function in areas other than their specific learning problems.

Notably, if effective educational interventions successfully address the child's learning problem, then it is unlikely to be SLD. It is important to recognise that as most SLD children have average IQ (or higher), the outcome can be good if they are effectively nurtured and given appropriate educational and other support.

> **Practice Point**
>
> The definitions used for SLD in clinical practice tend to be descriptive and refer to the child's learning problems as noted by teachers, psychologists and clinicians. A major difficulty in defining SLD is the lack of consistency with the terms that are used. The result is that researchers often do not have a common language in order to study the disorder effectively.[3]

TYPES OR CLASSIFICATION

Dyslexia

Dyslexia is characterised by weakness in verbal processing and is typically a consequence of phonological difficulties.[4] The condition is thought to fall on the continuum of language disorder where phonological processing is selectively impaired while other aspects of language like vocabulary and grammar can be normal.

These children often present with difficulties affecting reading and spelling, which is not surprising given that learning to read depends to a large extent on phonological skills. Learning to read is complex and incorporates visual perception and processing of shapes of letters; auditory processing of sounds associated with the symbols; and integration of this input through central processing systems which incorporate attention and memory skills. Therefore if breakdown occurs in any part of the system, the child will have difficulty with learning to read.

Children with dyslexia have problems with phonemic awareness, decoding and sound–symbol association. Some have problems with right–left confusion and many show reversals when writing words beyond the age where this finding is considered to be a normal phenomenon at approximately 5–6 years old.

The term dyslexia implies a homogeneous group of children who have similar presentation. However, there is variation in clinical presentation related to the extent of the problem so that individual differences are often observed. Problems with phonological awareness are common to all dyslexic persons. Children with dyslexia can have average or even above average cognitive skills in other domains apart from reading and spelling.

Learning to read is important and exposure to books from an early age plays a significant role in enabling this to become an automatic skill. The child first learns to read and then reads to learn. Difficulty with reading can have significant impact on all future learning.

Dyscalculia

Dyscalculia refers to impairment of arithmetic and mathematics skills out of keeping with the child's intellectual ability. The presentation of the disorder is varied in that the difficulties may extend from arithmetic computation to problems with reading and comprehending the maths questions. Clinically, it can sometimes be difficult to disentangle a reading from a maths difficulty, however this needs to be done in order to provide effective and targeted intervention.

Dysgraphia

Dysgraphia refers to specific disorder or impairment of writing skills out of keeping with the child's intellectual ability. The reasons may include fine motor problems due to functional motor impairment, such as motor dyspraxia (also referred to as developmental coordination disorder), or may be related to processing problems, where the child is unable to effectively record their thoughts in a written form (see Chapter 3 Motor and coordination problems). There is overlap with attention deficit hyperactivity disorder (ADHD), where processing difficulty also occurs and handwriting problems are common. In essence, ADHD and dysgraphia SLD are comorbid conditions.

Note that poor vision might also present with poor handwriting and must be considered in the differential diagnosis of handwriting problems. In addition, proprioception problems and cerebellar ataxia can affect coordination and handwriting skills, and should be excluded before diagnosing SLD.

Note: The use of the above terms (dyslexia, dyscalculia and dysgraphia) are not recommended in the new DSM-V criteria but will instead be considered under the overall term of specific learning disorders.

Language disorder

Preschool children may have delayed and/or disordered language skills that later present as SLD, which is predominantly language based. SLD appears to be part of the continuum of language disorder in that many children with SLD have a history of early language problems. They then go on to have difficulties with reading, spelling and comprehension at school where they are expected to perform these tasks. See Chapter 7 Language disorders for more on this topic.

Auditory processing disorder

Auditory processing disorder (APD) is defined by the American Speech-Language-Hearing Association (ASHA) Task Force on Central Auditory Processing Consensus Development (1996)[5] as difficulty in one or more of the following auditory behaviours:
- sound localisation and lateralisation
- auditory discrimination
- auditory pattern recognition
- temporal aspects of audition.

The report from the ASHA Working Group indicated that the disorder coexists with other disorders, like language disorders and specific learning disorders. Auditory attention and auditory memory problems are part of the clinical picture of APD and are also seen in ADHD, supporting the understanding that APD and ADHD are comorbid conditions.[6,7]

Some researchers have found a high prevalence of APD in children with learning disorders and believe that APD should be screened for in all children with learning difficulties and specific learning disorders.[8]

Clinically, these children have difficulty with making sense of information that is presented verbally, despite having good constructional or 'hands-on' skills. Bishop refers to this disorder as one where the child has problems with listening skills and performs poorly on tests that assess auditory processing, despite having a normal audiogram. Her recent paper also refers to the debate over whether APD is a separate diagnostic entity or whether it reflects a more general learning disability.[9] (See her blog access on APD at end of this chapter.)

The British Society of Audiology produced an interim position statement on APD in 2007 and the disorder was defined as 'impaired neural function characterised by poor recognition, discrimination, separation, grouping, localisation or ordering of non-speech sounds. It does not solely result from a deficit in general attention, language or other cognitive processes.'[10]

COMORBIDITY

Many developmental disorders are comorbid in childhood, and there are many developmental problems that are comorbid with SLD. One example is the child with SLD who has attention deficit hyperactivity disorder with significant concentration and memory problems that compound the learning difficulties. Unless attention difficulties are addressed, possibly with medication management, the child will continue to have problems with retention and show minimal improvement with educational support alone. (See sections on comorbidity in Chapter 7 Language disorders and Chapter 8 Attention deficit hyperactivity disorder.)

AETIOLOGY

In most instances the cause of the child's learning problems cannot be determined. There is often a family history of learning difficulties and there may be features in the history to suggest an increased risk, but aetiology is difficult to establish. While there is no research evidence to support a direct causal relationship, the factors below may be associated with increased risk.

Congenital
- chromosomal disorders
- CNS malformations such as neural tube defects, e.g. spina bifida, particularly myelomeningocele; Arnold-Chiari malformation that characteristically has other CNS malformations
- neuronal migrational disorders
- hereditary metabolic disease.

Acquired
- prematurity
- low birth weight
- maternal smoking or drinking alcohol in pregnancy
- medications in pregnancy that might affect the developing fetus, e.g. anticonvulsants
- maternal malnutrition in pregnancy
- malnutrition in child
- brain injury in early childhood: trauma; infection; malignancy; clotting disorder; toxic exposure, e.g. lead, mercury, other
- severe birth asphyxia injury resulting in hypoxic ischaemic encephalopathy (HIE)
- hydrocephalus and ventriculoperitoneal shunt infection.

There are many psychosocial factors that exacerbate the child's learning difficulties. They include poverty, disorganised home environment, lack of support or encouragement for schoolwork at home, and lack of support or intervention in the school environment. Important factors like child neglect can also play a part in increasing the negative academic effects of SLD. Thus SLD interacts with environmental factors such that problematic outcomes are amplified in the presence of one or more environmental risk factors.

> **Practice Point**
>
> Many risk factors mentioned above may be associated with cerebral palsy in their severe form. See Chapter 13 Cerebral palsy.

CLINICAL PRESENTATION

Many children with SLD are not seen by paediatricians because they are managed by teachers and school psychologists. Those who are referred to paediatricians usually present with behaviour and/or attention difficulties, or there may be concerns about their health. Their learning difficulties are subsequently detected when these issues are investigated.

Children who have SLD present with difficulties that are common to other developmental disorders. (See Chapter 7 Language disorders and Chapter 8 Attention deficit hyperactivity disorder.)

Some of these difficulties include:

- short-term memory problems with poor retention of information
- processing problems presenting as being slow to complete tasks and to grasp concepts
- inability to execute ideas effectively, e.g. in written form
- inability to express ideas verbally in a coherent manner and difficulties with clarity in thinking
- organisation difficulties with managing personal possessions
- poor time management when trying to execute tasks
- long time to complete schoolwork
- low self-esteem in relation to schoolwork
- tendency to give up and lose interest in schoolwork.

Children with SLD may have visual and/or auditory processing problems. These are complex and some children have a combination of problems. Clinical features that may be related to these problems are outlined in Tables 6.1 and 6.2 respectively.

TABLE 6.1 Visual processing problems

Difficulty experienced	May result in
Visual scanning and moving eyes across the page efficiently	Reading problems
Figure–background distinction	Spatial awareness problems
	Difficulty with writing words accurately, e.g. spelling
	Difficulty reading a blackboard or work projected onto screens
Spatial awareness and visual perception	Writing difficulty with spatial orientation of words or letters on the page
Spatial awareness and visual perception	Difficulty with orientation when reading maps or charts
Poor retention of visual information	Poor visual memory and recall of written information
	Poor recall of words leading to problems with reading and spelling
Visual sequencing and visual attention difficulty	Difficulty following worksheets that have too much written information resulting in task avoidance

TABLE 6.2 Auditory processing problems

Difficulty experienced	May result in
Tendency to tune out if given too much verbal information	Poor listening and poor following of verbal instructions
Poor retention of information which is given verbally	Poor memory for spoken word
Difficulty distinguishing sounds within words	Poor auditory discrimination of sounds for spelling and/or reading
Cannot easily distinguish sounds and focus on the relevant sounds only	Distracted easily in noisy classroom and busy environments
Problems listening to lectures and sessions where verbal information is given	Poor performance in subjects that are taught verbally with no visual input

Note: The table refers to difficulties that may be experienced by the child in the classroom situation. The list is not definitive or complete, and various combinations of difficulty may occur.

Practice Point

Each child's presentation is unique and children with similar SLD may have very different clinical presentations. The phenotype variability is likely to be related to genetic influences, intellectual ability and individual learning experience.

Children who present with learning problems present a diagnostic dilemma to the paediatrician because learning difficulties occur in relation to SLD, attention deficit hyperactivity disorder, language disorders, autism, emotional and behaviour disorders. The debate continues about whether these conditions should be considered under one category, e.g. executive dysfunction disorders.

DIFFERENTIAL DIAGNOSIS

There are many possible causes for learning difficulties in childhood and it is often difficult to determine whether the problem is truly SLD. This diagnosis should be made after a process of excluding other possible causes for poor school performance. Refer to Text Box 6.1 and also see Chapter 7 Language disorders, Chapter 8 Attention deficit hyperactivity disorder, Chapter 10 School refusal and truancy and Chapter 13 Developmental and intellectual disability.

ASSESSMENT

The paediatric medical assessment provides parents, teachers and allied health professionals with an overview of the child's developmental history, the medical background, a comprehensive physical with neurological examination, and recommendations for intervention.

The paediatrician's aim is to assess the overall health of the child, to exclude a medical cause and to give suggestions and recommendations for intervention

CHAPTER 6 Specific learning disorders   ■   119

> **TEXT BOX 6.1** Differential diagnosis for school failure
>
> These factors should be considered when diagnosing SLD: they do not cause SLD, their presence does not preclude SLD and they may occur concurrently in children who have SLD.
>
> **The child**
> - Medical illness involving any major system
> - Medications can result in side-effects that hinder learning
> - Neurological causes that hinder learning and attention, e.g. petit mal seizures, brain tumour, neurodegenerative disorders
> - Anxiety, depression or other emotional factors
> - Innate factors that hinder the child's learning, e.g. congenital problems, developmental disability
> - Sleep problems
> - Vision and hearing difficulties.
>
> **The family**
> - Poverty
> - Disorganisation within the family home
> - Dysfunctional family unit with poor relationships
> - Children not supported or encouraged to learn
> - Parental mental health problems
> - Drug-related problems, e.g. alcohol and illicit drugs
> - Child neglect and abuse.
>
> **The school**
> - Child bullied at school by peers
> - Unhealthy school environment, e.g. violent or aggressive students
> - Lack of support for children, i.e. educational and emotional
> - Vicious cycle of not doing well resulting in school refusal
> - Insensitive or intolerant teachers
> - Lack of facilities at school and children not encouraged to learn.

and support. There may be instances where treatment of a specific medical condition is needed, e.g. the child with learning difficulties who has sensory impairment or petit mal seizures that impact on learning.

The child is usually seen in the company of their parents or carers but where sensitive issues are discussed it may be necessary to talk to the parents alone. There are many instances where the doctor needs to speak to the child alone, and this is particularly important in the older child who may not wish to express feelings about school or bullying in the presence of their parents.

Involvement of the child in the process and explanation about what is being done helps management in the long term because the child who feels respected and considered is more likely to be cooperative.

Components of the history and examination familiar to doctors is given in Text Box 6.2.

> **TEXT BOX 6.2** History and physical examination
>
> **Current history**
> - What is the presenting problem?
> - Why is the child being seen at that time?
> - Who brings the child and who is most concerned about the child's problem?
> - What are the parent's particular concerns for the child?
> - When did concerns arise?
> - How does the child feel about the reported difficulties?
>
> **Pregnancy and perinatal history**
> - Any factors in the pregnancy that may affect the developing brain (smoking, alcohol, medications, maternal illness)?
> - Delivery, gestation, Apgar scores, any illness in neonatal period? Birth weight (can a be marker of placental insufficiency, and possibly chronic fetal hypoxia or malnutrition)?
> - Any treatments or investigations in the neonatal period? Feeding at discharge (regarding those children with dyspraxia and associated low oral tone)?
> - Ask about the birth process for the mother and 'bonding' after birth?
>
> **Developmental history**
> - Developmental milestones: any indication of general or global delay?
> - Regression or stagnation in development?
> - Early care history (mother working, child in day care, etc)?
> - Preschool attendance?
>
> **Family, social**
> - Family history of learning and school difficulties?
> - Family history of neurological problems?
> - Family history of behaviour, mood or other psychiatric problems?
>
> **General health and medical history**
> - Prior medical conditions, seizures, other neurological problems?
> - Immunisation, medication history, allergy to drugs?
> - Diet history: high intake of 'junk food', balanced diet?
>
> **Current abilities**
> - History of strengths and weaknesses? Social interaction skills?
> - History of basic language and learning skills: reading, writing, comprehension, maths?
> - History of motor function: fine and gross motor skills?
>
> **Physical examination**
> - General appearance: look for dysmorphic features or any indication of underlying medical problems (majority have no dysmorphic features)
> - Growth and percentile charts: ensure normal growth profile over time, compared with profiles in the parent-held child health record
> - Systems: respiratory, cardiac, abdominal, neurological, skeletal, ENT, endocrine, vascular, haematological.

Assessment of skills

The child's learning and behaviour is best assessed by the school counsellor or clinical psychologist. The doctor observes the child's behaviour and gains valuable information at the initial medical assessment. Screening tools can be used to examine learning, but the doctor will need training and experience to execute the tasks.

- **Social skills:** observe as soon as communication with the child commences, taking note of eye contact, responsiveness to questions and understanding of simple commands.
- **Language skills:** ability to understand simple commands and ability to follow a set group instruction (depending on the age of the child), expressive ability in describing interests or school experience.
- **Reading and comprehension ability:** simple clinical tests can be done using a children's book. Tools such as the Wide Range Achievement Test, Schonell Test and the Peabody Individual Achievement Test are examples of tests that may be helpful to the clinician.
- **Basic arithmetic task:** can be done as a simple task or using the above-mentioned tools.
- **Fine motor skills:** ask child to write name and age-appropriate words. Drawing a picture provides valuable information. Observe pencil control, writing posture and handwriting for fluency and letter formation.
- **Drawing a picture:** also allows the doctor to ask the child to describe the picture and its meaning, which gives further information about language and communication skills.

> **Practice Point**
>
> It is beneficial to the child and family if the paediatrician in sole practice has a working relationship with a team of experienced allied health colleagues (psychologists, special education teachers, occupational and speech therapists) who can carry out the necessary assessments and work collaboratively with the doctor. Ideally such support is available in multidisciplinary clinics but this may not be the case in private practice, particularly in rural areas. State and independent school education systems usually have trained counsellors and psychologists who are able to assist with assessments.

MANAGEMENT

The primary aim is to address the needs of the child within the family unit.
1. Assess and treat the medical condition, e.g. asthma or seizures. Where the condition falls outside the doctor's field of expertise, referral should be made to the appropriate specialists.
2. Ensure that the child's vision and hearing have been assessed.
3. Obtain information from the school (teacher and school counsellor) about the child's progress, with permission from the parents. Questionnaires (self-designed or others such as Child Behaviour Checklist and Connors Rating Scales) are helpful.
4. Obtain information from other professionals involved in providing therapy and support, i.e. occupational and speech therapists, special education

TABLE 6.3 Medical investigations

Clinical symptoms and signs	Investigation	May be related to
Pallor, lack of energy	FBC, serum iron	Anaemia
Pallor, history of home renovation or lead paint exposure	Serum lead level	Lead toxicity can adversely affect development
Tremulous, agitated, sweaty palms	Thyroid function	Hyperthyroidism
Sensitive to cold, slow, lack of energy	Thyroid function	Hypothyroidism (rare)
Major developmental delay with or without dysmorphic features suggestive of congenital condition, significant delay in learning skills	Chromosomes and karyotype	Fragile X syndrome
Klinefelter's syndrome
William's syndrome
Other rare syndromes
Absence episodes	EEG	Petit mal seizures
Poor listening and/or attention	Audiology	Deafness

These are rare causes of learning difficulties but should be considered where indicated.

teachers, after school care and other members of the family where appropriate.

5 Explanation of the findings to the child, parent and the school staff is very important. 'Demystification'[2] is a powerful tool for helping parents and carers to understand the child's difficulties. It essentially involves careful explanation of the child's difficulties and how it affects self-esteem, behaviour and social interaction at many levels. The aim is to give parents an understanding of how difficult it can be for the child to effectively learn and process new information.

6 Investigations may be required (see Table 6.3 for medical investigations; Table 6.4 for other investigations). Specific medical investigations are done when dictated by the clinical findings.

7 The child might need therapy assessment for language (speech therapist) or motor coordination problems (occupational therapist). Cognitive assessment by a psychologist through psychometric testing is likely to be necessary to assess the child's intellectual level of function, which provides a profile of their strengths and weaknesses, in order to effectively inform intervention. Behaviour support or counselling with a clinical psychologist might also be necessary.

8 Encourage the child's interests and areas of strength, e.g. sport and creative ability, as this protects self-esteem. Also remain aware of the importance of family and other supports that nurture self-esteem.

9 Where the child's presentation indicates comorbidity like ADHD, anxiety or mood disorder, the particular condition will need to be addressed.

10 The optimum strategies for helping the child depend on the child's individual needs (learning difficulty and associated processing problems) but may not always be possible due to funding or resource constraints.

TABLE 6.4 Other investigations

Clinical indication	Tests used
Reading problems	Schonell test
	Durrell test
	Wide range achievement test (WRAT)
	Wechsler Individual Achievement Test (WIAT)
	Neale Analysis of Reading Ability
Spelling problems	Schonell test
	Durrell test
	WRAT
	WIAT
Delay in many areas and slow at tasks	Psychometric assessments including:
	Stanford Binet
	Differential Ability Scales
	Wechsler Intelligence Scale for Children IV (WISC IV)
Fine motor problems	Beery test for visual–motor integration
Speech and language problems	Range of tests that assess language skills including the CELF, Lindamood
Poor social and self-help skills	Vineland's Adaptive Behaviour test

Note: It is not imperative that the clinician be familiar with these tests, because the tests are carried out by psychologists and therapists. The aim of providing the list is merely to indicate that specific skills can be assessed and some tools have greater specificity than others. The decision as to which tool is used rests with the professional who is trained to perform the assessment. Notwithstanding this, it does help if the paediatrician is conversant with the tests to interpret and detect any discrepancies that may occur.

11 The school's application for additional teacher support is enhanced by discussions with therapists. Therapist and doctor reports are often essential when schools apply for special funding for SLD children. These reports are also helpful with applications for Special Provisions for school examinations. Special Provisions can allow for extra time and a quiet room in which to do the exams. In special circumstances a reader and writer may be provided for the examinations.
12 The ultimate decision about services that the school can provide to support the child rests with the educators. However the medical, psychology and therapy input should not be underestimated.
13 Suggestions can be made by talking to the school via case conferences (directly or via teleconference) particularly for difficult cases. The suggestions in Text Box 6.3 and Text Box 6.4 are not directives and need to be done in collaboration with the teachers at school.

> **TEXT BOX 6.3** Suggestions to help the child with visual processing difficulties
>
> **Reading**
> 1. An auditory or linguistic system for reading may be helpful.
> 2. Use of a marker or window to focus attention on the word being read.
> 3. Contextual clues to aid the reading process.
> 4. Finger pointing to the word while reading may help in the early stages.
>
> **Spelling**
> 1. Encourage decoding by breaking words down into simple sounds.
> 2. Lined paper with widely spaced words helps to focus on the words being read.
> 3. Avoid too much information on worksheets. Keep them simple.
> 4. A multisensory approach helps; for example look at the word, pronounce the word, write the word in a sentence and then write the word from memory.

> **TEXT BOX 6.4** Suggestions to help the child with auditory processing difficulties
>
> 1. Keep verbal information and instructions short and simple.
> 2. The child will tend to 'tune out' if exposed to verbal overload.
> 3. Encourage the child to make eye contact and to listen to what is being said.
> 4. Visual representations when teaching are helpful, as these children are often 'visual learners'.
> 5. Visual aids, charts and presentations may be helpful.
> 6. Model good language techniques, like turn-taking and eye contact, as these children may have social interaction difficulty.
> 7. Older students can be encouraged to make notes to remind them of the subject content.

14. A medical follow-up appointment allows review of the child's progress with intervention, allows parents time to process the information and provides further opportunity for questions and clarification.

Practice Point

The clinician must remain sensitive to how advice is given so as not to appear patronising or inadvertently undermine good teachers. Suggestions should be given with the recognition that the teacher is working with the child on a daily basis, and has to manage the entire class not just one child. Direct discussion with the teacher where possible is often helpful.

Practice Point

It is not advisable to make a definitive diagnosis following a single assessment. A better approach is to review the child's progress after strategies or interventions have been put in place. Often there is pressure to reach a diagnosis, but a hurried approach might mean that the diagnosis is later found to be incorrect or inadequate.

Be aware that alternative therapies, like behavioural vision therapy and eye exercises for dyslexia or SLD, are not supported by evidence.[11] Parents may pursue alternative therapies in order to help their child and it is important that the paediatrician provide a balanced perspective with research evidence, while respecting parental decisions and the need to help their child.

Assessment allows early intervention to be implemented. Early intervention should be encouraged either through speech therapy or school-based learning programs, irrespective of the particular diagnostic category.[12]

MANAGEMENT OF COMORBID CONDITIONS

Children who initially present with learning difficulty and complex problems like poor short-term memory, attention and processing difficulties may have comorbid ADHD. In many instances treatment of the ADHD symptoms can result in significant improvement in the child's school performance. Therefore a broad understanding of the various conditions and how they can present in one child is important. (This chapter should be read along with Chapter 5 Autism spectrum disorders, Chapter 7 Language disorders, Chapter 8 Attention deficit hyperactivity disorder and Chapter 13 Developmental and intellectual disability.)

MEDICAL REPORTS

It is usual practice to give parents copies of the medical report, and it is helpful if the report is easy to follow and understand. The report can aid the school and other agencies involved in the care of that child because they can follow or question the approach and the suggestions made. This allows collaboration between various agencies that can be encouraged to make contact with the doctor if necessary.

Practice Point

The medical report may be read by teachers and other professionals. The provision of reports to others must be under the control of the parents, except for the report that is sent to the referring doctor. If there is a need to send reports to other parties, written consent must be obtained from the parents and the adolescent or young adult.

Where third party information is obtained for the child's medical history, the information should not be included in an 'open' report as consent will need to be obtained from that party. If the report is written in several sections, the parents can be encouraged not to provide the 'confidential' information section, e.g. family and pregnancy history, to other parties. It is important to always remain cognisant of confidentiality issues.

CONCLUSION

SLD and learning difficulty in children is complex and many factors require consideration. The clinician needs to remain aware of the differential diagnoses to ensure that appropriate investigations and assessments are done to allow targeted support and intervention.

REFERENCES

1. Dyck MJ, Hay D, Anderson M, et al. Is the discrepancy criterion for defining developmental disorders valid? Journal Child Psychology Psychiatry 2004;45(5):979–95
2. Levine MD, Brooks R, Shonkoff JP. A pediatric approach to learning disorders. Boston: Wiley Medical; 1980
3. Flanagan DP, Ortiz SO, et al. Integration of response to intervention and norm-referenced tests in learning disability identification: Learning from the tower of Babel. Psychology in the Schools 2006;43(7):807–25
4. Snowling MJ. From language to reading and dyslexia. Dyslexia 2001;7:37–46
5. American Speech-Language-Hearing Association. Central Auditory Processing: Current Status of Research and Implications for Clinical Practice 1996. DOI: 10.1044/policy.TR1996-00241. Online. Available: http://www.asha.org/docs/html/TR1996-00241.html; 22 Feb 2012
6. Sharma M, Purdy SC, Kelly AS. Comorbidity of auditory processing, language and reading disorders. Journal Speech Language Hearing Research 2009;52:706–22
7. Dawes P, Bishop D. Auditory processing disorder in relation to developmental disorders of language, communication and attention: a review and critique. International Journal of Language & Communication Disorders 2009;44(4):440–65
8. Lliadou V, Bamiou D, Kaprinis S, et al. Auditory processing disorders in children suspected of learning disabilities – a need for screening? International Journal of Pediatric Otorhinolaryngology 2009;73:1029–34
9. Dawes P, Bishop D. Psychometric profile of children with auditory processing disorder and children with dyslexia. Archives of Disease in Childhood 2010;95(6):432–6
10. British Society of Audiology: Auditory Processing Disorder Special Interest Group. Online. Available: http://www.thebsa.org.uk/index.php?option=com_content&view=article&id=72:apd&catid=21:apd&Itemid=29; 22 Feb 2012
11. American Academy of Pediatrics. Joint Statement – Learning disabilities, dyslexia and vision. Pediatrics 2009;124(2):837–44
12. Weindrich D, Jennen-Steinmetz Ch, et al. Epidemiology and prognosis of specific disorders of language and scholastic skills. European Child Adolescent Psychiatry 2000;9:186–94

RESOURCES

For Parents, Carers and Professionals:
http://www.ldaustralia.org/
http://www.dest.gov.au
http://www.ldc.org.au
http://www.cheri.com.au/
http://www.learningdifficulties.com.au/
http://www.learninglinks.org.au
http://education.qld.gov.au/studentservices/learning/

http://www.doctorg.org/faq.htm
http://www.auspeld.org.au
http://www.asha.org/

Dorothy Bishop's Blog on APD:
http://deevybee.blogspot.com/

For Teachers:
http://www.curriculumsupport.education.nsw.gov.au
http://www.doctorg.org/faq.htm

7 Language disorders

Sandra Johnson

DEFINITIONS

There is no clear consensus for the definition of language disorders. Earlier work by Rapin and Allen[1] defined language disorder on the basis of impairment that included phonological, lexical, semantic, syntactic and pragmatic aspects. The work of Bishop and Rosenbloom[2] provided a classification differentiating between cases of known, e.g. hearing loss or brain injury, and unknown aetiology. The Diagnostic and Statistical Manual of Mental Disorders of the American Psychiatric Association (DSM-IV) provides the more familiar classification, namely: expressive language disorder, mixed receptive–expressive language disorder and phonological disorder.[3]

Specific language impairment

The term 'specific language impairment' (SLI) is defined as delay in language skills with discrepancy between the child's language skills and their non-verbal functioning. The discrepancy is usually more than 1 standard deviation (about 15 points) between verbal and performance scores on psychometric testing. This discrepancy model has been challenged, particularly in children at the extremes of the normal distribution curve, e.g. children with superior performance IQ who have a large discrepancy between their verbal and performance scores, and yet their language score might be average or even above average. Rice et al. noted that the use of non-verbal IQ as an exclusionary criterion in the definition of SLI is flawed in that there are similarities and differences in children's language skills above and below the traditional cut-off in performance IQ of 85, so that the difficulties that they encounter with learning and language skills are similar.[4] In addition, both groups of children require intervention services and the IQ distinction is not helpful in guiding intervention. Also, there is a wide distribution of the differences between verbal and non-verbal skills in the normal population.

It is worth noting that children with language disorders or SLI form a heterogeneous group where the presentation varies widely, so that there is no clear phenotype for the disorder.[5] Bishop et al. found that children who meet language test criteria for SLI are not necessarily the same as those referred for speech and language therapy.[6] This phenomenon might in part be because of an inverse relationship between socioeconomic status and the point when parents become worried about their child's language, meaning that in poorer communities parents are more likely to present late with concerns about their child's language delay.

A simple approach is to define SLI on the basis of delayed language development that is out of keeping with the development of the child's other skills on clinical history, without using a performance IQ criterion of 85 as the threshold. Although the presentation is usually identified in preschool years, it can also be identified in children after they commence school.

The definition for SLI usually excludes neurological disease, mental retardation, autism and significant hearing impairment.[7] These exclusions are questionable as neurological impairments, mental retardation and autism often coexist with the language deficits in children with SLI.

Developmental language disorder

Hall and Aram state that the term 'development language disorder' (DLD) implies a developmental, rather than an acquired process in children who have language disorders.[8] They suggest that this term is more inclusive than specific language impairment and reflects the heterogeneous nature of the disorder. In addition, the disorder transcends the language domain and provides a neurological basis for classification. However the term DLD is not applied to children who have structural neurological lesions. Here the term 'developmental aphasia' is used instead.

Developmental aphasia

The term 'developmental aphasia' is usually applied where there is structural neurological injury resulting in an acquired aphasia, which affects language development in the young child. In adults this may occur as a result of a lesion in the dominant left hemisphere, but in children language development is not localised to one hemisphere and language development can be affected by diffuse injury. In addition, the right hemisphere in children can take over language function if the left hemisphere is damaged in early childhood. See Table 7.1 for causes of acquired aphasia.

Selective mutism

This is an acquired disorder where the child does not speak in one or more environments, such as school or to adults outside the home, and yet the child's speech at home is reported to be typical and average for age. However, a significant proportion of these children have articulation or language deficits and go on to have language-based learning difficulties at school. The onset is usually in preschool or early school years.

Some children who fail to speak may not have a language disorder but have features of childhood psychiatric problems. Anxiety has been noted to be a factor in children with selective mutism.

Neurological causes should also be considered, such as acquired epileptic aphasia (Landau-Kleffner syndrome) without overt seizures, mass lesion in the brain, and neurodegenerative disease.

An informative article is available for further study of this subject.[9]

TABLE 7.1 Some causes of acquired aphasia

Cause of acquired aphasia	Clinical presentation
Secondary to infections	Bacterial or viral resulting in encephalitis and/or encephalopathy
Secondary to hydrocephalus	Superficially the child has good language, but lacking in content ('cocktail party' syndrome)
Traumatic brain injury	Presentation depends on the lesion and area of brain affected
Tumour	Involving language-sensitive areas of brain
Vascular lesions or stroke	Involving language-sensitive areas of brain
Acquired aphasia with seizures (Landau-Kleffner syndrome)	Normal language development initially but then regress, either suddenly or over a few weeks, and may stop talking. Seizures occur at the onset or later. Mostly normal social behaviour or may be timid.
Degenerative disorders	Speech and language is lost as part of global loss of skills and function in children with degenerative brain disorders

Practice Point

The term disorder, although used in many conditions, is fraught with difficulty in that disorder implies abnormality or disease. In young children, where language development has a broad range of normal, it may not be clear at first that the language delay is permanent and therefore disordered.

For the purposes of this chapter, delay is used to imply that catch-up in language skills may occur at a later point in time. Disorder is used to imply that the development of language skills is disrupted or not occurring in the usual (typical) manner and is dysfunctional as well as being delayed.

This chapter will focus on specific language impairment as defined above. See the appendix at the chapter end for explanation of terms commonly used by language specialists.

FUNCTIONAL NEUROANATOMY OF SPEECH AND LANGUAGE

Language processing occurs predominantly in the left hemisphere in 95 per cent of right-handed persons and in 70 per cent of left-handed persons.[10]

The familiar and classical neuroanatomy of language includes involvement of Broca's area (the 'expressive motor area' at the inferior frontal area of the left cerebral hemisphere), Wernicke's area (the 'receptive sensory area' in the posterior superior temporal region) and the arcuate fasciculus (a connecting fibre tract).

Studies of adults with brain injury show that lesions involving Broca's area result in non-fluent, monotonous speech with phonemic paraphrasias (where words are mispronounced or syllables are out of sequence, e.g. 'treen' instead of 'train') and there is poor articulation of sounds. However, the comprehension of language is relatively good. Lesions involving Wernicke's area result in fluent, melodious and 'empty' speech, which includes semantic paraphrasias (where the substituted word is similar to the word intended, e.g. 'chair' instead of 'table' or 'television' instead of 'computer') and the comprehension of language is poor.[11]

Many researchers believe that this classical model is too simplistic in that it does not account for a range of aphasic syndromes and it is both anatomically and linguistically non-specific. New investigations, such as haemodynamic imaging, electromagnetic recording, transcranial magnetic stimulation and neuropsychological methods, support the following observations and hypotheses:[12]

- Fractionation of the superior temporal gyrus (STG) shows that this is a very active area in language
- There appear to be two parallel pathways: a dorsal pathway (for sensory–motor integration and mapping of sound to articulation) and a ventral pathway (for speech comprehension and linguistic processing of sound to meaning)[12,13]
- The middle and interior sectors of the temporal lobe are involved in word processing; the anterior STG is involved in construction of sentences; and the subcortical structures (basal ganglia and cerebellum) are involved in 'linguistic computation'
- Although the dominant left hemisphere plays a major role in language in most persons, the right cerebral hemisphere also plays a part as supported by imaging research.

The advances in anatomical tractography, as well as intraoperative cortico–subcortical electrical mapping in vivo in humans, has enabled study of the pathways that are involved in linguistic functions.[14] A further review of the functional neuroanatomy of language provides more detail on the subject.[15]

Note

Brain lesion distinctions are less clear in children and typical Wernicke's aphasia is rare in children. Lenneberg in 1967 put forward a theory that cortical control of language is at first bilateral and then gradually lateralises, usually to the left hemisphere as the child matures, which could explain the relatively better recovery in young children with acquired aphasia. Other theories have since been put forward. Further reading can be done on this subject.[16]

PREVALENCE

Prevalence varies and depends on the definitions used. In a study of preschool children, the prevalence of language delay was estimated to be 7.6 per cent[17] and Tomblin et al. found that 7.4 per cent of kindergarten-aged children met criteria for specific language impairment.[7] Language difficulties in children are not uncommon and many papers report long-term impact on social, communication and academic skills in individuals with language impairment. (See Prognosis later in the chapter.)

CLASSIFICATION

The simplest classification is that of the DSM-IV and this approach is most likely to be applicable in clinical paediatric practice.[3] However, the clinician might wish to be familiar with a classification system used by linguists and speech pathologists. One example is the classification for language disorders provided in Lees and Unwin,[18] which is based on the work of Rapin and Allen (see Text Box 7.1 for a summary: reproduced with permission).

DSM-IV classification

In clinical practice, the DSM-IV classification is more likely to be useful to the paediatrician, although it is somewhat limited compared to that used by linguists and speech pathologists:
- Expressive language disorder
- Mixed receptive–expressive language disorder
- Phonological disorder.

> ### Practice Point
> The distinctions described in Text Box 7.1 allow speech therapists to determine a therapy pathway, but may be difficult for the paediatrician to determine in clinical practice. Neurologists may find these terms helpful when considering specific lesions that cause particular language deficits.

AETIOLOGY

Most researchers agree that there is no clear aetiology for SLI. However there are many causal factors associated with language delay. See Text Box 7.2 for an approach based on texts by Lees and Unwin[18] and Bishop and Mogford.[19]

Neuropathological findings, such as loss of cortical tissue near the Sylvian fissure and dysplasia in the inferior left frontal cortex, have been reported in children with SLI.[20] Neuroimaging studies (MRI) have shown asymmetry of the cerebral cortex in frontal and parietal regions[21] and white matter volume loss with ventricular enlargement has also been reported.[22] The findings suggest that children with SLI have structurally different brains, but it is difficult to be certain as the findings may reflect a normal variation in the population.

Genetic factors are significant. *Nature* first reported a dominant mutation in the FOXP2 gene, which was associated with severe speech and language disorder in about half the members of the KE family in Britain.[23] The role of genes in SLI is important and is discussed by Dorothy Bishop.[24] The high concordance rate of SLI in monozygotic twins supports genetic influence, but environmental factors are also significant.[25]

Environmental factors were examined in a study in Florida. Factors found to be independently associated with increased risk of language impairment were short duration of maternal education, maternal marital status (being single) and late enrolment to antenatal care.[26] The work of Hart and Risley showed that what parents said and did with their children in the first three years had an enormous impact on how much language children learned and used.[27] The observers noted that the parents in low income families tended to talk less to their children and were inclined to give more negative feedback than those of professional and higher income families. It is prudent to say that many factors are at play in relation to low income families that may have impacted on these observations.

TEXT BOX 7.1 Subtypes of language disorder

1 Expressive sub-types

Developmental verbal dyspraxia
- Poor verbal output, speech is laboured
- Severe deficit in phonology and fluency
- Delayed onset of language development
- *Not* due to muscle weakness or pseubobulbar palsy (as in cerebral palsy).

Phonologic production deficit
- Impaired phonology and syntax which compromises intelligibility, but with preserved fluency
- Compatible with good vocabulary and appropriate pragmatics
- Comprehension normal or near normal.

2 Mixed receptive–expressive subtypes

Verbal auditory agnosia (word deafness)
- Severe impairment of ability to decode auditory information
- Severe comprehension and expressive deficits
- Sometimes thought to be deaf, but normal audiology
- Often need an alternative communications system (signs).

Phonologic–syntactic deficit
- Speech is dysfluent, speak in short utterances
- Make morphological errors (confusing tense, grammar and plurals)
- Comprehension impaired but less affected than expression
- Receptive skills may be equal or superior to expressive ability
- Can imitate words and simple phrases.

Lexical–syntactic deficit
- Main feature is severe word retrieval difficulty
- Child knows what they want to say but is unable to find the words to do so
- Employs strategies to overcome word-finding problem – gesticulation, using a general word like 'thing' to refer to object
- Comprehension is defective but better than expressive
- Immature syntax, severe anomia (difficulty recalling the names of everyday objects)
- phonology and intelligibility may be good
- child can imitate phrases, fluency varies.

3 Higher-order language subtypes

Semantic-pragmatic deficit
- Expressive skills better than receptive language
- May be hyperverbal, but lack comprehension
- Tendency to be literal in comprehending information
- Speech may be fluent
- Echolalia and perseverations may be a feature
- Poor pragmatic concepts, i.e. greeting behaviour, turn-taking and use of conversational tools
- Word retrieval deficits
- Circumlocution with tendency to talk around the subject without good content.

CHAPTER 7 Language disorders — 133

TEXT BOX 7.2 Factors that may be associated with language delay

Factors affecting language input
- Environment: bilingualism, social circumstances, neglect, institutionalisation
- Sensory deprivation: hearing and vision impairment (see Chapter 4 on Hearing and vision loss)
- Genetics or hereditary influences: affect language processing in that some disorders have a genetic basis (e.g. ADHD, autism).

Factors affecting language processing
- Cognitive deficits: mental impairment, cerebral palsy, congenital brain abnormalities
- Communication deficits: autism, selective mutism
- Attention deficits: ADHD, executive dysfunction (and associated learning difficulties).

Factors affecting language output
- Structural abnormalities: cleft lip and palate, CNS lesion leading to dysarthria (cerebral palsy), surgical (long-term tracheostomy)
- Disorders of oromotor control: focal or diffuse brain injury, aphasia
- Lesions involving Broca's and Wernicke's areas
- Congenital syndromes:
  - Down syndrome: large tongue with thrusting can affect expressive language and articulation
  - Moebius syndrome: with paralysis of soft palate and atrophy of the tongue
  - Worster-Drought syndrome (WDS): congenital pseudobulbar palsy resulting in difficulty with swallowing, feeding, speech and saliva control; non-progressive; possible abnormality in perisylvian cortex[47]
  - Congenital perisylvian dysfunction: thought to be on spectrum with WDS; perisylvian polymicrogyria on imaging; mild spastic tetraplegic cerebral palsy due to pyramidal tract involvement.[48]

The twin study by Thorpe, Rutter and Greenwood showed that twins and singletons differed in the observed patterns of mother–child interaction and that these differences accounted for the difference in their language level.[28] The burden on parents of twins is greater than with singletons because there are two babies to look after and their sleeping and feeding patterns may not coincide. The average language levels of twins lagged behind those of singletons by about 3 months measured at 36 months of age, and this lag was not related to obstetric factors. The conclusion was that environmentally-mediated family factors play a slightly greater role than genetics with respect to individual differences in language.

Bilingualism deserves mention. Bishop indicated that bilingual language development differs from monolingual development in superficial ways, but essentially development is the same in that bilingual children acquire the same strategies for learning language and they mix elements of the two languages in the early stages.[29] It is worth noting that this may be true of children growing up in a bi- or tri-lingual environment. However migrant or refugee children who have to 'place on hold' their half-learned primary language and start again may have more problems, especially if their parents do not speak the language of their adopted country. General cognitive abilities of bilingual children are the same as those of monolingual children.

Although not strictly causative factors, memory and processing deficits are often seen in children with SLI and may be involved in the causative pathway.[30,31] These deficits also occur in specific learning disorders, attention deficit hyperactivity disorder (ADHD) and autism, which again supports the importance of comorbidities in developmental conditions. (See Chapter 5 Autism spectrum disorders, Chapter 6 Specific learning disorders and Chapter 8 Attention deficit hyperactivity disorder.)

Neurological deficits as a cause for language disorders are important, but are excluded in the current criteria for SLI. The impact of focal neurological lesions,[32] traumatic brain injury,[33,34] epilepsy[35] and stroke[36] is discussed in various publications.

> **Practice Point**
>
> In an attempt to aid recall and understanding, Text Box 7.2 is likely to be an over-simplification, which might not reflect the complexity between factors. The causal associations are not linear and sometimes language development progresses normally without delay, despite the presence of the above-mentioned factors.

CLINICAL PRESENTATION

Children with language disorders form a heterogeneous group and the presentation largely depends on the type of language disorder. Refer to the classification to review the presenting features of children with expressive, mixed receptive–expressive and higher-order language difficulties.

The preschool child

There is variability in the development of language in young children and the rate of progress is dependent on many factors, particularly genetic (hereditary) and environmental. Delay in language acquisition in an otherwise typically developing child could be hereditary in a family of late talkers. Usually speech is delayed but not deviant in these children. Environmental factors, like poor verbal stimulation and child neglect, impact significantly on a child's language development.[19]

The young child might present with language delay in skills, such as babbling, use of single words and use of sentences. See Table 7.2 for milestones of language. The term 'delay' implies that 'catch up' might occur at a later point in time. The diagnosis of disordered or deviant development is made retrospectively in those cases where:

- It is clear that catch up has not occurred
- There is a scatter of skills with significant difference between expressive and receptive ability
- There is good expressive ability on formal testing, with poor pragmatic skills.

Behavioural difficulties, including aggression, can be a presenting feature in young children. Where young children are unable to express their desires effectively they may act out in unacceptable ways, e.g. a young boy with delayed

TABLE 7.2 Milestones in language development

Mean age	Pre-language and language skills
Birth	Baby makes eye contact with parent
4–6 weeks	Baby smiles at parent responsively
6–16 weeks	Baby coos in response to parental interaction and 'motherese' (intonations of voice that mothers use when talking to their babies)
4–8 months	Babbling; baby makes sounds that show early communicative intent and these occur in response to parent's verbal responses
9–12 months	Baby's babbling approximates the intonations of language, makes eye contact while interacting, begins to babble word approximations e.g. 'dadda'
12–14 months	First single words, pointing to objects
15–24 months	Increase in word vocabulary, up to about 50 words; but there is a large variability in normal development
24 months	First short 2-word phrases
3 years	Full sentences; may have grammatical errors; may not yet grasp concepts like 'under', 'next to', 'behind'
4 years	Complex sentences, and begins to grasp language concepts mentioned above

language skills appears aggressive and 'hits out' at others because he is unable to make verbal requests or to let others know what he wants. The adult, without understanding his inappropriate attempts at communication, might punish his behaviour that then reinforces the aggression.

The clinician needs to be aware of the importance of effective communication between parent and child, and how this interaction affects the child's behaviour. It is also worth noting that behaviour and language problems may coexist, so that it is often impossible to establish which problem came first. See more on Behaviour difficulties in Chapter 9.

Stuttering, which is a fluency disorder, occurs more commonly in boys and first presents between 3.5 and 5 years of age.[37]

The preschool child who stops talking

A history of cessation in language development in the child who also shows poor reciprocal social interaction should raise the suspicion of autism spectrum disorder. This diagnosis can be difficult to establish in the under three-year-old child, particularly after one clinical presentation. (See Chapter 5 on Autism spectrum disorders.)

The differential diagnosis should include:
- Landau-Kleffner syndrome: regression of language skills, seizures may not be clinically overt or may commence at a later point in time
- Degenerative brain diseases: includes storage and metabolic disorders, these are rare but should be considered. (Rett's syndrome is an important cause.)

- Child abuse
- Tumour or space-occupying lesion.

Note: The deaf child does not speak at all in the early years, rather than stops talking.

> **Practice Point**
>
> There is a broad range of normal for early language development. At one end of the spectrum is the child who speaks in short phrases or sentences by age 2.5 years (clearly typical) and at the other end is the child who is not using 2-word phrases by 4 years (clearly not typical), with a wide variation in between.

The school-aged child

There are various features that may present to the clinician, and many occur in other disorders as well (ADHD, specific learning disorders):
- Difficulty with following verbal instructions
- Appears not to listen or process verbal information
- Delay in or poor reading skills
- Poor reading comprehension
- Poor expressive language ability
- Problems with getting thoughts down in written form
- Takes a long time to complete written work
- Social interaction difficulty
- Unable to grasp idioms or other abstract language concepts
- Tendency to prefer own company rather than interact with peers
- Aggressive behaviour in the child who has difficulty communicating their needs.

Comorbidity

The features described above are common to many developmental problems, such as specific learning disorders, ADHD, developmental coordination disorders (motor problems), autism and related disorders, and intellectual disability. Therefore a comprehensive approach is needed when doing the medical assessment recognising the high rate of comorbidity between these disorders.

The comorbidities associated with SLI include reading disorder,[38] attention deficit hyperactivity disorder[39] and motor abnormalities.[40] The clinical presentation for these disorders overlaps in many cases and a common genetic basis has been postulated.[41]

The clinician must remain aware of the effect of anxiety or depression on the child's school performance and consider underlying contributing or environmental factors.

ASSESSMENT

The clinician or paediatrician's primary aim is to:
- Exclude a medical cause for language problems – normal hearing very important

- Determine that language delay or disorder is present to the extent that further assessment for language therapy intervention is required
- Consider emotional or environmental cause.

Ideally, assessment of language disorder occurs in a multidisciplinary setting with a speech therapist on the team of professionals. However the clinician in private practice, in a community clinic or in the rural practice setting might not have immediate access to speech therapy.

In some instances the speech therapist may be the first professional to assess the child, and then refer to the paediatrician where there is concern about the medical aspects of the child's development.

Exclude a medical cause

Hearing impairment
- Congenital deafness with sensorineural hearing impairment, especially high tone deafness which is easy to miss. (See Chapter 4 on Hearing and vision loss.)
- Chronic middle ear problems, e.g. suppurative otitis media can affect hearing and impair early language development. Suppurative otitis media with a damaged eardrum may result in significant hearing loss that affects language and learning at school. This is particularly relevant for Aboriginal children where this condition is not uncommon.
- Severe persistent glue ear in child with Down or Turner's syndromes may have a greater impact on language development.

Severe medical illness
Any young child with severe medical illness who requires regular hospital admissions might present with delay in early language skills.

Neurological disorders
Conditions that affect brain function impact on the development of language skills. Many central nervous system (CNS) causes are not likely to specifically affect language alone (except Landau-Kleffner syndrome), and are more likely to have a global effect on development. Consider these under the well-recognised headings in a clinical approach to diagnosis.

Prenatal
- Congenital syndromes: usually there are physical features to indicate a congenital or genetic disorder, e.g. Down syndrome
- Maternal infections: TORCH (toxoplasmosis, rubella, cytomegalovirus, herpes)
- Drugs or medications: alcohol and its effect on a developing fetus
- Prenatal causes for cerebral palsy.

Perinatal
- Infections during neonatal period that might hinder development
- Traumatic delivery and severe asphyxia.

Postnatal
- Infective: encephalitis, encephalopathy – various causes
- Traumatic: acquired brain injury
- Metabolic: associated encephalopathies
- Tumour: lesions affecting speech sensitive regions of the brain.

Determine that language delay or disorder is significant

Parental report is paramount in assessment. Parents spend more time with the child so that if parents are concerned then the clinician should take careful note of their concerns.

However parents of only or firstborn children may not recognise language delay or disorder because they have no point of comparison. In addition, there may be the issue of heritability, so that parents who also have a degree of SLI may not recognise the child's language delay at first. Parents from lower socioeconomic areas may not recognise the extent of the child's language delay where their gold standard is other children in the neighbourhood, who may also have delayed language skills compared to children from higher socioeconomic areas.

Language test scores, although important, should not be relied on solely when assessing delay or disorder. Clinical suspicion together with parental report of difficulties must be taken into account. There is research to support the value of parental report.[6]

Checklists can be used when assessing language to aid determination of delay or deviance in the clinical setting (see Table 7.3). The assessment tools (Table 7.4) are usually administered by speech therapists rather than by paediatricians. The list is not complete but serves to indicate there are several tests that can be used to assess language abilities in children. Where delay or deviance is suspected early referral to speech pathology services is recommended.

Consider emotional causes

Emotion and environmental influences, with respect to nurturing the child's learning and language skills, are important considerations. In clinical practice this can be difficult to assess but the clinician should remain aware of the potential impact.

The general practitioner, social worker and/or community clinic nurse can provide valuable information about the child's early years and the family or home environment.

The impact of abuse or neglect on a child's development and language acquisition cannot be overestimated. A review article on this subject found that neglect was more damaging than abuse with regard to language development.[42]

TABLE 7.3	Checklists
Test	**Useful for assessing the following**
Ages and Stages Questionnaire (Paul H Brookes Publishing 2004)	Checklist of development for ages 4 mo to 5 yr old
PEDS (Parent's Evaluations of Developmental Status) (Ellsworth & Vandermeer Press) 2002	Questions that determine parental concerns and may help to monitor development
MacArthur-Bates Communicative Development Inventories Level III (CDI-III)	Parent questionnaire about child's language skills For children up to 43 mo, also two versions (Words and Gestures)

TABLE 7.4 Assessment tools

Test	Useful for assessing the following
CELF (Clinical Evaluation of Language Functions) Semel & Wiig 1987	Age range 6–18 yr Assesses linguistic concepts, sentence structure, semantics, sentence recall and listening Assesses receptive and expressive language
REEL (Receptive and Expressive Emergent Language Scale) Bzoch & League 1970	Observational checklist, suitable 1 mo to 3 yr old Scores language behaviour observed by examiner and parent
McCarthy Scales of Children's Abilities (MCSA)	Assesses word knowledge
Peabody Picture Vocabulary Test, 4th edn (PPVT-4)	Receptive vocabulary
Test for Auditory Comprehension of Language, 3rd edn (TACL-3)	Receptive grammar, vocabulary and syntax

Practice Point

The paediatrician should not feel compelled to make a specific diagnosis of the type of language disorder, because this requires assessment by a speech and language therapist experienced in assessing language difficulties. However the doctor and therapist should aim to reach a working diagnosis, which may take several sessions, to ensure that all areas of the child's development are taken into account. Caution and review of the child's progress over time is best, rather than making a hasty diagnosis that subsequently has to be withdrawn.

Parental report and the paediatrician's interpretation of language tests based on the background of their broader clinical experience is a valuable tool rather than relying on test scores alone.

The term specific language impairment should only be used where neurological deficit, intellectual impairment, significant hearing impairment and autism have been excluded, according to the current definition of SLI.

MANAGEMENT

Management of the child with language disorder, irrespective of cause, is long term, and monitoring the child's progress over time will allow targeted intervention to be implemented.

When the problem is detected in the preschool child, it is likely that the child will need regular review during early school years because there is a high incidence of language-based learning difficulties in children who present with early language delay.

Language therapy intervention should commence as soon as delay or disorder is suspected. The therapist will assess the child's language deficit and provide intervention accordingly. Regular therapy will be required over a period of time. Therapists usually provide parents with exercises that are done at home and that complement therapy sessions. Ideally intervention should involve all the key communication partners in a child's life, e.g. home, preschool, and community.

Intervention can focus on training parents to be the primary intervention provider, e.g the Hanen program developed by the Hanen Centre in Canada.[43] This is a parent-only program and is not used in conjunction with clinical therapy sessions with the child. The program teaches parents new ways of communicating and playing with their children in order to facilitate language development.

The importance of therapy intervention for children with language delay or disorder is well recognised. Cochrane review involving meta-analysis of results from 25 studies showed that speech and language therapy is effective for expressive phonological and expressive vocabulary difficulties, with less evidence that interventions are effective for receptive difficulties. Heterogeneity in the results was noted and further investigation was recommended.[44]

Contact with the educators during the preschool years will assist implementation of language support programs when the child commences school.

School-aged children with language disorder or SLI need educational support at school. They require individualised goals for intervention based on collaborative assessment involving the family and the school personnel. These goals can be tailored to the child's immediate needs, incorporating strengths and weaknesses, and should be revised over time as needs change. Learning programs like Fast ForWord, Lindamood, Multilit and others may be useful to assist these children.

Reading recovery programs in the early years of primary school may aid children with language deficits who also have early reading difficulties. However reading recovery alone may not benefit language-disordered children, as they are more likely to need multi-faceted targeted support for reading comprehension, word attack, word recognition and contextual reading. (See Chapter 6 Specific learning disorders for an approach to helping these children.)

Early psychometric assessment will provide information about the child's cognitive ability, strengths and weaknesses profile, and will enable educational intervention to be planned in relation to specific difficulties. The school psychologist or the clinical psychologist of a multidisciplinary team can perform the assessment.

The child with SLI, despite having no neurological or obvious medical cause, should continue to be monitored by the paediatrician with respect to general health, height, weight, academic progress and emotional response to the problem. These children are often bullied by other children and are at risk for emotional difficulties such as anxiety and/or depression.

Academic difficulty places these children at risk for social interaction problems with peers and others, poor self-esteem, lack of motivation and tendency to give up in relation to schoolwork. Intervention and support should be long term as their difficulties are likely to continue throughout their school years.

It is vital to encourage the child's natural ability and talents in non-academic areas, because this helps to protect self-esteem and foster achievement in areas other than schoolwork, e.g. the child who does poorly academically but who does well at sport.

Accommodations and adjustments may be required for children with persistent language learning difficulties in later school years to enable them to more effectively access the school curriculum. Early withdrawal of educational support in primary school without proper review and follow-up, due to apparent improvement with educational and therapy intervention, is unwise because these individuals may go on to have learning and comprehension difficulties in the more complex language environment of high school.

Support from parents, therapists, educationalists and doctors goes a long way to help children with language disorders cope with their difficulties. (See Chapter 6 Specific learning disorders, Chapter 8 Attention deficit hyperactivity disorder and Chapter 10 School refusal and truancy, as these conditions are often comorbid with language disorders.)

PROGNOSIS

As mentioned, children with language disorder form a heterogeneous group and therefore it is not possible to predict prognosis quantitatively. The outcome depends on the type and severity of the language disorder; the presence of associated learning difficulties or other comorbid conditions; and environmental factors such as the extent of intervention and support for the child. As in many developmental conditions, genetic influence and vulnerability play a part in the outcome for the individual child.

Bishop and Edmundson studied speech-impaired preschool children and found that 37 per cent had resolution of their language impairment at 5.5 years (18 months after initial testing).[45] Those who had persistent language impairment at age 5.5 years had poor prognosis with respect to literacy, continued language development and educational progress in later school years.

Further studies are reviewed by Simms.[46] Tomblin et al. found that children diagnosed with SLI at 8 years old had residual language deficits as adults. Clegg et al. followed children with normal intelligence who had severe language impairment, and found that persistent language difficulties were associated with poor outcome on cognitive, academic and social–emotional measures. Poor outcome in emotional, behavioural and social areas has been reported for young adults who had language disorder as children.

Therefore children who have persisting language deficits by the time they start school, irrespective of aetiology, are at risk long term. They require continued support and intervention from many agencies throughout their school years and possibly also into adulthood.

APPENDIX: TERMS USED IN LANGUAGE DISORDERS ASSESSMENT AND MANAGEMENT

Terms relating to the form of language
- Phonology: system of speech sounds that constitute a language; includes phonetics
- Syntax: rules that govern arrangement of words in sentences; grammar
- Lexical: the vocabulary of the language.

Terms relating to the content and function of language
- Semantics: the meaning of words, phrases or sentences
- Pragmatics: the function of communication, e.g. request, reject, share information. Also refers to contexts in which language is used, e.g turn-taking, conversation.

Other terms

- Dyspraxia: problems with planning motor–movements and coordination; affects motor planning for large muscle groups and also for muscles of speech, i.e. oro-motor control
- Dysarthria: difficulty with articulation of sounds due to weakness or incoordination of the muscles of speech; may be due to structural defect involving the speech system, e.g. cleft palate, or CNS–supratentorial lesion, e.g. brain injury, tumour, cerebral palsy, CNS haemorrhage
- Dysrhythmia: problems with the rhythm of speech, e.g. stutter, stammer
- Aphasia: difficulty with receptive and/or expressive language usually acquired as a result of brain damage.

REFERENCES

1. Rapin I, Allen DA. Syndromes in developmental dysphasia and adult aphasia. Language, Communication and the Brain. New York: Raven Press; 1988. p. 57–75
2. Bishop D, Rosenbloom L. Childhood language disorders: classification and overview. In: Yule W, Rutter M, editors. Language Development and Disorders. Clinics in Developmental Medicine 101/102. Philadelphia: JB Lippincott; 1987. p. 16–41
3. American Psychiatric Association. Diagnostic and Statistical Manual of Mental Disorders, edn 4 (DSM-IV). Washington DC: APA; 1994
4. Rice ML, Tomblin JB, et al. Grammatical tense deficits in children with SLI and nonspecific language impairment: relationships with nonverbal IQ over time. J Speech, Lang & Hearing Research 2004;47:816–34
5. Tager-Flusberg H, Cooper J. Present and future possibilities for defining a phenotype for specific language impairment. J Speech, Language & Hearing Research 1999;42(5):1275
6. Bishop DVM, McDonald D. Identifying language impairment in children: combining language test scores with parental report. International Journal Language & Communication Disorders 2009;44(5):600–15
7. Tomblin JB, Records NL, et al. Prevalence of specific language impairment in kindergarten children. J Speech Lang Hear Res 1997;40:1245–60
8. Hall N, Aram DM. Classification of developmental language disorders. Clinics in Developmental Medicine 1996;139:10–20
9. Stein MT (ed.) Selective mutism. Journal Developmental & Behavioral Pediatrics 2001;22(2):S123–6
10. Lurito JT, Dzemidzic M. Determination of cerebral hemisphere language dominance with functional magnetic resonance imaging. Neuroimaging Clinics North America 2001;11:355–63
11. Smits M, Visch-Brink E, Schraa-Tam CK, et al. Functional MR imaging of language processing: an overview of easy-to-implement paradigms for patient care and clinical research. RadioGraphics 2006;26:S145–58
12. Poeppel D, Hickok G. Towards a new functional anatomy of language. Cognition 2004;92:1–12
13. Saur D, Kreher BW, Schnell S, et al. Ventral and dorsal pathways for language. Proc Nati Acad Sci USA 2008;105(46):18035–40. Online DOI:10.1073/pnas.0805234105
14. Duffau H. The anatomo-functional connectivity of language revisited. New insights provided by electrostimulation and tractography. Neuropsychologia 2008;46:927–34
15. Hickok G. The functional neuroanatomy of language. Physics of Life Reviews 2009;6:121–43
16. Bishop D, Mogford K. Language development in exceptional circumstances. Ch 13 Language development after focal brain damage. London: Churchill Livingstone; 1988
17. Silva PA. A study of the prevalence, stability and significance of developmental language delays in preschool children. Dev Med Child Neurol 1980;22:768–77
18. Lees J, Urwin S. Children with language disorders. Ch 1 The language impaired child. London: Whurr Publishers; 1991

CHAPTER 7 Language disorders ■ 143

19 Bishop D, Mogford K. Language development in exceptional circumstances. London: Churchill Livingstone; 1988
20 Cohen M, Campbell R, Yaghmai F. Neuropathological abnormalities in developmental dysphasia. Ann Neurol 1989;25:567–70
21 Jernigan TL, Hesselink JR, et al. Cerebral structure on magnetic resonance imaging in language- and learning-impaired children. Arch Neurol 1991;48:539–45
22 Trauner D, Wulfeck B, et al. Neurological and MRI profiles of children with developmental language impairment. Dev Med Child Neurol 2000;42:470–5
23 Lai CS, Fisher SE, Hurst JA, et al. A forkhead-domain gene is mutated in a severe speech and language disorder. Nature 2001;413:519–23
24 Bishop DVM. The role of genes in the etiology of specific language impairment. Journal Communication Disorders 2002;35:311–28
25 Bishop DVM. Genetic and environmental risks for specific language impairment in children. International Congress Series 2003;1254:225–45
26 Stanton-Chapman TL, Chapman DA, Bainbridge NL, et al. Identification of early risk factors for language impairment. Res Dev Disabil 2002;23:390–405
27 Hart B, Risley T. Meaningful differences in the everyday experience of young American children. Baltimore: Paul H Brookes Publishing; 1995
28 Thorpe K, Rutter M, Greenwood R. Twins as a natural experiment to study the causes of mild language delay. II: Family interaction risk factors. Journal Child Psychol Psych 2003;44(3):342–55
29 Bishop D, Mogford K. Language development in exceptional circumstances. Ch 4 Bilingual language development in preschool children. London: Churchill Livingstone; 1988
30 Baird G, Dworzynski K, et al. Memory impairment in children with language impairment. Develop Med Child Neurol 2010;52(6):535–40
31 Cardy JE, Tannock R, et al. The contribution of processing impairments to SLI: Insights from attention-deficit/hyperactivity disorder. Journal Communication Disorders 2010;43:77–91
32 Avila L, Riesgo R, et al. Language and focal brain lesion in childhood. J Child Neurol 2010;25(7):829–33
33 Sullivan JR, Riccio CA. Language functioning and deficits following pediatric traumatic brain injury. Applied Neuropsychology 2010;17(2):93–8
34 Klein SK, Masur D, et al. Fluent aphasia in children: definition and natural history. J Child Neurol 1992;7:50–9
35 Caplan R, Siddarth P, et al. Language in pediatric epilepsy. Epilepsia 2009;50(11):2397–407
36 Martins IP, Loureiro C, et al. Grammatical dissociation during acquired childhood aphasia. Develop Med Child Neurol 2009;51(12):999–1002
37 Guitar B. Stuttering: an integrated approach to its nature and treatment. New York: Lippincott Williams & Wilkins; 2006
38 Catts HW, Fey ME, Tomblin JB, Zhang X. A longitudinal investigation of reading outcomes in children with language impairments. J Speech Lang Hear Res 2002;45:1142–57
39 Tannock R, Brown TE. Attention deficit disorders with learning disorders in children and adolescents. In: Brown TE, editor. Attention deficit disorders and cognitive comorbidities in children, adolescents and adults. Washington DC: American Psychiatric Press; 2000
40 Webster RI, Erdos C, Evans K, et al. The clinical spectrum of developmental language impairment in school-aged children: language, cognitive and motor findings. Pediatrics 2006;118:e1541–9
41 Bishop DVM. Motor immaturity and specific language impairment: Evidence for a common genetic basis. Am J Med Genetics 2001;114:56–63
42 Law J, Conway J. Effect of abuse and neglect on the development of children's speech and language. Developmental Medicine and Child Neurology 1992;34(11):943–8
43 Pennington L, Thomson K, et al. Effects of It Takes Two to Talk: the Hanen program for parents of preschool children with cerebral palsy: findings from an exploratory study. J Speech Lang Hear Research 2009;52:1121–38

44 Law J, Garrett Z, Nye C. Speech and language therapy interventions for children with primary speech and language delay or disorder. Cochrane Database of Systematic Reviews. Online: 12 May 2010. DOI: 10.1002/14651858.CD004110
45 Bishop DVM, Edmundson A. Language-impaired 4 year olds: distinguishing transient from persistent impairment. J Speech Hear Disord 1987;52:156–73
46 Simms MD. Language disorders in children: Classification and clinical syndromes. Pediatric Clinics of North America 2007;54:437–67
47 Clark M, Harris R, et al. Worster-Drought syndrome: poorly recognized despite severe and persistent difficulties with feeding and speech. Develop Med Child Neurol 2010;52(1):27–32
48 Clark M, Chong WK, et al. Congenital perisylvian dysfunction – is it a spectrum? Develop Med Child Neurol 2010;52(1):33–9

FURTHER READING

Lees J, Urwin S. Children with language disorders. London: Whurr Publishers; 1991
Bishop D, Mogford K. Language development in exceptional circumstances. London: Churchill Livingstone; 1988
Capute AJ, Accardo PJ. Developmental disabilities in infancy and childhood. Baltimore: Paul H Brookes Publishing; 1991

RESOURCES

These resources available 23 Feb 2012.
The Hanen program: http://www.hanen.org
http://www.nidcd.nih.gov/health/voice/speechandlanguage.html
http://www.speechpathologyaustralia.org.au/

8 Attention deficit hyperactivity disorder

Sandra Johnson

DEFINITION

Attention deficit hyperactivity disorder (ADHD) is a descriptive term and refers to observed behaviour, which includes inattention with or without hyperactivity and impulsivity. The behaviour is perceived as a persistent problem by parents, teachers and carers in that the child's behaviour is at variance with normal or unaffected children at the same age.

Although many young children display some of the behaviours described in this condition, the difference is that in the child with ADHD the behaviour is more severe, persistent and disruptive not only to the child's social interaction and learning, but potentially to the child's educational and socioeconomic outcome in the long term.

In clinical practice there are two main subtypes of the condition, and the third is less common:

- **Combined subtype** where the child presents with inattention as well as hyperactive–impulsive symptoms.
- **Predominantly inattentive subtype** where inattention is the main presenting symptom and hyperactive–impulsive symptoms may be present, but are less significant.
- **Predominantly hyperactive–impulsive subtype** is rarely seen in clinical practice without symptoms of inattention.

PREVALENCE

The condition is common in childhood and is reported to be 6.8 per cent of children in Australia.[1] Fairly recent systematic reviews indicate a prevalence of 5–10 per cent, with percentages higher in some countries. A total of 50 studies were examined; 20 from the United States and 30 from other countries including the United Kingdom, New Zealand, Australia, Hong Kong, Germany, France, China, India and Sweden. Earlier suggestions that the prevalence was different between the United States and the United Kingdom was found not to be a true difference, but was related to the use of different criteria to define the condition.[2,3]

There has been some debate in the literature about the different criteria used to define ADHD and the differences between DSM-III, DSM-IV, ICD 9 and ICD10. The reader needs to be aware that DSM-V and ICD 11 are currently being developed.

AETIOLOGY

There is no definite causal agent in ADHD but there are many important genetic and environmental factors that play a part. The condition is heterogenous, so that a single aetiological cause is unlikely. A review on the subject examines current understanding of risk factors that influence ADHD.[4]

Genetics

Several studies show a genetic link and heritability to ADHD.[5] The risk of having ADHD is four to five times more likely where there is a first-degree relative with the condition.[6] Twin and adoption studies show a definite heritability to the condition, and data of twin studies from various countries estimate a heritability rate of 76 per cent.[7]

It is thought that multiple genes contribute to the predisposition to develop the condition, where genes and environmental factors interact in some way, and studies involving epigenetics may provide answers in the future. In clinical practice we do observe phenotype variability in members of the same family. Some postulate that the condition might include multiple disorders each having a different aetiology, possibly with different genes having small individual effects.[8]

Molecular genetics has focused on the genes that code for the neurotransmitters involved in brain pathways, namely dopamine, serotonin and noradrenalin. Meta-analysis of the various studies has shown significant association between susceptibility for the condition and gene variants.[9] Gene variants include dopamine receptors (D4 & D5) and transporter genes, serotonin transporter gene and synaptosomal-associated protein 25 gene (SNAP-25).[7,10]

Recently, chromosome deletions and duplications, known as copy number variants (CNVs), were found to be significantly increased in 410 ADHD children compared with 1156 matched controls from the 1958 British Birth Cohort. The locus at chromosome 16p13.11 showed a significant excess of CNVs, which provides a focus for research in the future. These findings give further support to a genetic basis of the condition. In this group CNVs were also increased in unexplained intellectual disability, schizophrenia and autism. The last finding suggests a common biological basis between ADHD and autism, supported by studies showing comorbidity between these two conditions. Research so far does not show a similar comorbidity with schizophrenia.[11]

Environment

There are environmental factors associated with increased risk for ADHD but they are difficult to study, as there are many confounding variables.[12] Some of these factors are:
- Maternal smoking and alcohol intake during pregnancy – while it is difficult to establish causation, it has been suggested that with smoking it may be the genetic predisposition to addictive behaviour in the mother with ADHD that is more relevant than smoking alone[13]
- Maternal stress – postulated to occur through stress effect on the hypothalamic-pituitary-adrenal axis and the production of cortisol, which in turn affects neuronal development and the neurotransmitter pathways[14]
- Prematurity and low birth weight for gestation
- Brain injury resulting in attention and processing deficits[15]

- Toxins – lead, mercury and polychlorinated biphenyl exposure in pregnancy. Children exposed to lead show a dose-dependent relationship between serum lead level and ADHD diagnosis
- Diet and sensitivity to certain foods has been postulated. In practice, many parents report that diet plays a role, but this is difficult to study[16]
- Psychosocial factors – family dysfunction, conflict and abuse have been linked to this disorder.[17] This may relate to similar neurobiology where the parent has ADHD as well, and might be less able to cope with the stress of child-rearing. Children who have been raised in institutional care also have a higher risk for the condition.

Epigenetics

As discussed in Chapter 1 Normal development, epigenetics means 'beyond or outside genetics' and is an emerging field that examines changes to DNA or associated proteins in relation to environmental exposures and factors. There is growing evidence for a link between environmental factors and gene expression, where factors like nutrition, stress, ageing, smoking, infections and other toxins impact on the genome. The mechanism through which this occurs is referred to in Chapter 1. The interaction between genes and environment is likely to be relevant in ADHD as well as in other medical conditions.[18]

NEUROBIOLOGY OF ADHD

In relation to the neurobiology of ADHD it is helpful to review normal brain development. Our present knowledge based on research is that over 90 per cent of total brain volume is reached by five years of age. MRI studies show that expansion between ages five and 11 years occurs predominantly in the prefrontal cortex. Sex differences in development reveal larger cerebrum and cerebellum in boys and larger caudate in girls. Increases in white matter volumes occur in children over time, and is likely to indicate increased myelination, but there is variability in grey matter growth. Reduction in grey matter from early childhood to adolescence might be due to selective pruning, with grey matter volumes peaking at around 12 years old in frontal and parietal lobes and then declining in post adolescence.[19,20]

There is evidence to show that children with ADHD have significantly smaller brains than healthy children throughout childhood and adolescence.[21] Meta-analysis of studies show overall reduction in total brain volume and cerebral volumes compared to controls. White matter volumes are also significantly reduced in ADHD. Changes have also been reported in basal ganglia, involving the caudate nucleus and putamen, but these findings are not consistent.[22]

The challenge of comparing results of neuroimaging studies is related to small sample sizes, no direct comparison with healthy controls, and the use of different methodology when interpreting results. ALE (activation likelihood estimation) meta-analysis aims to give quantitative analysis that is unbiased and objective. Findings across 16 peer-reviewed neuroimaging studies showed frontal hypoactivity as a consistent finding in ADHD patients compared with controls.[23] This work suggests that despite ADHD being a heterogeneous disorder commonality exists in these patients, which has implications for future research.

Other meta-analyses of structural imaging findings in ADHD show that regions beyond frontal or frontal-striatal areas are involved. The cerebellum, particularly the posterior inferior vermis, and the splenium of the corpus callosum appear to be significant so that there is growing support for abnormalities in the cerebellar-prefrontal-striatal network in ADHD.[24]

Maturational delay is thought by many to underpin the clinical findings of ADHD. This hypothesis is supported by longitudinal data using neuroimaging techniques that detail changes in cortical thickness, where the age of reaching peak cortical thickness is significantly delayed in ADHD children compared to controls. This delay is most marked in prefrontal regions that are important in cognitive processes like motor planning and attention.[25] Clinically, many patients with ADHD show improvement of symptoms with age and clinicians often find that children show less symptomatology as they move into adulthood. So far the finding of delayed structural maturation seems to be specific to ADHD, and in conditions like autism the finding appears to be that of deviance rather than delay.[26] In one clinical study MRI correlations of reaction times and grey matter volumes showed changes in keeping with delayed maturation in ADHD.[27] These results could guide further research into the notion of delay rather than deviance in cortical development of the brain in children with ADHD.

DIAGNOSTIC CRITERIA

The diagnosis of ADHD is made on the basis of observed behaviour outlined in the DSM-IV criteria and/or ICD10. Text Box 8.1 (with permission) outlines the essential criteria that are common to both and the reader is encouraged to refer to the tables provided in the Guidelines.[12] *DSM-V and ICD 11 are currently being developed, and should be released in 2013. It appears that the threshold for the presenting age will change (to 12 years old) in DSM V and symptoms will be included that mirror what is seen in clinical practice, e.g. emotional dysregulation and inflexibility. Criteria for diagnosis in adolescents and adults are likely to be included. Also information obtained from teachers and parents will be emphasised, which is what most clinicians do in practice anyway.*

Important factors in the assessment of a child for ADHD is to distinguish between behaviour considered to be in keeping with ADHD, and behaviour that represents normal variation in development. In ADHD the symptoms need to be present for at least 6 months, should occur in more than one environment and must be out of keeping with the child's developmental level. As such the condition can be diagnosed in children of above, at or below average intellectual potential, although caution is required in the last to ensure that the behaviour is not an expression of the developmental or intellectual disability.

The assessment process takes time and information must be obtained from multiple sources: the parents, other carers, teachers and other professionals who know the child well. Questionnaire reports and checklists may help to achieve this aim (see Text Box 8.2).

Where uncertainty about the presentation exists, time and review of the child's progress is recommended rather than pressure to reach a diagnosis at the initial assessment. ADHD symptoms are persistent for at least 6 months. Often it will be necessary to refer the child for psychological, speech or occupational therapy assessment before any conclusions can be inferred.

CHAPTER 8 Attention deficit hyperactivity disorder

TEXT BOX 8.1 Summary of criteria for diagnosis of ADHD based on DSM-IV and ICD10

A Inattention: six or more symptoms persisting for at least 6 months, maladaptive and inconsistent with child's developmental level
- Fails to give attention to details, makes careless errors
- Fails to sustain attention to tasks or play activities
- Appears not to listen when spoken to directly
- Fails to follow through on instructions
- Poor organisation with tasks and activities
- Often avoids or dislikes homework or tasks that require sustained mental effort
- Often loses things needed for tasks
- Easily distracted by noise
- Forgetful in daily activities.

B Hyperactivity or impulsivity: six or more symptoms persisting for at least 6 months, maladaptive and inconsistent with child's developmental level
- Hyperactivity
  - fidgets with hands and feet, or squirms in seat
  - often leaves seat in classroom
  - runs or climbs excessively where inappropriate
  - difficulty playing or doing activities quietly
  - often 'on the go' as if 'driven by a motor'
  - often talks excessively
- Impulsivity
  - often blurts out answers
  - difficulty awaiting turn
  - interrupts or intrudes on others, e.g. butts into conversations or games.

Either A or B required together with the following
- The behavioural symptoms must be present before 7 years of age
- The behaviour must be present in two or more settings, i.e. home, school or work
- There must be evidence of significant impairment in school, social or work functioning
- The symptoms should not occur only during the course of a pervasive developmental disorder, psychotic disorder or schizophrenia and the symptoms are not due to another mental disorder, such as mood disorder or personality disorder.

Note: DSM-V and ICD 11 are currently being developed and some criteria for ADHD might change. Please see comment under Diagnostic criteria.

> **TEXT BOX 8.2** Checklists and rating scales
>
> - Connor's Rating Scales (parent and teacher information)
> - ADHD Rating Scale based on DSM-IV criteria (parent and teacher)
> - Achenbach Behaviour Checklist
> - CBCL (Child Behaviour Checklist)
>
> Note: These tools are generally used by school psychologists and the information is then provided to the doctor. However the DSM-IV rating scales can be used by the paediatrician or medical officer doing the assessment.

Once the diagnosis of ADHD is made, regular follow-up is important as the child's needs change over time. At follow-up, information is again gathered from multiple sources as at the initial assessment.

EXECUTIVE DYSFUNCTION

Brain functioning is complex. Attention requires a coherent set of mental functions, including the ability to focus on a task, sustain focus over a period of time, encode the information, disengage and shift focus. Executive functions (EF) regulate behaviour and include the ability to inhibit, shift, set, plan, organise, use working memory and to problem solve. Many higher order cognitive functions are controlled by complex neural networks and involve the cerebellum, basal ganglia, thalamus, frontal and prefrontal cortex.

Brown describes a model of six clusters of cognitive functions that are impaired in children with ADHD and these include: activation, focus, effort, emotion, memory and action. He also refers to the 'situational variability' of the symptoms of ADHD, which is well recognised in clinical practice. That is, a child might be able to focus well on a specific task of interest but not be able to apply such attention to other tasks especially when feeling pressured to perform.[28]

A comprehensive theory of ADHD with deficient inhibitory control as the core deficit that disrupts other executive functions has been proposed.[29] While executive dysfunction, such as planning, vigilance, working memory and response inhibition, are important in the neuropsychology of ADHD, EF deficits are not present in all cases of ADHD.[30]

Recent work proposes an integrative model with neuroanatomical pathways involving cortico-striato-thalamo-cortical circuits and various parallel pathways that play a role in ADHD, which may account for the heterogeneity of the disorder.[31]

Interest in the role of working memory in children with developmental disorders is growing, particularly as working memory, which is defined as the ability to hold or retain information in the mind while modifying and changing it over brief periods of time, appears to impact significantly on learning in children. One group showed that working memory, rather than IQ alone, is a greater predictor of learning and academic achievement in children with learning difficulties.[32,33] This finding is likely to be significant in children with ADHD as well, because they often report having difficulty with holding information in the mind while doing new tasks.

IMPORTANCE OF COMORBIDITIES

Comorbidity in ADHD is now accepted as the rule rather than the exception. Recent Australian data show that 43 out of 64 children referred to a multidisciplinary paediatric clinic were diagnosed with ADHD and 74 per cent of these were diagnosed with at least one comorbid condition.[34]

Comorbidities that commonly occur with ADHD include specific learning disorders (SLD), oppositional defiant disorder (ODD), conduct disorder (CD), anxiety and autism spectrum disorder (ASD).

Language and specific learning disorders are not uncommon in children with ADHD, although prevalence cannot easily be estimated due to variations in the type of learning–language difficulties. Willcutt et al. found significant weaknesses in processing speed, working memory, phonemic awareness and response inhibition in children with ADHD; with mathematics and reading disability supporting common genetic influences in these disorders.[35] See Chapter 6 Specific learning disorders and Chapter 7 Language disorders.

There are varying reports for autism spectrum disorder (ASD) with studies reporting up to 50 per cent ASD children having symptoms of ADHD. One study showed that ADHD and autism are easily distinguishable, and although ADHD symptoms are common in autism, autistic symptoms are not common in ADHD.[36]

ODD is a common psychiatric comorbidity in children with ADHD, occurring in about 60 per cent of ADHD patients. Comorbid CD is noted in about 20 per cent of patients with ADHD.[37] Barkley reported that approximately 24–35 per cent of clinic-referred adults diagnosed with ADHD have ODD and 17–25 per cent have CD.[38] Anxiety disorder occurs in approximately 25–50 per cent of children with ADHD.[39] Comorbid anxiety was found in one study to aggravate behavioral dysregulation (e.g. adjustment to new environments, emotional control and inhibition) in children with ADHD.[40]

With respect to other psychiatric problems, some families of children with ADHD appear to have a higher rate for antisocial personality disorder, alcoholism and substance abuse.[12]

Learning and attention involves integration of various pathways in the brain, therefore it is not surprising that ADHD children are more likely to have learning difficulties due to their attention, working memory and processing deficits. The complexity of integrated functioning is evident where similar deficits occur across many disorders, e.g. writing, processing and attention problems in children with ADHD, autism, ODD, anxiety and depression.[41]

ADHD children are also more likely to have language disorders due to poor listening, comprehension problems and difficulty with processing verbal and also visual information.[42]

CLINICAL PRESENTATION

The child with ADHD can present with a variety of symptoms, and it is important that the clinician is aware of the comorbidities discussed. The core symptoms of inattention, hyperactivity and impulsivity must be present from a young age, prior to seven years old. Refer to DSM-IV criteria for making the diagnosis, but recognise that there may be changes and additions to these criteria in DSM-V to be released in 2013.

As a result of the symptoms mentioned in the criteria, the child may present with a variety of symptoms:
- Learning difficulties: affecting reading, spelling, writing and/or maths
- Problems retaining and recalling information due to working memory deficits
- Difficulty with listening skills and following instructions, such that repetition is needed
- Language comprehension problems for both oral and written language
- Requires more parental or teacher direction to perform tasks compared to other children of the same age
- Tends to be forgetful and somewhat disorganised with possessions, often loses things
- Difficulty with task application and completing work effectively
- Poor or lack of attention to social cues, so that the child is awkward in social situations or may blurt out comments inappropriately and offend others
- Poor attention to detail and thus tends to make careless errors
- Social interaction difficulty and lack of empathy for feelings of others, sometimes viewed as self-centred
- May seem socially or emotionally immature compared with peers
- Academic underachievement despite having the intellectual capacity to do the work.

When taking the complete history be aware of stressors in the child's life that might be contributing to the presentation and result in symptoms very similar to that of ADHD and its comorbidities. See Differential diagnosis below.

ADHD predominantly inattentive type

This subtype is easy to miss because the symptoms of hyperactivity and impulsivity are less obvious and less intrusive to others. It appears to be more common in girls, but occurs in boys as well.

These individuals often have problems with self-esteem and confidence. Learning difficulties may be the main presentation to teachers and parents. Significant memory and retention difficulties impact on their learning. Comorbidity with specific learning disorder and/or anxiety disorder must be considered.

Individuals with this subtype are also more prone to anxiety and internalisation of their feelings, with a tendency to fears and phobias. It may be difficult to tease out these symptoms, but it is important to be aware that they may occur in this subtype of ADHD.

THE INITIAL ASSESSMENT

The standard paediatric assessment is carried out with a few adjustments in relation to learning and attention problems. The assessment takes time and parents need the time to tell their story. Time should also be given to the child to allow him to express his views about his difficulties. It is often necessary to see the parents and then the child on their own. The doctor needs to remain sensitive to the child's feelings and perceptions during the interview with the parents.

Ideally, this assessment should be carried out in a multidisciplinary team setting, e.g. through a paediatric teaching hospital. However in Australia these problems often present to paediatricians in private practice, as access to hospital clinics can be difficult because of the demand for services and limited resources in the public health sector. Many community paediatricians in child health or similar clinics regularly do these assessments and they may have the support of allied health professionals on their team.

Prior to the assessment, questionnaires and behaviour checklists can be sent to the parents and school (via the parents) so that information is obtained from various settings, i.e. school, home and social situations. See Text Box 8.2 for tools that may be helpful.

A CLINICAL APPROACH

Current history
- Includes information about the child's problems; who is concerned and why?
- When did difficulties first start and when did parents first become concerned?
- What have the parents or school done to address the problems?
- (*Obtain history from multiple informants by use of questionnaires or direct communication where possible.*)
- Do parents agree on the issue being presented?
- If the mother is most concerned, what is father's perception of the problem? Does he see the child's behaviour as a problem?
- (*Note the pervasiveness of symptoms across several situations, home, school and social settings.*)
- History of therapy and educational intervention?
- What assessments have already been done?
- Any prior medical intervention for the presenting problem?
- History of alternative interventions or complementary medicines?

Background history
- What is the child's early history in terms of the presenting concern?
- Any clear precipitating event?
- Any changes or stressors within the family unit?
- If this is a recent problem, is there a previous history of similar problems?

History of strengths and weaknesses
- What are the child's strengths? (*Knowledge of the child's natural abilities helps to focus on self-esteem and confidence, allowing a discussion point to establish communication with the child.*)
- What are the child's weaknesses? (*Sometimes asking this question helps parent and child to appreciate the perceived weakness more clearly.*)

Social skills and peer relationships
- How does the child relate to his peers?
- Possibility of being bullied or the child bullying others?
- What about the child's turn-taking skills; how do they reciprocate or share with their friends?
- Do they enjoy the company of others?

- Do they have friends and do they enjoy being with them and seek or invite them out?
- What about lunch breaks at school? What does the child do during the morning tea and lunch break?
- How does the child spend time at weekends?

Family history
- What is the child's position within the family?
- How does the child relate with siblings and with their parents?
- Family history of other members who have had similar developmental problems or difficulties at school?
- Family history of medical or psychiatric illness?
- History of neurological problems, e.g. epilepsy or other neurological disorders?

Pregnancy and perinatal history
- Was this a planned pregnancy?
- Maternal health during the pregnancy?
- Maternal exposure to smoking, alcohol or medications during the pregnancy?
- Gestation and delivery; spontaneous or caesarean?
- Birth weight, Apgar scores, condition of baby at birth?
- First few days: established feeds? bonding with baby?
- Early infancy: feeding, weight gain, baby's general progress? History of maternal postnatal depression?
- Paternal support for mother during and after pregnancy?

Developmental history
- Milestones and any unusual pattern of development, e.g. bottom shuffling that might suggest disordered development?
- Clumsiness? Fine motor skills?
- History of early social and listening skills?
- Early child care? Parent at work?
- Toilet training, progress and problems?
- History indicating regression of skills?

Preschool history
- Did the child attend preschool?
- Social interaction with others during this time at home and preschool?
- Development of independent skills; personal hygiene, dressing etc?

Medical history
- Any medical illness, particularly if it impinges on development in some way?
- History of ear infections?
- Diet history:
  - Appropriate diet for age? *(Note: young toddlers tend to graze during the day rather than eat at set meal times.)*
  - Intake of junk food? Balanced healthy food intake?
- Medication and immunisation history?

Physical examination

- Examine height, weight and head circumference and plot on percentile charts
- Examine vision and hearing; examine visual fields, visual acuity and do fundoscopic examination. If there is any concern formal testing by an ophthalmologist and ENT is recommended. Audiology referral should be considered if there is concern about hearing.
- General appearance; exclude dysmorphic features, neurocutaneous stigmata
- Examine all systems: general, cardiovascular, upper and lower respiratory, gastrointestinal, endocrine, skin, central nervous system (CNS)
- Pay attention to CNS, exclude neurological cause for attention or learning difficulties (rare but important):
  o Subtle seizures, absence or petit mal seizures
  o Gradual decline in cognitive skills, e.g. neurodegenerative disorders, metabolic disorders (may be hereditary)
  o Decline in previously well child, e.g. encephalopathy (infective or other), brain tumour.

Screening of learning skills

This is an option for the paediatrician who may wish to do specific tasks to assess the child's skills clinically. See the tools used in Chapter 6 Specific learning disorders.

Observe the child's attention and approach to doing these tasks. Also note the child's interest and exploration of their environment, their interaction with the clinician and the quality of their eye contact.

Preschool child

Note the young preschool child's ability to following instructions, simple and complex:
  o Simple one-part instruction for toddler (around 2 years old) – ask to give you a toy which is visible to the child
  o Simple two-part instruction (around 2.5–3 years old) – give you a toy and take another object to mother (two consecutive actions required)
  o Complex two-part instruction (around 3–3.5 years old) – includes language concepts like next to, behind, in front of
  o Complex three-part instruction (around 4–5 years old) – includes language concepts and three consecutive tasks linked together.

Note fine motor and pencil control:
  o Hand dominance begins to emerge at 12 months old, but is not clearly established until about 18 months to 2 years old. *(Note: obvious dominance on one side at 12 months should alert examiner to possible weakness on the other side.)*
  o Total grasp of pencil in young toddler and scribbles on the page
  o Early tripod grip by 3 years old, copies a line, begins to copy a circle
  o Copies a cross by 4 years old, begins to copy a square
  o Should have good pencil control and grip when the child starts school at 6 years old.

School-aged child

- Short-term memory task – recall for sequence of numbers, objects and/or pictures

- Note the older child's listening and conversation skills. Ask simple questions and note the response. Complex questions that require detailed explanations can be given to gain impression of the child's language skills.
- Ask the child to perform a reading, spelling and writing task
- Observe the child's behaviour and approach while doing these tasks.

> **Practice Point**
>
> The doctor may not feel comfortable about doing the reading, spelling and writing tasks in the school-aged child. The teacher and/or psychologist can test these skills by means of an academic assessment, so that it may be easier to request this information from the school.

DIAGNOSTIC TOOLS

There is no specific test for the diagnosis of ADHD. It remains a clinical assessment made on the history from many sources (parents, carers, teacher, others who work with the child), rating scales and behavioural observation. Neuropsychological assessment, neuroimaging and electroencephalogram might aid the process of diagnosis and planning for intervention. It is worth noting that some doubt the accuracy of these tests and question whether it aids the diagnostic process in children with ADHD.[12]

Technological advances in neuroimaging techniques, particularly functional MRI (fMRI) but also magnetic resonance spectroscopy, PET scans, diffusion tensor imaging (DTI) and electrophysiology studies, might become more useful in clinical practice in the future.[43] Interpretation of fMRI findings is complex and currently there is no consistent evidence available regarding the use of this tool. However, there appears to be some evidence for reduced activation in the striatum in patients with ADHD.[44]

Despite the promise of these new technologies it is wise for the clinician to remain aware of the cost-effectiveness of these investigations and to be alert to the sensitivity, specificity and variability in the results of these investigations. A report on the role of imaging in diagnosis and assessment of ADHD cautions the clinician about the use of present research tools that claim to evaluate ADHD.[45]

> **Practice Point**
>
> The Guidelines suggest that the use of neuropsychological measures may be of limited or no benefit in the routine assessment of ADHD. However where the child has functional deficits, such as learning and organisation problems, the assessment can give information about strengths and weaknesses that can aid educational intervention and support.
>
> Tools like the Continuous Performance Task (CPT) and the Test of Variable Attention (TOVA) can be helpful, especially when parents want an objective measure of the child's attention skills. However these tests are costly and are not required to make the diagnosis of ADHD. More importantly they do not replace the diagnostic process of a comprehensive medical assessment by an experienced clinician.

DIFFERENTIAL DIAGNOSIS

- Consider vision and hearing impairment as potential causes for learning, attention and/or behaviour problems.
- Pay particular attention to possible mood disorders like anxiety and depression.
- Consider comorbid conditions that occur together with ADHD: anxiety, depression, specific learning disorders, autism, and other psychiatric conditions.
- Exclude neurological disorders that may present with cognitive decline together with attention and/or behaviour problems (complex partial seizures; encephalitis; acquired brain injury; neurodegenerative disorders; brain tumour; metabolic or endocrine disorders that affect brain function, e.g. hypoglycaemia; hypothyroidism; hyperthyroidism).
- Consider sleep disorders as a cause for sleep disturbance and daytime attention or behaviour problems.
- Consider chronic medical conditions affecting major organs resulting in lethargy with secondary decline in learning and/or behaviour.
- Consider family dynamics and environmental factors that may contribute to the child's attention and/or behaviour problems.

MANAGEMENT

Initial medical management

1. Ensure that vision and hearing have been assessed.
2. Arrange medical investigations to exclude medical conditions where indicated by the clinical signs and history.
3. Refer for psycho-educational assessment. See below.
4. Refer for therapy assessments where indicated.
5. Explain your approach and plan to the parents; give reasons for your clinical impressions.
6. Do not rush to making a diagnosis at the initial assessment. Obtain more information from others (family members, school and other carers) and wait for allied health assessment results.
7. Provide the family and referring doctor with a management plan and outline for review and follow-up. Discuss suggestions for assisting the child in the classroom environment while further information is gathered.
8. The information is given to the parents and can be shared with the class teacher. Teachers are usually keen to be involved in the management process to help the child. See Text Box 8.4 for suggestions to help the child who has attention problems. Resources for teachers are also provided at the end of the chapter.

Educational assessment

- By special education teacher: academic profile and learning skills
- By school psychologist or guidance counsellor: to assess reading, comprehension, spelling, mathematics and attention skills.

Psychometric assessment

- Provides information about the child's cognitive ability, short term or working memory and processing skills

- Is not diagnostic for ADHD, but gives a comprehensive overview of the child's learning potential as well as the child's strengths and weaknesses. This information can help with educational planning of intervention.
- The assessment can be done by the team or clinic psychologist, school counsellor or by a psychologist in the private sector who has been trained to carry out these assessments.

Therapy assessment

- Assessment of language skills by speech therapist: indicates where difficulties with receptive and expressive language skills noted. Should also be considered if there are problems with written narrative, which may be the result of language processing problems.
- Assessment of fine and gross motor skills: by occupational therapist and/or physiotherapist where indicated by the physical examination.

Psychiatry assessment

May be needed if there is suspicion that the presenting symptoms reflect a psychiatric disorder or significant family dysfunction.

Follow-up and medical review appointment

1. Obtain information through reports and assessments from all sources to gain a bigger picture about the child's learning, social and behavioural progress since the initial assessment.
2. Discuss progress and strategies that have helped the child and family. Further explanations to parents may be required.
3. Where a clearer picture for the diagnosis of ADHD emerges, develop a new management plan:
   - The approach for helping the child with ADHD is multimodal and involves the treating doctor, GP, therapists, educators, counsellors and parents.
   - Educational support for learning difficulties is important as these children often have associated learning problems. This intervention is best coordinated through the school, but sometimes children prefer not to attend special classes at school to avoid being different to their peers. Private special education teachers may be able to assist, but it is important that these teachers work closely with the schoolteacher.
   - Therapy intervention may be needed if assessments confirm specific problems, e.g. speech, motor coordination and handwriting difficulties.
   - Psychological counselling support should occur alongside medical, educational and therapy intervention.
   - Medication management may be an option and should be discussed with the child and family. Some families prefer not to pursue this path and

Practice Point

Therapy should be targeted to the child's specific needs. Endless physiotherapy sessions for a child who has no particular interest in sport or who is disinterested in the activity being addressed might not be the best use of family time and resources.

their decision must be respected, provided that they have been informed about medication management based on the best available evidence. Parents need time to do their own research about medication and they need information to do this effectively.

School involvement

Involvement of the school personnel is important for effective management of ADHD as these children need understanding, behaviour support and educational intervention at school. Parents often report having difficulty with the school's understanding of their child's ADHD. However, such reports vary and limited resources to schools might be a valid reason. Many schools provide support programs for children, particularly if there is associated comorbidity like autism spectrum disorder, language and learning disorder. Ongoing communication with the school and doctors' reports being available to the school, via the parents, with explanation of the child's difficulties can be helpful. A study using a questionnaire survey to parents showed that many perceived that teachers do not have adequate understanding of ADHD and that there are insufficient resources to assist students.[46]

New intervention approach

An intervention approach that involves training to improve working memory (WM) function is of interest because poor WM is seen in children with ADHD, learning disorders and language disorders, and it appears to be a limiting factor in academic performance and daily activities for many patients. However, this is an emerging field of study that is yet to produce consistent and repeatable results.[47]

For a website providing information about working memory training see the resource list.

Medication management

Medication management is an option for treating ADHD and not all patients will require medication. Once interventions are put in place to address the behaviour and attention difficulties as discussed above, many parents and teachers report improvement in the child's symptoms.

When medication is considered it is important to discuss the plan and side-effects of the particular medication to be trialled. A trial of treatment for about 4 to 6 weeks is recommended, which gives the child, parents and teachers an opportunity to see if there are any benefits in the child's attention, learning and behaviour.

The available medications licensed in Australia for children over six years old with ADHD are: methylphenidate in immediate release (Ritalin® 10 mg and Attenta® 10 mg) and dexamphetamine 5 mg; extended release formulations (Ritalin® LA and Concerta®), dexamphetamine (compounded slow release) and atomoxetine (Strattera®). There are other medications that have been proposed for use in ADHD, but they are not licensed in Australia.[48] See Table 8.1 for the common medications used to treat ADHD.

There are regulations for prescribing stimulant medications (methylphenidate and dexamphetamine) in Australia as they are Schedule 8 drugs and the regulations vary depending on the state. It is important that the prescribing doctor is aware of the regulation within their particular state, and information can be obtained from the Health Department of that state.

TABLE 8.1 Medications most commonly used to treat ADHD

Medication	Dose	Treatment approach
Ritalin® 10 mg (immediate release)	Start with ½ (5 mg) tablet morning and lunchtime; or early morning, mid-morning recess and afternoon top-up dose	For initiating treatment and to determine effect Start low and increase dose slowly This preparation is used as a 'top-up' dose in afternoon when Ritalin® LA is given in morning
Ritalin® LA 10 mg, 20 mg, 30 mg, 40 mg (extended release)	Once a day in morning (usually lasts about 5–7 hours, less in some and longer in others)	After trial treatment shows positive effect, the ongoing dose is usually 0.5–1 mg/kg/day Be aware that some children will have side-effects even on relatively low dose for weight Dose will need to be increased or titrated as the child grows to the recommended maximum dose of 60 mg/day Many do well on lower doses, while some need higher doses Adolescents may need a top-up dose of immediate release Ritalin® 10 mg after school
Concerta® 18 mg, 27 mg, 36 mg, 54 mg	Once a day in morning (lasts 8–10 hours but this varies in different individuals)	Same approach as for Ritalin® LA
Dexamphetamine immediate release 5 mg, extended release 10 mg	Once a day in morning, may need top-up of immediate release in afternoon	Beneficial in some patients when methylphenidate is not effective (Author experience: somewhat more appetite suppression and sleep disturbance)
Atomoxetine (Strattera®)	10 mg, 18 mg, 25 mg, 40 mg, 60 mg single day dose	Useful for patients who have side-effects on stimulants and particularly those with comorbid anxiety Start with low dose and increase weekly. Dose of 0.5–1.2 mg/kg/day. Stop at the dose where effect is observed as some require lower doses Takes a few weeks to obtain effect. Be aware of suicidal ideation as a potential side-effect. Not recommended for children under 6 years old.

Note: There are many potential side-effects with these medications. Caution and careful monitoring is recommended when the medication is used for the first time.
Main contraindications to using stimulants are:
- Psychiatric disorder (particularly psychosis)
- Cardiac disorder
- History of substance abuse
- Glaucoma
- Be familiar with pharmaceutical product precautions.

CHAPTER 8   Attention deficit hyperactivity disorder

TEXT BOX 8.3 More common side-effects of stimulant medications

- Appetite suppression
- Sleep difficulties
- Gastrointestinal (GIT) side-effects: nausea or abdominal discomfort
- Headache
- Mood changes: feeling irritable, tearful or 'down' in mood
- Agitation or jitteriness
- Cardiovascular: tachycardia, slight rise in BP is some individuals
- Dry mouth
- Tics: particularly important where family history of Tourette's syndrome
- Be aware of suicidal risk: caution with Atomoxetine®, but this is a factor irrespective of the medication in individuals with comorbid depression.

Side-effects of medication

Side-effects should be discussed with the child and family. It is helpful to give them notes to take away regarding the side-effects of treatment. As with all medications, there are many adverse effects related to drugs reported in the package inserts containing the patient information. It is important to be aware of these, although many are extremely rare. It is essential to discuss the common side-effects and encourage the family to read more about medication and side-effects before you commence treatment.

See Text Box 8.3 for the common side effects of stimulant medications. The doctor is encouraged to review the side effects for any medication prescribed.

Parental concerns

When medication is commenced, parents are naturally concerned about side-effects and long-term effects. The paediatrician can provide information based on results in the Guidelines[12] and it is worth referring to side-effects that may be of particular concern. Referring to literature on subjects like growth,[49] cardiac effects[50] and substance abuse[51–54] can be helpful and reassuring for parents. In the child with cardiac disease, special cautions are required.[55]

Concerns in the community about doctor's management of ADHD in children was addressed in the Special Review of ADHD in Children and Adolescents in New South Wales, which found that medical prescribing practices are cautious and conservative, where only 1.5 per cent of 4–17-year-old individuals received approval for stimulant treatment during the study period.[56] This is conservative, particularly when the prevalence of the disorder is considered.

TREATMENT APPROACH

Preschool

Medication is not advised as first-line treatment in preschool children and other strategies (behaviour and psychosocial interventions) should be tried initially. The Guidelines support the use of medication in children between three and five with severe symptoms that impact on the child and family, and where there has been poor response to behaviour and psychosocial therapy. If the doctor has limited experience in the use of medication in young children, then it is advisable to

> **TEXT BOX 8.4** Suggestions for helping the child who has attention difficulties
>
> **At home**
> - Keep instructions simple and make eye contact or touch the child when giving an instruction to ensure that they are listening
> - Give information while you are in the same room as the child, yelling from one room to the child in another room might lead to the child not responding
> - Stay positive in communicating with your child, even when their behaviour is difficult or unacceptable
> - Be clear about what you expect from your child in terms of their behaviour and keep encouraging their efforts
> - Avoid comments like 'you never listen', as this undermines the child's ability to even try to do the right thing resulting in the child giving up and not bothering to listen next time
> - Encourage the child's talents, which helps to protect self-esteem and confidence
> - Praise for good effort and for trying their best, rather than giving praise only when a 'good' result is achieved
> - Be sure to make time to have fun with your child, as this builds a healthy relationship and leads to good communication with your child.
>
> **In the classroom**
> - The child might be easily distracted by noise, so it may help to have them sit closer to the teacher
> - Most children cope better with routines and clear guidelines regarding expectations, and even more so if they have attention problems
> - Keep instructions short and clear; written notes might help with retention of important information
> - Keep worksheets as simple as possible, otherwise the child might feel overwhelmed and tend to give up at the task
> - It helps to break the tasks up so that the child has an ability to achieve one step at a time, allowing breaks or time to move about if necessary
> - The child may find it difficult to sit at a desk for too long; give them tasks to do in class that allow them to get up and move about; tasks to assist the teacher can also enhances a sense of responsibility
> - To help with organisation difficulty encourage the child to carry a diary and to write reminders for work that needs to be done
> - Remain positive with the child, avoid making comments that focus on their attention or learning problems especially in the company of peers
> - Avoid a punitive or authoritarian approach, particularly with adolescents as they are likely to respond negatively and not cooperate
> - Always respect the child as an individual who has some choice with respect to their needs in the learning environment.

obtain a second opinion to ensure that this is the best treatment approach for that child.

It is wise to bear in mind that more research is needed regarding our understanding about the use of medications in ADHD for very young children. Therefore a conservative approach is encouraged, while ensuring that children and families are provided with the intervention and support that they need.[57]

School age

Where the symptoms of ADHD are mild and have no major impact on the child's social interaction, learning and behaviour, medication is not necessarily indicated.

The child who has moderate to severe ADHD may benefit from medication and methylphenidate or dexamphetamine are the first line of treatment. The approach is to start with a low dose of the immediate release formulation, and titrate the dose slowly until effect is obtained. Change to the extended release preparation after the trial period. This avoids the need to use medication during the school day.

A clinical approach example

With methylphenidate (MPH), start at about 0.25–0.5 mg/kg, depending on the child's age and increase up to 0.9 mg/kg if necessary. The first dose is given around breakfast at about 7.30 am (to be working well on arrival at school), the second dose at mid-morning recess (to be effective in the later part of the school morning and in the playground), and a third dose given on arriving home (to assist with homework). If medication is only given just before leaving home, there may be symptoms at home before the medication has taken effect, compromising the start of the day. The first dose may wear off for the last hour of the class (when all are tired) and may not work in the playground where processing behaviour and self-regulation demands are considerable. The second dose given at the beginning of lunch begins to work when returning to the class.

The dose is increased from two doses to three doses a day, with observation of effect of when individual doses wear off, noting that the initial doses may be too low or infrequent to be effective. This is titrated over about a week, then add two or three doses, whichever is most effective, increasing the doses over the next week or so to gain optimum benefit with the least adverse effects if they occur.

Close contact with the paediatrician is important, particularly if there are symptoms that are of concern. It is invaluable to have the teacher's observations on the relative effectiveness of different dosages and timing. The duration of action depends on the individual child's metabolism, in that some report a shorter response time, which supports the notion of titrating the dose in the individual child.

After the trial period establishes an optimum dose for immediate release preparation, with best response and no significant side effects, the medication can be compared with the sustained release preparation in the most effective dose. Ritalin® LA releases more of the dose immediately than Concerta® that tends to last longer. The specific extended-release preparation needs to be chosen depending on the individual's needs and responses.

Practice Point

The dose response is different for each individual in that some children have a good response on low doses while others need higher doses. This might relate to differences in drug metabolism and some evidence suggests that genetic influences may play a role in response to medication.[58,59]

The MTA titration trial found that the best dose distribution across all subjects for MPH was 10–50 mg/day.[60] They established a total daily dose limit of 35 mg for children weighing less than 25 kg and a full range of doses up to 60 mg/day. Clinical practice shows that the doses used in the MTA trial are somewhat conservative and may result in medication considered to be ineffective, where possibly a higher dose could produce improvement in attention and behaviour, particularly in combined ADHD.

Many experienced clinicians find that higher doses of medication are needed to achieve effect. Dose titration is important while noting that in some children higher doses lead to more side-effects, while others tolerate high doses well. Anecdotally, in some children with more severe ADHD symptoms, higher doses may be needed to reach optimal effect. In New South Wales the figures on naturalistic prescribing show that the dose is generally prescribed up to 1 mg/kg/day.

Importantly, in some children higher doses do not benefit learning and may lead to the occurrence of side-effects. One study reported decline in learning and increasing tachycardia at higher doses around 1 mg/kg.[61] Therefore it is important to monitor the child's response and review the child's learning profile while on treatment. Teacher reports are valuable and academic testing on treatment may be needed in some circumstances.

Many teachers or schools are reluctant to give medication at school. This is only necessary during the trial period when the immediate release medication is used. After the trial period the child can be placed on the extended release preparation, which requires a morning dose only. Alternatively, during the trial on immediate release the medication can be given in the morning and after school. This means that there will be a difference between the morning and after lunch behaviour during the school day, which can inform effectiveness during the trial period.

Ongoing management

Regular follow-up is important for optimal management. Obtain reports:
- From teachers and other educators to provide information about the child's school progress.
- From allied health professionals that provide intervention.
- From parents about the child's behaviour, approach to schoolwork, demeanor and social interactions.

Remain aware of comorbidities as children with ADHD may have anxiety, learning disorders and/or behaviour disorders, and all these areas need to be addressed in ongoing management.

If the child is on medication, monitor any side-effects:
- Determine the side-effects from the parent's and the child's point of view.

- Some side-effects are minimal, transient and tolerable, for example appetite suppression and mild irritability. Often these side-effects abate with change to the extended release preparations.

Physical examination should include height and weight profile, being aware of any weight loss. Check the heart and blood pressure (BP) on each occasion. Sometimes tachycardia and even slight increase in BP may occur with stimulants. Significant change in heart rate and BP might require reduction in dose or change of medication. If any cardiac symptoms occur, such as palpitations, dizziness or other, while on stimulant medication best practice is to refer to a cardiologist.

While on medication:
- The dose may need to increase as the child grows and gains weight, but aim to stay within the recommended dose range. Children with a larger build may need higher doses, therefore dose titration is important.
- For the child on extended preparation, e.g. Ritalin® LA, there might be the need for a top-up dose of immediate release Ritalin® 5–10 mg in the afternoon, as the LA medication generally lasts for the school-day hours and wears off in the afternoon. The top-up dose reduces the chance of 'rebound' difficult behaviour when the dose wears off after school
- Balance the extent of the side-effects with the positive effect on the child's behaviour and learning.
- Weight loss and lack of sleep as a result of the medication should not be tolerated.
- If side-effects occur, the first step would be to reduce the dose, but if they persist it may be necessary to stop that particular medication and try an alternative. It is worth noting that medication can produce intolerable side-effects in some children and should be ceased.

Sometimes a change of medication is needed, as one medication might work better for that individual child than another. For example, where Ritalin® results in side-effects of appetite suppression the child might tolerate Concerta®, and vice versa. Sometimes the change needs to be from the stimulant to the non-stimulant medication, such as atomoxetine (Strattera®). The reader is encouraged to read the Guidelines on ADHD management.

Bear in mind that the management of ADHD is a long-term relationship with the child and family. The child's learning, emotional and social needs will change over time. Paediatricians who treat children have longstanding relationships with their patients. It is good practice to involve the child early in the process to foster a positive relationship so that they feel comfortable about reporting their concerns directly to the doctor during the management process. There might come a time when the child–adolescent wants to stop treatment and open

Practice Point

It is helpful to parents and to the management of the child that the doctor is available for parents to contact if they have concerns, both while the child is on the trial and during ongoing treatment with medication. It is easier to address concerns immediately, rather than have the family wait until the next follow-up medical appointment. Parents find that a contact phone number is both helpful and reassuring.

discussion should be encouraged. Sometimes short breaks off treatment result in the student requesting that the medication be resumed, and this allows the patient to feel involved in management. Long-term management requires tailoring the dosage and schedule to meet the individual's needs.[62]

THE ADOLESCENT PATIENT

Adolescence is a period of individualisation, increasing self-awareness and questioning of the 'status quo'. Therefore it is not surprising that the adolescent patient might question their treatment and the need for taking medication. If the doctor has established a relationship with the adolescent at a younger age, they are more likely to cooperate in discussion about their treatment. It is important to respect the adolescent's views and concerns about medication.

An adolescent might request that their medication be stopped or might even refuse to take medication. It is helpful to discuss this in a positive manner. The patient can be given a trial off medication so that they can see their response in terms of learning and behaviour off treatment. It is not unusual for the patient to request to go back on treatment after a break of a month or so, as they might find a decline in their concentration and ability to complete work at school off medication. The patient who feels that they are listened to and respected is more likely to cooperate with medical opinion and return to using medication, particularly if they can see that there has been some value in using the treatment.

Alternatively, as students develop and brain pathways mature, an improvement in their reasoning ability and focus in relation to their schoolwork may occur. This is more likely to be the case in the milder forms of ADHD. In this instance, it is appropriate that the medication be ceased anyway. This gives the doctor and the family an opportunity to see how the patient progresses off medication.

It is important to note that the apparent reduction in the prevalence of ADHD in young adults may be related a decline in the hyperactive–impulsive symptoms while the symptoms of inattention and disorganisation persist. This might account for an underestimation of persistence of the condition in young adults.[63]

An observation by many clinicians is that often adolescents and young adults require lower doses than they needed in prior years. This might relate to them developing strategies for dealing with their condition, thereby requiring less medication, and there could be a contributory neuromaturational effect.

Medication management

In terms of dosage it may be necessary to increase the dose of medication as the adolescent grows and gains weight. However, in some adolescent individuals mood change may occur on the background of mood changes related to hormonal effects of puberty. Sometimes decreasing the dose of the medication when mood change becomes evident is appropriate to determine if this symptom improves. If mood change persists it may be necessary to cease the medication or try an alternative.

If medication is ceased at one point in time because of mood change, it is sometimes possible to resume treatment at a later point in time, e.g. when the individual reaches major examinations and is having difficulty with focus and task application. In this instance, resuming a lower dose of the medication, which helps the individual's focus and memory without the side-effect of mood change, is prudent. An observation by many clinicians is that often adolescents and young adults require lower doses than they needed in prior years. This might relate to them developing strategies for dealing with their condition, thereby requiring less medication, and there could be a contributory neuromaturational effect.

TRANSITION TO ADULTHOOD

The adolescent should be given the opportunity to graduate to psychiatric care for ongoing management of ADHD into young adulthood. In Australia, adult ADHD patients are managed by psychiatrists. Paediatricians who have managed ADHD children may look after them until they reach 25 years of age. However the choice as to when to graduate to psychiatric care rests with the patient, and some may choose to do so earlier rather than later.

It is helpful to involve a psychiatrist during this transition period while the paediatrician is still involved, so that the patient can establish a relationship with the psychiatrist. In this way the paediatrician and psychiatrist can work together on medication and behaviour management, until the patient is ready for the psychiatrist to take over ongoing care into adulthood.

Adults with ADHD find support groups, conference workshops, group programs by psychologists and individual counselling with life coaching to be extremely beneficial as they live with and come to better understand their condition.

In many instances individuals with ADHD find that they can come off medication once they leave school, particularly if they are doing a job or career that utilises their strengths and interests. ADHD patients who feel motivated often find that they are able to cope within the work environment. However many individuals continue to experience symptoms of ADHD, such as short-term memory difficulty, concentration over long periods and problems with organisation skills. Some individuals report that the early behaviour intervention during their paediatric years has skilled them with strategies for dealing with these difficulties as adults.

Many patients who have had ADHD in childhood, particularly at the moderate to severe end of the spectrum, will continue to need medication management into adulthood. It is important to remain aware of the effect of ADHD on driving skills in those young adults where symptoms persist. It is recommended that these individuals continue to take their medication when driving and also when operating machinery of any kind. The reader is directed to the Guidelines for more about driving and ADHD.

Practice Point

Young adults who continue study through college or university may find that they need the medication for lectures and/or study. These students often prefer flexibility in the use of medication and may not need to use the treatment daily, as they did during school years.

Instead, they might choose to use treatment for study or for certain lectures only. In practice this seems to work well for many patients, particularly those who have the predominantly inattentive sub-type of ADHD. Some individuals find that the immediate release medications work well in these situations, but others prefer the slower onset of the extended release formulations. The young adult is very much part of the management process and is given choice about the best way to manage their symptoms.

NATURAL HISTORY AND OUTCOME

ADHD is a common condition in childhood, and research has shown that symptoms can persist into adulthood in the majority of cases. An analysis of the data from 32 follow-up studies of ADHD showed that about 15 per cent of individuals diagnosed with ADHD as children had persisting symptoms at 25 years of age, and meta-analysis showed 'partial remission' with some symptoms persisting in up to 65 per cent of patients at age 25 years.[64]

The MTA study results at eight years, a prospective follow-up of children with combined-type ADHD, showed that despite initial symptom improvement during the treatment period children with combined type continued to have significant impairment in adolescence. This work also suggested that behavioural intervention and socio-demographic advantage provided the best long-term prognosis for children with combined-type ADHD.[65] Whether the dosage used or the treatment time frame in this study was a factor in determining long-term outcome is not clear, especially as many clinicians find that higher doses are often needed in practice than those used in the MTA trial. However, what is clear is that other intervention strategies are important and that medication alone is unlikely to produce optimal outcome.

Some adults report ongoing symptoms, such as short-term memory and organisation problems, but they also report having developed strategies to help them cope with their symptoms. Consequently these patients are not on medication in adulthood.

It is worth noting that individuals with ADHD are often very creative and have the ability to put their mind to many interests. The challenge for them is to see the tasks to completion and to be focused in their application of their creative talents. Those adults who continue to have significant symptoms that impair their daily functioning, their social interaction and their family life are likely to require ongoing medical management. These individuals need ongoing support with psychologists and counsellors for behaviour strategies and stress management, and may also require medical management by psychiatrists.

It appears that genetic influences play a part in persistence of the symptoms of ADHD.[66] Psychosocial supports also play a significant role in long-term outcomes for these individuals.

REFERENCES

1. Graetz BW, Sawyer MG, Hazell PL, et al. Validity of DSM-IV ADHD subtypes in a nationally representative sample of Australian children and adolescents. J Am Acad Child Adoles Psychiatry 2001;40(12):1410–17
2. Faraone SV, Sergeant J, Gillberg C, Biederman J. The worldwide prevalence of ADHD: is it an American condition? World Psychiatry 2003;2(2):104–13
3. Skounti M, Philalithis A, Galanakis E. Variations in prevalence of attention deficit hyperactivity disorder worldwide. European Journal of Pediatrics 2007;166(2):117–23
4. Thapar A, Cooper M, Jefferies R, Stergiakouli E. What causes attention deficit hyperactivity disorder? Archives of Disease in Childhood 2011. Online. DOI: 10.1136/archdischild-2011-300482
5. Levy F, Hay DA. Attention, genes and ADHD. Hove: Brunner Routledge; 2001
6. Albayrak O, et al. Genetic aspects in attention-deficit–hyperactivity disorder. J Neural Transm 2008;115(2):305–15
7. Faraone SV, Perlis RH, Doyle AE, et al. Molecular genetics of attention deficit–hyperactivity disorder. Biol Psychiatry 2005;57(11):1313–23

8 Tripp G, Wickens JR. Neurobiology of ADHD. Neuropharmacology 2009;57:579–89
9 Mick E, Faraone SV. Genetics of attention deficit hyperactivity disorder. Child and Adoles Psychiatr Clinics North Am 2008;17(2):261–84, vii–viii
10 Goldstein S. Current Literature in ADHD. Journal of Attention Disorders 2011;15:176–8
11 Williams NM, Zaharieva I, Martin A, et al. Rare chromosomal deletions and duplications in attention-deficit hyperactivity disorder: a genome-wide analysis. Lancet 2010;376:1401–8
12 National Health and Medical Research Council (NHMRC) Draft Guidelines on Attention Deficit Hyperactivity Disorder (ADHD). Royal Australasian College of Physicians. Draft June 2009. Online. Available: http://www.nhmrc.gov.au/publications/synopses/adhd_draft.htm; 1 Mar 2012
13 Ball SW, Gilman SE, Mick E, et al. Revisiting the association between maternal smoking during pregnancy and ADHD. Journal of Psychiatric Research 2010;1–5. DOI:10.1016/j.jpsychires.2010.03.009
14 Talge NM, Neal C, Glover V. Antenatal maternal stress and long-term effects on child neurodevelopment: how and why? J Child Psychol Psychiatry 2007;48(3–4):245–61
15 Catroppa C, Anderson V. Children's attentional skills 2 years post-traumatic brain injury. Dev Neuropsychol 2003;23(3):359–73
16 Bateman B, Warner JO, Hutchinson E, et al. The effects of a double blind, placebo controlled, artificial food colourings and benzoate preservative challenge on hyperactivity in a general population sample of preschool children. Arch Dis Child 2004;89(6):506–11
17 Biederman J, Milberger S, Faraone SV, et al. Impact of adversity on functioning and comorbidity in children with attention-deficit hyperactivity disorder. J Am Acad Child Adolesc Psychiatry 1995;34(11):1495–503
18 Groom A, Elliott HR, Embleton ND, Relton CL. Epigenetics and child health: basic principles. Archives of Disease in Childhood 2011;96:863–9
19 Giedd JN, Blumenthal J, Jeffries N, et al. Brain development during childhood and adolescence: a longitudinal MRI study. Nature Neuroscience 1999;2(10):861–3
20 Wozniak JR, Lim KO. Advances in white matter imaging: a review of in vivo magnetic resonance methodologies and their applicability to the study of development and aging. Neuroscience and Biobehavioral Reviews 2006;30:762–74
21 Castellanos FX, Lee PP, Sharp W, Jeffries NO, et al. Developmental trajectories of brain volume abnormalities in children and adolescents with attention deficit–hyperactivity disorder. Journal of American Medical Association 2002;288:1740–8
22 Krain AL, Castellanos FX. Brain development and ADHD. Clinical Psychology Review 2006;26:433–44
23 Dickstein SG, Bannon K, Castellanos FX, Milham MP. The neural correlates of attention deficit hyperactivity disorder: an ALE meta-analysis. Journal of Child Psychology and Psychiatry 2006;47:1051–62
24 Valera EM, Faraone SV, Murray KE, Seidman LJ. Meta-analysis of structural imaging findings in attention-deficit–hyperactivity disorder. Biol Psychiatry 2007;61:1361–9
25 Shaw P, Eckstrand K, Sharp W, et al. Attention-deficit–hyperactivity disorder is characterized by a delay in cortical maturation. PNAS (Proceedings of the National Academy of Sciences, USA) 2007;104:19649–54
26 Rubia K. Neuro-anatomic evidence for the maturational delay hypothesis of ADHD. PNAS 2007;104:19663–4
27 McAlonan GM, Cheung V, Chua SE, et al. Age-related grey matter volume correlates of response inhibition and shifting in attention-deficit hyperactivity disorder. British Journal of Psychiatry 2009;194:123–9
28 Brown TE. ADD/ADHD and impaired executive function in clinical practice. Current Psychiatry Reports 2008;10:407–11
29 Barkley RA. Behavioral inhibition, sustained attention and executive functions: constructing a unifying theory of ADHD. Psychological Bulletin 1997;121:64–94
30 Willcutt EG, Doyle AE, Nigg JT, Faraone SV, Pennington BF. Validity of the executive function theory of attention deficit–hyperactivity disorder: A meta-analytic review. Biol Psychiatry 2005;57:1336–46

31 Castellanos FX, Sonuga-Barke EJS, Milham MP, Tannock R. Characterizing cognition in ADHD: beyond executive dysfunction. Trends in Cognitive Sciences 2006;10(3):117–23. DOI:10.1016/j.tics.2006.01.011
32 Alloway TP. Working memory, but not IQ, predicts subsequent learning in children with learning difficulties. European Journal of Psychological Assessment 2009;25: 92–8
33 Alloway TP, Rajendran G, Archibald LMD. Working memory in children with developmental disorders. Journal of Learning Disabilities 2009;42:372–82
34 Efron D, Sciberras E. The diagnostic outcomes of children with suspected attention deficit hyperactivity disorder following multidisciplinary assessment. J Paed Child Health 2010;46:392–7
35 Willcutt EG, Pennington BF, Duncan L, Smith SD, et al. Understanding the complex etiologies of developmental disorders: Behavioral and molecular genetic approaches. J Dev Behav Pediatrics 2010;31:533–44
36 Mayes SD, Calhoun SL, Mayes RD, Molitoris S. Autism and ADHD: Overlapping and discriminating symptoms. Research in Autism Spectrum Disorders (2011) in press. DOI:10.1016/j.rasd.2011.05.009
37 Connor DF, Steeber J, McBurnett K. A review of attention-deficit–hyperactivity disorder complicated by symptoms of oppositional defiant disorder or conduct disorder. J Dev Behav Pediatric 2010;31:427–40
38 Barkley RA, Murphy KR. Comorbid psychiatric disorders in adults with ADHD. The ADHD Report 2007;15:1–7
39 Vloet TD, Konrad K, et al. Impact of anxiety disorders on attentional functions in children with ADHD. Journal of Affective Disorders 2010;124:283–90
40 Sorensen L, Plessen KJ, Nicholas J, Lundervold AJ. Is behavioral regulation in children with ADHD aggravated by comorbid anxiety disorder? Journal of Attention Disorders 2011;15:56–66
41 Mayes SD, Calhoun SL. Learning, attention, writing, and processing speed in typical children and children with ADHD, autism, anxiety, depression and oppositional defiant disorder. Child Neuropsychology 2007;13:469–93
42 Cardy JE, Tannock R, et al. The contribution of processing impairments to SLI: Insights from attention-deficit–hyperactivity disorder. Journal Communication Disorders 2010;43:77–91
43 Bush G. Neuroimaging of attention deficit hyperactivity disorder: Can new imaging findings be integrated in clinical practice? Child and Adolescent Psychiatric Clinics of North America 2008;17:385–404
44 Paloyelis Y, Mehta MA, Kuntsi J, Asherson P. Functional MRI in ADHD: a systematic literature review. Expert Review of Neurotherapeutics 2007;20:1337
45 Zametkin A, Schroth E, Faden D. The role of brain imaging in the diagnosis and management of ADHD. The ADHD Report 2005;13:11–14
46 Efron D, Sciberras E, Hassell P. Are schools meeting the needs of students with ADHD? Australasian Journal of Special Education 2008;32:187–98
47 Klingberg T. Training and plasticity of working memory. Trends in Cognitive Sciences 2010;14:317–24
48 McBurnett K, Weiss N. New drug treatments for ADHD. Psychiatric Annals 2011;41:16–21
49 Faraone SV, Biederman J, Morley CP, Spencer TJ. Effect of stimulants on height and weight: a review of the literature. Journal Am Acad Child Adolescent Psychiatry 2008;47:994–1009
50 Schelleman H, Bilker WB, Strom BL, et al. Cardiovascular events and death in children exposed and unexposed to ADHD agents. Pediatrics 2011;127:1102–10
51 Greenhill L. The science of stimulant abuse. Pediatric Annals 2006;35:553–6
52 Williams RJ, Goodale LA, Shay-Fiddler MA, et al. Methyphenidate and Dextroamphetamine abuse in substance-abusing adolescents. American Journal on Addictions 2004;13:381–9
53 Wilens TE, Faraone SV, Biederman J, Gunawardene S. Does stimulant therapy of attention-deficit–hyperactivity disorder beget later substance abuse? A meta-analytic review of the literature. Pediatrics 2003;111:179–85

54 Volkow ND, Swanson JM. Does childhood treatment of ADHD with stimulant medication affect substance abuse in adulthood? (editorial). Am J Psychiatry 2008;165:553–5
55 Vetter LV, Elia J, Erickson C, Berger S, et al. Cardiovascular monitoring of children and adolescents with heart disease receiving medications for attention deficit–hyperactivity disorder: a Scientific Statement from the American Heart Association Council on Cardiovascular Disease in the Young Congenital Cardiac Defects Committee and the Council on Cardiovascular Nursing. Circulation 2008;117:2407–23
56 Attention Deficit Hyperactivity Disorder in children and adolescents in NSW: Final report of the Special Review. Clinical Excellence Commission, 2007. Online. Available: http://www.health.nsw.gov.au/pubs/2008/adhd_report.html; 1 Mar 2012
57 Posey WM, Bassin SA, Lewis A. Preschool ADHD and medication: More study needed? (report). Journal of Early Childhood and Infant Psychology Annual 2009:57
58 Levy F. Dopamine and noradrenaline theories of ADHD and drug response. The ADHD Report 2009;17:9–16
59 Levy F. Dopamine vs noradrenaline: inverted-U effects and ADHD theories. Australian and New Zealand Journal of Psychiatry 2009;43:101–8
60 Greenhill L, Swanson J, Vitiello B, et al. Impairment and deportment responses to different methyphenidate doses in children with ADHD: The MTA Titration Trial. J Am Acad Child Adolesc Psychiatry 2001;40(2):180–7
61 Sprague RL, Sleator EK. Methylphenidate in hyperkinetic children: differences in dose effects on learning and social behavior. Science 1977;198:1274–6
62 Powell SG, Thomsen PH, Frydenberg M, Rasmussen H. Long-term treatment of ADHD with stimulants: a large observational study of real-life patients. Journal of Attention Disorders 2011;15:439–51
63 Hazell P. Pharmacological management of attention deficit hyperactivity disorder in adolescents: special considerations. CNS drugs 2007;21(1):37–46
64 Faraone SV, Biederman J, Mick E. The age-dependent decline of attention deficit hyperactivity disorder: a meta-analysis of follow-up studies. Psychological Medicine 2006;36(2):159–65
65 Molina B, Hinshaw SP, Swanson JM, Arnold LE, et al. MTA at 8 years: prospective follow-up of children treated for combined-type ADHD in a multisite study. J Am Acad Child Adolesc. Psychiatry 2009;48:484–500
66 Larsson JO, Larsson H, Lichtenstein P. Genetic and environmental contributions to stability and change of ADHD symptoms between 8 and 13 years of age: a longitudinal twin study. J Am Acad Child Adolesc Psychiatry 2004;43(10):1267–75

FURTHER READING

ADHD management today. Arch Dis Child Feb 2005;90(supp. 1)
Barkley RA. Take Charge of ADHD. Dingley, Victoria: Hinkler Books; 2005
Guevara J, Stein M. Evidence-based management of attention deficit hyperactivity disorder. BMJ 2001;323:1232–5
Royal Australasian College of Physicians. Draft Guidelines on Attention Deficit Hyperactivity Disorder (ADHD). 2009. Currently under review with the development of Clinical Practice Points based on this document. Online. Available: http://www.nhmrc.gov.au/guidelines/publications/ch54; 2 Mar 2012
Pelham WE, Fabiano GA, Massetti GM. Evidence-based assessment of attention deficit hyperactivity disorder in children and adolescents. J Clin Child Adolesc Psychol 2005;34(3):449–76
Curatolo P, Paloscia C, D'Agati E, et al. The neurobiology of attention deficit–hyperactivity disorder (review). European Journal of Paediaitric Neurology 2009;13:299–304
Seidman LJ. Neuropsychological functioning in people with ADHD across the lifespan. Clinical Psychology Review 2006;26:466–85
Taylor E. Syndromes of overactivity and attention deficit, ch 26. In: Rutter M, Hersov L. Child and Adolescent Psychiatry, 2nd ed. Oxford: Blackwell Scientific; 1990

RESOURCES

These websites available 1 March 2012.
Fact sheet on ADHD for parents: http://www.rch.org.au
Understanding ADHD: http://www.adhd.org.au
General information about ADHD: http://www.cheri.com.au/index.html
ADHD guidelines: http://www.nhmrc.gov.au/publications/synopses/adhd_draft.htm
Website for professionals, especially teachers, and parents: http://physicalasanything.com.au/
Information for parents about children and adults with ADHD: http://www.chadd.org
Living with ADHD: http://www.livingwithADHD.com.au
Fitness to drive for adolescents: See http://www.austroads.com.au/aftd/hp.html
Support through Relationships Australia: http://www.relationships.com.au/resources
UK information for parents and professionals: http://www.addiss.co.uk/
Information on developmental and other medical conditions: NSW Government Education, Communities and Children's Hospital Westmead website: http://www.physicalasanything.com.au
Putting evidence into practice to reach and teach ADHD: CHERI Conference, 2007: http://www.cheri.com.au/PuttingEvidenceintoPracticetoReachTeachADHD.htm
TEACHADHD home page: http://research.aboutkidshealth.ca/teachadhd
Collaborative management: http://www.wraparoundkids.com/index.htm
Working Memory: http://www.cogmed.com/

9 Behaviour difficulties

Sandra Johnson

INTRODUCTION

Paediatricians, whether they are working in child development or general paediatrics, often encounter children who present with behaviour difficulties for a multitude of reasons. The challenge for the doctor is to determine the underlying cause and extent of this sometimes-troubling presentation.

Many general paediatricians report that this problem is not uncommon in their practices and is a concern for parents, carers and the referring professionals. The referral might come from the general practitioner because the parents have presented the child to the doctor or it might come from other professionals, like teachers and therapists, who are concerned about the child's behaviour.

Irrespective of the referral pathway, behaviour difficulty in childhood needs careful attention because its presence usually means that the child, the parents or both are in distress. Alternatively, the parent may be responding to concerns expressed by the school.

DEFINITIONS

Behaviour difficulty in childhood is not a clearly defined entity, and there are many patterns of behaviour that could be perceived as a problem by parents, carers and other adults who work with or relate to children. DSM IV-TR and V include diagnostic criteria for a number of behaviours like anxiety, mood, sleep, eating, impulse control and other disorders, but these criteria refer to the severe end of the 'spectrum' for behaviour difficulty and usually the term 'disorder' is applied here.

Many problems that are of concern to parents relate to misunderstanding of normal stages of development, e.g. the demands that the young toddler who needs close supervision makes on parents, or the defiance of the young adolescent trying to assert their will over that of their parents. Many parents manage these problems as they arise and often 'move through' the difficult period without needing to consult a professional. However others do consult professional support because raising children can be hard and challenging for busy parents who want the best for their children and who may have other demands on their time. Also they may have had little experience of children prior to becoming parents.

For the purposes of this chapter, behaviour difficulty refers to any behaviour that parents find difficult, demanding, cannot manage, are overwhelmed by or that they are concerned about. The aim is to provide an individual-, family- and child-centred approach rather than a medical diagnostic one, which generally deals with distinct symptoms and characteristics of a disorder.

PREVALENCE

Research to determine prevalence is immediately met with the problem of defining what we consider to be a problem in the child's behaviour. Notwithstanding, limited research has been done to determine prevalence within certain populations.

Cullen at al. in Western Australia looked at the prevalence of behaviour disorders in children of 1000 families. The behaviours examined included fears, withdrawal, negativism, aggression, school difficulties, habits and problems related to feeding, elimination, sleep and antisocial behaviour (stealing, lying and running away from home or school). The results showed that boys experienced more defiance, destructiveness, dislike of school, reading problems, head-banging and problems with antisocial behaviour, while girls showed more lethargy, thumb-sucking and habit disorders. The number of children with behaviour disorders reached a peak at six years old for boys and seven years old for girls, and remained fairly steady until after 12 years old for boys and 14 years old for girls.[1]

Prevalence of behaviour problems has also been examined in low birth weight (LBW) infants. In the United Kingdom a case-controlled study of 233 LBW infants examined at eight to nine years of age showed a higher prevalence of behaviour disorders in this group.[2] Although further work needs to be done to replicate results, it means that LBW infants warrant careful follow-up as they move into school years. LBW infants may also have other risk factors, such as poor maternal nutrition, maternal smoking and socioeconomic disadvantage.

In a special report on child mental health in the United States, the authors grapple with the difficulty of estimating prevalence, given the lack of standard definitions.[3]

Recent work done by the Australian Paediatric Research Network (APRN), yet to be published, showed that one in two children seen in paediatric outpatient clinics have a developmental–behavioural component to their presentation. This is a growing area of demand for services in the community and consequently it is essential that paediatricians and other doctors who work with children have a clinical approach to the problem.

Practice Point

It will be clear to the reader that there are a vast number of behaviours that are of concern to parents, that are difficult to define and where research results cannot easily be replicated, particularly when parental perception is the key variable that is being measured. Importantly, however, if it is a problem for the parents, it is a problem for the paediatrician.

CLASSIFICATION

Similar issues arise in relation to the classification of behaviour disorders. As mentioned, DSM criteria deal with the severe end of behaviour problems, yet not all problems are so clearly defined. The Child Behaviour Checklist (CBCL) was examined in a multi-centre study in Melbourne to determine the applicability of CBCL scores to an Australian population, and found that this is a useful tool for assessing childhood behaviour disorders in this population.[4]

In the United States, the Substance Abuse and Mental Health Services Administration (SAMHSA) adopted the term 'serious emotional disturbance' to identify children who have significant emotional and behaviour problems. The term refers to:

> *persons from birth to age 18 who currently or at any time during the past year had a diagnosable mental, behavioral, or emotional disorder of sufficient duration to meet diagnostic criteria specified within the DSM-III-R and that resulted in functional impairment … in family, school or community activities … it is a legal term that triggers a host of mandated services to meet the needs of these children.*[3]

Individuals with behaviour difficulties suffer significant morbidity in daily function and social adjustment, and these individuals often require long-term support and intervention.

Irrespective of classifications, the clinician is required to assess and support the family of the child who presents with behaviour difficulty, and this chapter aims to provide a practical approach.

PRACTICAL CLINICAL APPROACH

The paediatrician faced with helping families and children, where behaviour difficulty is the presenting problem, finds that the 'art' rather than the 'science' of medicine comes into play.

All clinicians are trained to gather information in a systematic manner to gain an overview of the presenting difficulties so that the problems can be addressed. This clinical skill should not be underestimated, especially if the underlying approach is one of taking the time to listen to parental concerns, to be objective, to take all factors into account, to collate the information, and then to provide a child- and family-centred framework for dealing with the difficulties. A published paper by an experienced paediatrician is available to guide clinicians on this path.[5]

History

Obtain the history from parents, teachers and other adults familiar to or working with the child. Questionnaires can be helpful (e.g. Child Behaviour Checklist (CBCL))[6] which has good cross-cultural generalisability, and the Strengths and Difficulties Questionnaire (SDQ)[7] which is a screening tool for behaviours of 3–16-year-old children (see http://www.sdqinfo.org/).

Take a history of the particular troublesome behaviour. The 'ABC' approach is a standard way of finding out the circumstances in which the behaviour occurs (see Table 9.1).

There may be several behaviours in one child that are of concern. Parents can be encouraged to rate the behaviours so that the most troublesome can be addressed initially and others dealt with later. Also, rating the behaviour allows the parent to discover that some behaviours are in fact minor and less troublesome than first thought. Attention can then be given to the worrying behaviours. With more difficult behaviour problems that are intractable, the opposite order is recommended. Begin with the do-able and the tractable, then move towards the more difficult.

TABLE 9.1	History of the behaviour
Antecedent (A)	What events precede the behaviour? Is there a pattern to the behaviour – time of day, level of tiredness, etc? Are there any events or circumstances in the environment that predispose to the behaviour episode?
Behaviour (B)	Describe the behaviour? Who is around when it occurs? When is it most likely to occur? Where does it occur? How does the parent react while the behaviour is occurring?
Consequences (C)	What happens as a result of the behaviour? What is the parent's immediate response? What is the usual outcome, e.g. does the parent 'give in' to the child? Does the child learn about consequences and is there age-appropriate reprimand, e.g. removal of privileges, time out?

Practice Point

When taking the history, the following points should be considered:
1. The clinician needs to decide if the problem is sufficiently severe to seek the involvement of specialist professionals.
2. A core task is to try and understand why the problems are appearing or being brought to the attention of the paediatrician at this point in time.
3. In relation to (2), it is important to remember that the same problem can arise for different reasons and that different problems can arise from the same underlying reason.

The child's point of view

It is important to find out how the child sees the problem. Time spent talking with the child alone can be very valuable and can give the doctor insights that are not at first evident. The self-report form of the SDQ may be helpful here.

The age and developmental ability of the child is very relevant. The young toddler who is willful, active and difficult for parents to manage is a very different presentation to the young teenager with similar symptoms. The history that is taken by the doctor will also place different emphasis on the symptom depending on the age of the child. For example, in the former there is a need to clarify for parents what normal behaviour is for toddlers, where typically children are active and demanding, while the doctor remains sensitive to parental perception of the problem. The child who has delayed development and who is therefore immature socially might present with behaviours long after the age where these are considered typical.

The child presenting with behaviour problems may do so due to specific or general learning difficulties, for instance subtle language problems (therefore they do not always understand what is being said), or dyspraxia (where they are excluded from sports or find writing difficult and frustrating due to motor problems). It is important to exclude these factors, and specialist assessment may be necessary. (See Chapter 6 Specific learning disorders and Chapter 7 Language disorders.)

The child's temperament will affect how that child responds and reacts in different situations. It helps to obtain an impression of the child's early temperament as an infant, if possible, in order to understand the fit between the parents' expectations and the child's temperamental leanings – the so called 'goodness of fit'.[8] Personality traits and temperament influence how individuals think, behave and feel, and is discussed in a chapter by Caspi and Shiner.[9]

The child's medical condition might lead to irritability due to pain, immobility, medication effects and symptoms related to the illness, and any of these factors understandably can result in negative behaviours. It is important to ask if there is a history of head injury, as there can be long-term effects, which may emerge slowly after a number of years.

The position of the child within the family is relevant. The eldest male child within certain cultures is regarded as special. He may be allowed to 'get away with' unacceptable behaviour. The youngest child, who is somewhat indulged and regarded as cute, could also be given an unfair advantage within a family unit.

Attachments also influence behaviour. The relationship that the child has with the parent or carer will impact on behaviour, and is worth considering when assessing difficulties.[10] This is particularly relevant in situations of emotional abuse.[11]

Other factors in the child's environment may dominate the clinical presentation. Poverty and lack of resources within the family and/or the community; attitudes of adults towards children in general; respect for children within the family unit; neglect and abuse (physical, emotional, sexual); the child's experiences at home (e.g. marital difficulties and/or domestic violence); and at school (e.g. playground bullying): all have a powerful impact on behaviour.

Boundaries and expectations of behaviour set at home and cultural expectations of children are important, e.g. some cultures do not believe in letting a child cry.

Early communication with children is significant, as shown in an Australian study where mothers with clinical depression and life difficulties reported significantly more behaviour problems in their children. This work also found that the child's temperament affected communication within the mother–child interaction.[12]

In situations where the behaviour is entrenched, time and resources are needed, e.g. visits to the family home by a team member in order to assess the behaviour within the home environment is often very valuable.

Examination

Physical examination should place emphasis on health concerns that may accompany the behaviour in order to exclude a physical cause, e.g. ear problems, irritating skin rash, headaches.

Vision and hearing difficulty must be excluded, as undetected problems may present with behaviour difficulty.

Physical examination must be mindful of physical manifestations of inflicted injury. Also see Chapter 14 Child abuse and neglect.

The interaction with the child gives an enormous amount of information:
- The child who is distant and who shows little emotion
- The child who inappropriately climbs on the doctor's lap with little display of personal boundary
- The child who is overtly angry, either directed to the parents or the doctor during the session
- The child who is passive and appears fearful
- The child who is disrespectful and who ignores adult conversation.

There are several behaviours that may be observed during the doctor–patient interaction and each should be carefully noted.

Examination also includes impressions gained about the child's development:
- Receptive and expressive language
- Sense of empathy and mindfulness to the needs of others
- General knowledge about issues, relevant to the child's age
- Child can be given learning tasks to determine approach to schoolwork
- Assessment of the child's cognitive ability, language, social skills, emotional skills and educational progress is important – this component of the assessment can be done by the psychologist on the team or can be obtained by collateral history, i.e. from school or other community organisations.

Consider important causes of difficult behaviour

1. Exclude medical reasons for difficult behaviour:
   - Illness and pain – might cause irritability and non-compliance
   - Side-effects of medication – might cause difficult behaviour
   - Sleep disorders – sleep apnoea or sleep disturbance can lead to tiredness and irritability during the daytime and result in difficult behaviour
   - Vision and hearing problems
   - Any signs of central nervous system pathology must be noted:
     - sub-clinical or missed seizures – may result in irritability, unusual or worsening behaviour
     - neurodegenerative disease may be associated with decline in behaviour
     - brain tumour
     - traumatic brain injury – behaviour, learning and attention difficulties may occur secondary to brain injury[13–15]
     - severe traumatic brain injury is often associated with behaviour problems and might not be due to the organic injury alone, but environmental factors (such as poor family functioning, lower socioeconomic status and lack of family resources) can also play a role.[16,17]
2. Other factors to consider as causes for difficult behaviour:
   - Adverse environment – child abuse (physical, emotional, sexual)
   - Special circumstances that may be contributing and where careful consideration of all the factors is needed:
     - Indigenous communities
     - Social disadvantage
     - Family displacement – refugees, migrant families, families displaced for other reasons.

MANAGEMENT

There are many reasons why a child might act in a particular way in a particular circumstance and there are many ramifications of difficult behaviour. The challenge for the doctor is to determine the 'what, why, when and how' of the behaviour – no easy task. See the practice point above.

Multiple sessions might be needed to get close to the core of the problem. Alternatively, the paediatrician might feel that the issue is best dealt with through referral to a paediatric mental health colleague, such as a psychiatrist or clinical psychologist. Early referral, if possible, is preferable where the doctor senses that the behaviour is entrenched and that simple techniques will not address the problem.

Where behaviour difficulties are severe, multimodal and multidisciplinary intervention is the ideal. In this setting the team consisting of the paediatrician, psychologist, therapist and clinic nurse all play a role in support and behaviour intervention for the child and family. In some clinics psychiatry trainees are also involved. These clinics are found in teaching hospitals, community child health clinics, and in clinics that support and assess children with developmental problems and disabilities.

In the community, rural or private practice setting, the doctor in solo practice needs to collaborate with others who can assist the family. These professionals include general practitioners (GPs), therapists, counsellors, teachers and psychologists in the community and educational setting. The work can be demanding and challenging, so that it is wise to collaborate with other colleagues early in the process to avoid feeling overwhelmed when the family are in crisis, e.g. when dealing with the aggressive, demanding child.

The initial assistance for parents might come from close relatives, community leaders, church counsellors and close friends. All supportive persons involved in the child's life play a role. Where behaviour goes beyond that with which the family can cope, they may seek professional help.

GPs provide support and counselling to families over many appointment sessions for a variety of health-related problems. They usually know the family well and appreciate the stressors and problems facing the family. Hence input from the family GP is invaluable in providing behaviour support and intervention. In more complex situations or due to shortage of clinic time, the GP might refer the child and family to the paediatrician or other mental health professional.

Underlying difficulties such as learning problems, bullying, intellectual difficulties, adjustment difficulties and parental mental illness should be taken into account in overall management.

In milder behaviour difficulties simple techniques for parents are helpful, in particular with respect to their communication with the child. If parents are authoritarian, give little reward for 'good' behaviour and focus attention on 'bad' behaviour, they can be guided in principles of behaviour modification and positive communication with the child. (See Text Box 9.1 for suggestions). In addition, it helps to put parents in touch with websites and resources so that they can do their own research on simple behaviour management strategies. (See Resources for Parents at the end of the chapter.)

Parent training and support

Parents often blame themselves for their child's difficult behaviour or feel that they are being blamed. It helps to give them an understanding about the influence

> **TEXT BOX 9.1** Positive communication with the child
>
> Suggestions to parents for improving communication with their child:
> - Maintain a calm attitude when dealing with difficult behaviour
> - Avoid becoming overly emotional, keep a clear calm pattern to your voice because the angry child is likely to react adversely to high-pitched shouting
> - Maintain a 'matter of fact' approach while listening to the child and avoid giving the child the impression that you as the parent are overwhelmed by the situation
> - Be clear when communicating, using short sentences and avoid verbal overload or long sentences as the child is likely to 'tune out'
> - Respect the child's reasons for the particular behaviour (if they have view), try to see the situation from the child's point of view
> - Parental self-awareness is important as the tired, exhausted parent is less likely to be able to deal with difficult behaviour; seek help from a partner or other family members
> - 'Pick the battles' as minor issues can be ignored while dealing with the more difficult and unacceptable behaviours; targeting all perceived difficult behaviours is not only exhausting, it undermines success for dealing with the tough ones
> - Avoid name-calling and negative comments like 'you *never* listen', 'you are *always* annoying' because the child then has no experience of success or acknowledgement of effort, even when they try to change
> - Emphasise that it is the behaviour which is unacceptable, not the child
> - Ultimately, respect and love for the child means that the parent makes an attempt to act in the best interests of the child
> - When parents make mistakes they should apologise to the child so that the child learns about fairness, learns to say sorry and learns that we all make mistakes
> - When behaviour is entrenched the parent can be encouraged to seek formal counselling, where many of these principles are discussed during regular sessions (usually with a clinical psychologist)
> - The approach used must be maintained for a sufficient period: many parents give up on an approach too early, particularly as behaviours often get worse when changes are instituted, long before they improve
> - Importantly, parents must work *together* on the problem or they run the risk of undermining each other, thereby impeding success.

of individual temperament. Temperament is evident early and babies from birth have the ability to engender feelings towards them through their reactions to their parents. As children develop differences in temperament become more obvious, e.g. the shy, withdrawn child versus the outgoing, friendly child. Discussions with parents about the interactive process of communication and how the child contributes to the relationship can help parents to understand the behaviour, which might aid their perception of themselves as effective parents.[18]

Parent training techniques are beneficial in many instances and provide parents with tools for dealing with difficult behaviour. There is evidence for effectiveness of parenting programs in promoting positive discipline techniques in order to enhance children's social skills, self-regulatory skills and problem-solving ability.[19]

Mindfulness in parent-training techniques, which include facilitative listening (on the part of the clinician, being attentive to parental concerns and remaining non-judgmental), distancing (from parent's past learned ways of coping) and motivated action plans (that help parents to work on effective goals with specific plans to reach those goals) have been shown to reduce the automaticity of reacting in families with disruptive children.[20]

Positive parenting programs run by community health clinics and some private agencies can be of enormous benefit to families in that they provide guidance and support for dealing with children and their behaviour. The Triple P parenting program and programs run through the Child and Youth Mental Health Services (CYMHS) are examples, and families can be referred to these organisations.

Counselling

Where the difficulties are entrenched and where ongoing support over time is needed, it is best to refer the family for counselling with a clinical psychologist who has experience in helping families. The techniques used will depend on the developmental age of the child.

Counselling techniques can include:
- Behaviour management: essentially involves rewards for acceptable behaviour, use of reward or star charts, attention given to 'good' behaviour and ignoring of 'bad' behaviour or removal of privileges for unacceptable behaviour. Punishment is not recommended, as it is rarely effective and may become abusive. This method is often helpful for younger children.
- Counselling: about attitudes and motivation, focus on the reasons for the child acting in a particular way, encourage the child to think about the effect of their behaviour on others, encourage the parents to consider issues from the child's point of view.
- Cognitive behaviour techniques: where the child or parent holds a belief about a particular act or issue that is not based on reality, they can be encouraged to challenge and redirect their thinking regarding the issue. This method is often useful when the child has fears or anxiety about particular situations, and is more likely to be effective in the older child, usually beyond 8 years of age.

Activity-based support

Informal techniques that encourage the child to do an activity which directs attention away from the behaviour and enables therapists or counsellors to intervene in a positive way with respect to attitudes, beliefs, anxieties and fears. Examples of such intervention are:
- Sport or physical activity that the child enjoys: the coach might develop a relationship with the child and nurture good thinking and better attitude to improve the child's interaction with others
- Music therapy: enjoyment of music can be relaxing and can also help to divert energy from a worrying issue, e.g. in the anxious child

- Other outdoor activities: there are many techniques that therapists, educators and counsellors can use to engender positive behaviour and that also enhance self-esteem.

> **Practice Point**
>
> Intervention approaches in Parent training and support and Counselling above are evidence based, whereas Activity-based support is not; but nonetheless it is a useful approach in many instances.

Medication management

Medication is not the first-line approach and is used in circumstances where the behavioural change or improvement does not occur despite the interventions discussed, and where the consequences of non-treatment put the child in jeopardy.

Where the child has a comorbid condition like ADHD, medication management to allow better focus and 'tuning in' to others and their feelings needs to be considered. Anxiety or depression in the child warrants the same approach. In this circumstance, involvement with a child psychiatrist in overall management is encouraged.

Children with autism spectrum disorder and severe behaviour problems may require medication management to deal with anxiety and/or aggressive behaviour. See Table 9.2 for medications that are used more commonly to treat difficult behaviour. There are other medications used by child psychiatrists depending on assessment and the child's needs.

> **Practice Point**
>
> When prescribing medications, side-effects must be closely monitored. Where raised blood pressure and tachycardia occur, the medication dose should be reduced. If signs persist or if any cardiac symptoms occur, it is advisable to refer to a cardiologist for assessment.

CONCLUSION

Behaviour difficulty occurs in childhood for many reasons. If severe and not addressed it can result in long-term morbidity with respect to social interaction, adaptability, education and even future employment.

Support for parents and children with behaviour difficulties is important whether the problems are mild and managed by solo practitioners (GPs, paediatricians or clinical psychologists) or severe and requiring multidisciplinary assessment and intervention. In either case the work involves collaboration with parents, extended families and involved community members in order to provide family-centred treatment and support.

Where the clinician assesses the problem to be beyond their skill, it is advisable to refer to mental health professionals (psychologists and child psychiatrists) for more intensive management and support.

CHAPTER 9   Behaviour difficulties   **183**

TABLE 9.2   Medications for treating difficult behaviour[21]

Medication & dosage	Indication	Main side-effects
Omega-3 1 standard capsule bd for prepubertal children 2 standard capsules bd for adolescents	Over activity ADHD Depression and anxiety-based behaviour disturbance	Indigestion Increased clotting time Worsening acne
Atomoxetine Initial dose 0.5 mg/kg/day Maintenance dose up to 1 mg/kg/day	ADHD where diversion of medications or addictions are present in other family members Is also the first-line treatment in comorbid anxiety	Sedation (usually temporary) Fatigue (usually temporary) Tachycardia (usually mild) Hypertension (usually minimal) QT interval prolongation (usually mild) Headache, abdominal pain and urinary hesitancy (usually temporary)
Stimulants (methylphenidate and dexamphetamine) For dosages see Ch 8 ADHD	ADHD	See Ch 8 ADHD for detail Sleeplessness Weight loss Triggering psychosis, mania or depression
Clonidine Initial dose 2 mcg/kg/day nocte single dose Maintenance 5 mcg/kg/day in divided doses with loading in evening	Traumatised children with aggression and hyper-arousal states	Sedation Hypotension Bradycardia Heart block Rebound hypertension on cessation (should be withdrawn slowly)

REFERENCES

1   Cullen KJ, Boundy CAP. The prevalence of behaviour disorders in the children of 1000 Western Australian families. Medical Journal of Australia 1966;2(17):805–8
2   Pharoah POD, Stevenson CJ, Cooke RWI, Stevenson RC. Prevalence of behaviour disorders in low birthweight infants. Archives of Disease in Childhood 1994;70:271–4
3   Boydell Brauner C, Bowers Stephens C. Estimating the prevalence of early childhood serious emotional–behavioral disorders: challenges and recommendations. Public Health Reports 2006;121:303–10
4   Nolan TM, Bond L, Adler R, et al. Child Behaviour Checklist classification of behaviour disorder. Journal of Paediatrics and Child Health 1996;32(5):405–11
5   Parry T. Assessment of developmental learning and behaviour problems in children and young people. Medical Journal of Australia 2005;183:43–8
6   Heubeck BG. Cross-cultural generalizability of CBCL syndromes across three continents: from the USA and Holland to Australia. Journal of Abnormal Child Psychology 2000; 28(5):439–50
7   Goodman R. The Strengths and Difficulties Questionnaire: A research note. Journal of Child Psychology and Psychiatry 1997;38:581–6
8   Thomas A, Chess S, Birch HG. Temperament and Behavior Disorders in Children. New York: New York University Press; 1968

9. Caspi A, Shiner R. Temperament and personality, ch 14. In: Rutter M, Bishop D, Pine D, et al, editors. Rutter's Child and Adolescent Psychiatry. 5th ed. Oxford: Wiley-Blackwell; 2008
10. Rees CA. Thinking about children's attachments. Archives of Disease in Childhood 2005;90:1058–65
11. Rees CA. Understanding emotional abuse. Archives of Disease in Childhood 2010;95:59–67
12. Prior M, Bavin EL, Cini E, et al. Influences on communicative development at 24 months of age: Child temperament, behaviour problems and maternal factors. Infant Behavior and Development 2008;31:270–9
13. Middleton JA. Psychological sequelae of head injury in children and adolescents. Journal of Child Psychology and Psychiatry 2001;42:165–80
14. Taylor HG, Yeates KO, Wade SL, et al. A prospective study of short- and long-term outcomes after traumatic brain injury in children: Behavior and achievement. Neuropsychology 2002;16(1):15–27
15. Anderson VA, Catroppa C, Dudgeon P, et al. Understanding predictors of functional recovery and outcome 30 months following early childhood head injury. Neuropsychology 2006;20(1):42–57
16. Schwartz L, Taylor HG, Drotar D, Yeates KO, et al. Long-term behavior problems following pediatric traumatic brain injury: Prevalence, predictors and correlates. Journal of Pediatric Psychology 2003;28(4):251–63
17. Yeates KO. Traumatic brain injury, ch 5. In: Taylor HG, Pennington BE, editors. Pediatric Neuropsychology: Research, Theory and Practice, 2nd ed. New York: Guilford; 2010
18. Berger M. Temperament and individual differences, ch 1. In: Rutter M, Hersov H, editors. Child and Adolescent Psychiatry: Modern Approaches. Oxford: Blackwell Scientific; 1985
19. Bauer NS, Webster-Stratton C. Prevention of behavioral disorders in primary care. Current Opinion in Pediatrics 2006;18(6):654–60
20. Dumas JE. Mindfulness-based parent training: Strategies to lessen the grip of automaticity in families with disruptive children. Journal of Clinical Child & Adolescent Psychology 2005;34(4):779–91
21. Lask B, Taylor S, Nunn KP. Practical Child Psychiatry: The Clinician's Guide. London: BMJ Press; 2003

FURTHER READING

Rutter M, Bishop D, Pine D, et al. Rutter's Child and Adolescent Psychiatry. 5th ed. Wiley-Blackwell; 2008
Kagan J. The temperamental thread. How genes, culture, time, and luck make us who we are. New York: Dana Press; 2010

RESOURCES FOR PARENTS

These websites available 2 March 2012.
http://www.kidsmatter.edu.au/uploads/2009/09/serious-behaviour-overview.pdf
http://raisingchildren.net.au/
http://www.mumsnet.com/
http://www.community.nsw.gov.au/docswr/_assets/main/documents/researchnotes_parenting_programs.pdf
http://www1.triplep.net/
Child and Youth Mental Health Services (CYMHS) http://www.health.qld.gov.au/childrenshealth

10 School refusal and truancy

Sandra Johnson

INTRODUCTION

School refusal and truancy are not uncommon. They can be caused by, result in or exacerbate emotional, educational and socioeconomic morbidity. The prevalence of school refusal is approximately 5 per cent of school-aged children, with peaks at around 5–7 years, then again at 11 years and 14 years of age. Overall, it is more likely to occur between the ages of 5–6 years and 10–11 years, which appears to be related to the transition points in the child's school experience.[1] There is no apparent gender predominance.

BACKGROUND

The fear of attending school was first termed 'school phobia' in 1941 in a paper by AM Johnson et al. The term 'school refusal', later described in 1960 in a paper by Hersov, became the accepted term used in Britain[2] and elsewhere. In the United States, the term 'school refusal behaviour' is used to encompass various subsets of problematic absenteeism, such as truancy, school phobia and separation anxiety.[3]

More recently there have debates in the literature as to whether school refusal and truancy should be regarded under the umbrella term of 'school absenteeism', because the risk factors, assessment and management approach is similar for both.[4] For the purposes of this chapter the definitions are given for each, however a unified management approach is given as an overview for both presenting problems.

DEFINITIONS

School refusal

A commonly accepted definition is 'a child motivated refusal to attend school and/or difficulties remaining in classes for an entire day'.[1] Emotional distress and anxiety are usually part of the presentation in school refusal but tend to be less obvious in truancy. It appears that these children prefer both to stay home and avoid the school environment. They tend not to conceal their distress from their parents.

Truancy

The truant child absconds from school during school hours but does not necessarily want to stay at home. In contrast to school refusal, truant children tend not to show anxiety or fear about attending school. There may be elements of delinquent behaviour in their presentation.

RISK AND ASSOCIATED FACTORS

There are many reasons for school refusal and truancy and these factors are relevant in both, maybe with different emphasis in each.

The family environment

Dysfunction and anxiety within the family might lead to the child wanting to stay home, subconsciously wishing to reduce the anxiety. The child might wish to stay home to be with a parent whom the child perceives to be vulnerable in some way. The parent might have a medical or psychiatric illness and the child is reluctant to leave the parent.

There might be an over-anxious attachment to the parent and the child may not want to leave that particular parent alone for a variety of reasons. Usually these children display separation anxiety in their early preschool and school years.[5]

Poverty and homelessness can be a significant factor where the child stays away from school to help the parent. The child might need to earn money to help to support the younger family members. Examples include countries where child labour occurs and some financial benefit is paid to the families of these children. Even in Western countries young teenagers may be expected to work to support the rest of the family, which can be a factor in school absenteeism.

Families that move frequently, for reasons of job relocation or other reasons, can be a contributing factor. The child in this situation is required to repeatedly adapt to a new school setting and this might be stressful for the child, particularly if predisposed to anxiety.

The lack of parental involvement and supervision is also noted to be a significant factor.[6] Children who are disinterested in school are more likely to have parents and older siblings who were disinterested in school. A lack of value placed on education within the family occurs more frequently in the truancy group.

The school environment

The school environment is relevant. If the child feels unsafe at school for any reason or where the child is exposed to bullying, which is not adequately managed by the school, the child might refuse to attend school. Overt violence at school is uncommon but is a factor, which needs to be addressed if children are to feel safe about attending school. Violence and gangs at school are noted to be a significant factor in relation to school absenteeism.

If the child feels isolated in a school environment where little support, emotional or educational, is given to students they might feel unhappy within that environment.

The learning environment

The child might find the academic environment stressful and become very anxious at examination and assessment times. Children who have learning difficulties and who cannot keep up with their peers might display anxiety about attending school (see Chapter 6 Specific learning disorders).

The child might have poor relationships with one or more teachers, which can significantly influence the child's unwillingness to attend school.

Where there is inadequate educational support for students, the child with learning problems will find the school environment particularly difficult.

The social environment

Communities with a gang culture and where drug use is prevalent will have an impact on children's school attendance. The child might stay home out of fear and uncertainty for their safety.

If the social environment, often as a result of poverty and poor socioeconomic circumstance, is such that education is not valued and is one where most adults in that society have not completed school and/or are chronically unemployed, then there might be less desire to learn and less impetus for attending school in the younger members of that society. The circumstances of Indigenous people are complex and must be considered when working in these communities.

After a major natural disaster a child may refuse to return to school long after the disaster has abated. This was reported in Sri Lanka in the aftermath of the tsunami in 2004.[7] The psychological stress and mental health impact on families after Hurricane Katrina in the United States has also been reported.[8] These disasters leave their mark on children within families and the schools that they attend.

The cultural attitudes about education and conforming to the needs of the society must be considered. Some have suggested a mismatch between the Western education system and other cultures' learning styles. For example, sitting in a highly structured classroom of twenty or more students for extended periods of time with all students expected to do the same task in the same manner, so typical of Western education, might not suit the learning style of Indigenous children. This is particularly true for those from traditional communities who are more familiar with learning in small groups or individually from their elders in practical, hands-on, and obviously relevant and applicable ways.

Social or civil unrest in situations of society breakdown, such as in riots or wars, is an important consideration in countries where this is an issue.

THE FUNCTIONS OF SCHOOL REFUSAL BEHAVIOUR

Kearney in the United States who has studied the subject gives a description of the functions of school refusal behaviour that provides an approach to aid the

Practice Point

While the model described might help clinicians to understand the problem, it is necessary to say that in some circumstances school refusal and truancy might be a rational response on the part of the child to deal with a negative school experience. These include bullying by peers, poor interactions with teachers, lack of educational support, inadequate learning experiences and unhappy school environments. Thus, the clinician needs to take account of the student's experiences and reasons for wanting to avoid school.

> **TEXT BOX 10.1** Functions of school refusal behaviour
>
> **1 Avoidance of school-related stimuli that provoke anxiety, fear or depression**
> This situation usually occurs in younger children who may have difficulty identifying the cause of their distress, but they experience discomfort at school and want to avoid it. The child might complain of somatic symptoms. Kearney describes these children as being of anxious disposition.
>
> **2 Escape from aversive social or evaluative situations at school**
> This situation is typically seen in older children and adolescents who have difficulty interacting with peers or others at school. They may have difficulties with oral presentations, recitals and examinations. These children may be ostracised at school for various reasons, which may be a contributing factor.
>
> **3 Pursuit of attention from significant others**
> This presentation occurs more often in younger children who prefer to stay home with their parents or others. They usually have tantrums, non-compliance and tend to run away from school. Kearney reports that this presentation is likely to be associated with separation anxiety disorder and oppositional defiant disorder.
>
> **4 Pursuit of tangible reinforcers outside the school setting**
> This presentation is more often seen in older children and adolescents. These children might refuse school because of activities outside school that they find more attractive; such as computer or electronic games, television, and time with friends. Kearney reports a strong association with family conflict, delinquency and substance abuse in this traditional truancy group.

clinician in understanding the problem so that effective, individualised treatment and management can be provided.[9] The School Refusal Assessment Scale (SRAS) is a measure developed by Kearney's research team in order to assess school refusal.[10] Factor analysis of the revised version (SRAS-R) revealed four possible functions of school refusal behaviour discussed see Text Box 10.1 (reproduced with permission).

CLINICAL PRESENTATION

School refusal

The problem might commence with an illness where the child has been at home for a short period of time, usually a mild viral infection, and thereafter refuses to return to school. Alternatively, the presentation can be insidious and over time the child reports reluctance to attend school. This can then escalate to the point where the child shows extreme anger, tantrums and distress about attending school. When the child is taken home, they relax and seem happier. The longer the child stays away from school the harder it is for them to return to school, thus setting in train a problematic and increasingly entrenched cycle.

These children are distressed and anxious about attending school and they may have other symptoms like abdominal pain, headaches, muscular pains or dizziness. As a result of these distressing symptoms they are likely to be kept home from school, a further factor or process contributing to the problematic cycle.

Truancy

Children who are truant attempt to conceal their absences from their parents. They generally do not show distress or anxiety about going to school. They will go to school but will not attend school for some or all of the day. These children often show disinterest in schoolwork or any activities associated with the school environment. They are at risk for delinquent and antisocial behaviour. Truancy is often accompanied and sustained by a negative peer influence.

Comorbid psychiatric symptoms and disorders

Many researchers have noted high comorbidity of anxiety (separation anxiety disorder), depression and oppositional defiant disorder (ODD) in those who present with school refusal and high comorbidity of conduct disorder, ODD, depression and substance abuse in those who present with truancy.

MANAGEMENT APPROACH

In many instances of school refusal and truancy paediatricians are not involved at all, because the problems are dealt with through the school, teachers and psychologists. The paediatrician might be consulted because the concerned parent has sought medical involvement, via the general practitioner, who then refers to the paediatrician. The following is a management approach that involves the paediatrician.

The management and treatment of the condition, like many areas in child development, is multi-modal. The paediatrician who does the assessment needs to collaborate with the child, the parents, teachers, psychologists, general practitioners and other therapists who work with the child. In many circumstances child psychiatrists are involved as well. The initial assessment is important, as in other aspects of child development.

The paediatric assessment

1 History and nature of the event
- When did the problem start?
- What were the circumstances at the time: illness, stressors, medications?
- What happens when the child is taken to and left at school?
- Who is most concerned? Whose idea was it to see the paediatrician?
- Is the child attending school at all?
- What has been done so far to remedy the situation?
- Who has been helping the child and parents with the problem?

2 Educational history
- How is the child coping with learning?
- History of specific learning difficulties; if present, what support is given at school?
- How is the child progressing academically?
- What about school reports?
- Is this an acute decline in performance in an otherwise high achiever (suggestive of some emotional factor) as opposed to a child with longstanding learning difficulties?

- What are the child's peer relations like?
- Is bullying a contributing factor?

3 Perinatal and early development, including preschool experience
- Pregnancy history: was this a planned pregnancy?
- Birth history: traumatic delivery? Bonding with the baby?
- Early developmental milestones?
- Preschool development: development of autonomy and early social interaction skills?

4 Medical history
- Acute or chronic medical illness?
- History of somatic symptoms to indicate anxiety or distress?
- Is the child on any medications?
- Immunisation history?

5 Family and social history
- Family history of medical illness (current or past)?
- Is there a current illness in a family member that could be distressing to the child?
- Is there a history of learning difficulties or school refusal for other members of the family?
- Family history of mental illness, including anxiety, depression and other psychiatric disorders?

6 Physical examination
- Complete physical examination of all systems
- Examination of specific areas where somatic symptoms are a factor
- Thorough examination can be reassuring that the child does not have a medical condition and helps to exclude an organic problem.

7 Investigations
- These are done only where clinically indicated.
- Clinical findings may indicate that a particular test should be done, e.g. FBC and serum iron studies if clinical pallor and poor diet.
- Refrain from doing unnecessary tests to avoid the sense that the child has a valid reason for not going to school, where such a reason does not exist.
- The School Refusal Assessment Scale-Revised developed by researchers in the United States to assess the functions of school refusal behaviour may be a useful tool in assessment.
- The Child Behaviour Checklist (CBCL), or the subsequent Achenbach Behaviour Checklist and Connor's Rating Scales, may be helpful in giving an overview of the child's behaviour in various settings. The CBCL has been applied in various national settings.[11] The clinician should choose tools that are validated in the relevant national context.
- Psychological and educational assessment may be indicated to assess school performance and abilities (see Chapter 6 Specific learning disorders) and to give a second opinion on anxiety, self-esteem and depression. The school counsellor, psychologist or special education teacher would be able to give feedback about the child's progress within the school environment.

8 Clinical impressions and diagnosis
- Once the clinical assessment is complete, a summary of findings is given to the parents and child with an explanation that no physical cause can be found,

if this is indeed the case. Where tests are necessary these are discussed and explained.
- The diagnosis is provisional and if medical illness is found then the treatment and intervention plan is implemented.

> **Practice Point**
>
> The history and physical examination should be thorough. Avoid reassuring the family that there is no medical reason if you have not been thorough.
>
> There are rare instances of organic disease contributing to somatic symptoms and school refusal behaviour, for example headache and brain tumour.[12]

TREATMENT AND INTERVENTION

The overall aim is to get the child to return to school as soon as possible, because the longer the child remains away from school the more difficult it will be to reach attendance.

Collaboration between the family and school is important to achieve this aim.

Initial approach

1. Discussion between the parents and the school is necessary so that a collaborative approach is reached.
2. The child's input is important so that they feel involved with the process. The child might have very valid reasons for not wanting to go to school.
3. Where anxiety is a key component, psychological intervention with the school counsellor and/or clinical psychologist is indicated. Cognitive behaviour therapy, including imagery and relaxation techniques, is helpful to enable the child to deal with the scenarios at school that they find stressful.[13]
4. Introduce the child to the school environment through graduated re-integration and re-exposure over several days until full day attendance is achieved.
5. Educational and emotional support within the school environment allow this process to work more smoothly.
6. Peer support for the child might also work, but this depends on the child's presentation and their personality. The child might work better with a supportive teacher rather than a peer.
7. Address other factors that influence the situation, for example, family counselling and support if the family unit is dysfunctional, psychological support for one or both parents where indicated.
8. Educational and support sessions for teachers at school about the vulnerabilities of students, for example, students who do not feel supported or who are the subject of bullying.

Secondary approach

1. Medication management may be indicated where anxiety or depression is present.
2. Medication management for attention deficit hyperactivity disorder (ADHD) might be necessary where the clinical presentation is in keeping with this

diagnosis. Chronic underachievement and behavioural problems associated with ADHD might also lead to truancy (see Chapter 8 Attention deficit hyperactivity disorder).

3   In the child suspected of being depressed, it is wise to obtain the opinion of a child psychiatrist who will need to assess the child and family, and who will make recommendations as part of the treatment plan.
4   Where success is not achieved with the initial approach, a multidisciplinary team assessment is recommended so that intervention can be provided at different levels and with the assistance of a variety of professionals, such as social worker, special educator, therapists (occupational and speech where indicated by the child's learning problems), psychologist and medical personnel.
5   Alternative school programs may need to be considered as a last resort if factors within the school system cannot support the intervention.
6   Broader factors involving the community might be relevant where school safety and violence is an issue.
7   Recognise the importance of working with other agencies and professions where indicated to assist the child and family.
8   The paediatrician often acts as an advocate for the child where the school is not addressing concerns or facilitating the child's education.
9   In rare circumstances home schooling might be considered, but this needs to be weighed up against the child's need for peer interaction and the parent's ability to support home schooling.

PROGNOSIS

The outcome depends on the severity, but intervention and management by a team of professionals go a long way to producing a better outcome. The best outcome is achieved by early return to school with support from various agencies as discussed.

There are long-term morbidities associated with school refusal and these include anxiety, depression, social phobia, underachievement in employment and poorer career prospects.[14] Thus early intervention and support for these students at various levels can alleviate their stress, so that they can have a better long-term outcome through to adulthood.

REFERENCES

1   King NJ, Bernstein GA. School refusal in children and adolescents: A review of the past 10 years. J Am Acad Child Adolesc Psychiatry 2001;40(2):197–205
2   Hersov LA. Refusal to go to school. J Child Psychol Psychiatry 1960;1:137–45
3   Kearney CA. Dealing with school refusal behavior. A primer for family physicians. Journal of Family Practice 2006;55(8):685–92
4   Kearney CA. School absenteeism and school refusal behavior in youth: a contemporary review. Clinical Psychology Review 2008;28:451–71
5   Egger HL, Costello EJ, Angold A. School refusal and psychiatric disorders: a community study. J Am Acad Child Adolesc Psychiatry 2003;42(7):797–807
6   Orfield G. Dropouts in America: Confronting the graduation rate crisis. Cambridge, MA: Harvard Education Press; 2004
7   Nikapota A. After the tsunami: a story from Sri Lanka. International Review of Psychiatry 2006;18(3):275–9

8. Picou JS, Hudson K. Hurricane Katrina and mental health: A research note on Mississippi Gulf Coast Residents. Sociological Inquiry 2010;80(3):513–24
9. Kearney CA. Forms and functions of school refusal behavior in youth: an empirical analysis of absenteeism severity. J Child Psychol Psychiatry 2007;48(1):53–61
10. Kearney CA, Silverman WK. Measuring the function of school refusal behavior: The School Refusal Assessment Scale. Journal of Clinical Child Psychology 1993;22:85–96
11. Heubeck BG. Cross-cultural generalizability of CBCL syndromes across three continents: from the USA and Holland to Australia. Journal of Abnormal Child Psychology 2000;28(5):439–50
12. Stein MT. School refusal and emotional lability in a 6-year-old boy. J Develop Behav Pediatrics 2001;22(2):S29–32
13. Doobay AF. School refusal behavior associated with separation anxiety disorder: A cognitive–behavioral approach to treatment. Psychology in the Schools 2008;45(4):261–72
14. Prabhuswamy M, et al. Outcome of children with school refusal. Indian Journal of Pediatrics 2007;74:375–9

11 Mood disorders in children and adolescents

Kenneth Nunn

INTRODUCTION

Conditions, illnesses and disorders that predominantly present with troubled mood and feeling states have been documented since ancient times, including alternating mood states that may afflict the young. In the early 20th century Kraepelin,[1] the great German psychiatrist, noted in relation to manic depressive illness that:

> In rare cases the first beginnings can be traced back even to before the tenth year … The greatest frequency of first attacks, however, is in the period of development with its increased emotional excitability between the fifteenth and twentieth year.[1]

While this statement has largely been born out by epidemiological studies, concerns abound about over-diagnosis, on the one hand, and the delay in diagnosis of childhood and paediatric mood disorders with consequent long-term cognitive and psychosocial sequelae, on the other. Largely, but not exclusively, the concerns about over-diagnosis have been directed towards pre-pubertal cases of bipolar disorder. Concerns about delay in diagnosis have arisen from longitudinal studies indicating that most cases commencing in the adolescent years remain undiagnosed, or misdiagnosed, for an average of 10.1 years.[2] For a substantial period of time during the early twentieth century psychoanalytic influence suggested that children and adolescents were too immature to experience bipolar-type conditions and senior paediatric clinicians, such as Leo Kanner at Johns Hopkins, removed the diagnosis from his textbook of child psychiatry to avoid controversy. The growing evidence for both white matter, grey matter and functional changes in activation in key areas of the brain in those with mood disorders have shifted these formulations to a pathological and neurobiological understanding rather than developmental, and purely psychological, explanations.

Whatever the current state of diagnostic practice, it is now evident that depression in childhood and adolescence lasting greater than twelve months is likely to endure into adulthood.[3] Carefully constructed longitudinal epidemiological studies[2] indicate that a third of all bipolar disorder commences prior to 20 years of age. There are a significant number of adults with both depression and bipolar disorder who trace their disease onset to the pre-pubertal period. The intuitions of concern centre around the notion that children and young people ought not to be afflicted with such serious conditions; that 'normal' untoward behaviour is being medicalised into psychiatric disorder, along with the use of other diagnoses such as attention deficit hyperactive disorder (ADHD) and autistic spectrum disorder (ASD). Over expansion of diagnoses renders any diagnostic system increasingly suspect. Beneficial response to treatment, in even a significant minority who are severely functionally impaired, is likely to keep the diagnostic debate alive.

BACKGROUND

Feeling depressed in an enduring, persistent manner, which approaches insidiously and relentlessly and lifts slowly over time, is the most usual picture in clinicians' minds of depression. Depression that is associated with sudden, precipitous depressive feelings that come and leave equally suddenly within hours or days, as part of a volatile turmoil of feelings that may include waves of irritability, anger, ebullience and driven desperation, is a less common understanding but very characteristic of mood disorders in adolescents. This chapter presents these two very different clinical entities, which are frequently indistinguishable in cross-section and often only become extricated with time and treatment. Each has the accompanying sub-threshold conditions:
- Depression
- Sub-threshold depression
- Bipolar disorder
- Sub-threshold bipolar disorder.

Despite many recommendations from the literature, experienced clinicians can find that in distinguishing these conditions, time and treatment prove us wrong commonly enough to maintain clinical humility. What appears to be a simple decision ushers in one of two treatment processes, which have quite different goals, methods of management and adverse outcomes if directed to the wrong condition. Treating bipolar disorder as depression can be as problematic as treating anaphylaxis as if it is asthma. Failing to distinguish may sometimes work out without a major negative consequence, but there is a significant risk that it will not. Treating depression as bipolar disorder is less problematic, but means exposing the patient to a wider variety of medications and delaying full treatment response. Fortunately there are some simple principles that can guide treatment to minimise unwanted outcomes.

In pre-puberty, the point prevalence of all mood disorders combined is 4.5–5.4 per cent. This corresponds to rates found in large clinical samples with carefully defined diagnostic criteria.[4] At this stage we do not have accurate lifetime prevalence for pre-pubertal disorders. Lifetime prevalence estimates overall for mood disorders in 13–17 year olds is 21.9 per cent.[5]

Differences between adult and adolescent presentation

In recent years, characteristics (e.g. mixed features) thought to be more common in adolescents and children have been re-examined in adults and the original descriptions of adults have been found wanting. Despite this tendency for paediatric psychiatry to wag the diagnostic dog, there is agreement that emerging mental illness is less clear-cut, less complete and more frequently changes form (so called pleomorphism) of clinical presentation in comparison to adult presentations. The prominence of concentration difficulties, executive dysfunction and neurocognitive impairment[6] in adolescent samples, and the place of irritability as a symptom, remain at the forefront in most clinical discussions. A significant number of adolescents with any major mental illness will present with features of borderline personality disorder, because their personalities are forming, but these features usually do not persist beyond early adulthood. This is the reason that the Diagnostic and Statistical Manual of Mental Disorders (DSM) has consistently discouraged the use of personality disorder as a diagnosis in adolescence.

In relation to bipolar disorder, the possibility of a predominance of irritability, no established history of enduring mania–hypomania, ultradian mood variation (i.e. sudden, major shifts in mood within the same day), rapid cycling, afternoon worsening of symptoms, and unexplained violence, remain prominent in the clinical literature. The terms 'elated and euphoric' are frequently better replaced with 'driven and desperate' and periods of full remission are less common.

Differences between child and adolescent presentation

Childhood or peri-pubertal presentations will have more motor activity changes (hyperactivity and/or underactivity), concentration impairment and oppositional features, coloured by the fears and desires of the developmental phase through which they are moving. It is not surprising then that sleep, elimination disorders, ADHD, oppositional defiant disorder (ODD) and separation anxiety, figure highly in the longitudinal development of their mood difficulties. Histories of trauma, family conflict and struggling at school (especially with mathematics and non-dominant hemisphere functions) may all be present because these may all reach prominence because of the children's sensitivity to adversity, criticism and social rejection. The presence of suicidal ideation, especially ideation and desire to harm oneself, in the pre- and peri-pubertal period are all much less prominent in ADHD and ODD. Potentially lethal attempts to commit suicide in children must always raise the issue of a serious mood disorder, especially in the presence of a family history of depressive illness, bipolar disorder, maternal alcoholism or substance abuse.

DEPRESSION

Defining characteristics

Distress

Feeling 'down', 'a heaviness to one's whole body', sad, empty and unable to think about the future without dread and an immobilising paralysis, an inability to enjoy or feel interested in all those things that usually capture thought and impel to action, are just some of the ways of describing depression. Young children often do not have the words and so may just not say anything at all but become preoccupied with sad themes (especially in the news), withdraw from spontaneous activities, or begin to think about dying or loved one's dying.

Boys are more likely to have angry or violent themes in their thoughts and play. Both boys and girls may express deep preoccupation with having done the wrong thing and having let people down, especially friends and family. Suicidal thoughts of wishing never to wake up, wanting to die, specific plans to hurt themselves and attempts to do so, may all occur in very young children.

Adolescents are likely to say they feel 'crap', or 'like shit', rather than more elaborate formulations. The more adult verbal content of them feeling worthless about themselves, hopeless about their futures and that the world is meaningless may or may not be verbalised. Sometimes this is because of linguistic limitations, or a developmental inability to distinguish between what is happening inside versus outside of themselves. Hopelessness and irritability in adolescents can be more profound than at almost any other time of life because of the increased intensity of all emotions during the teenage years.

Dysfunction

Movement and mood: watching the way children and young people move rather than what they say is helpful. Movement and mood neurocircuitry are intimately bound up with each other. The simultaneous appearance of autonomic arousal, social withdrawal and internal preoccupation is very common and much more reliable than verbal content. Tearfulness is a helpful indicator, if present, but frequently disappears as depression becomes more severe. Autonomic arousal may tip over into anxious restlessness or agitation. Covert self-harm to gain relief or to express self-loathing are common, especially in middle- and late-adolescent girls and young women.

Social impact: angry and combative fighting against the world are more common with boys and young men. Both boys and girls are likely to seek out social groups that reinforce their own view of themselves and the world, until they withdraw more completely. Substance abuse is common to deal with distress, to forget troubles and life's conflicts, to join with like-minded friends and to overcome the anxiety of intimacy seeking, when intimacy is sorely wanted. Poor judgments about who to trust and distrust are common, along with risk-taking. Sensitivity to criticism and bullying are all more pronounced making them easier targets for the critical and the bullying. Uncharacteristic shoplifting, petty crime or obsession with a 'love object', known or admired from afar, are minor themes on the major story.

Physical complaints: of inability to get off to sleep, interrupted sleep and early morning wakening can all be seen. Extreme phase shift in adolescents is very common with 'awake all night and asleep most of the day' type patterns occurring as an exaggeration of the normal phase – lag sleep problems of adolescents. Marked weight gain or loss (generally greater than 10 kilograms in three months) both may reflect the hypothalamic shift of depression. Changes in menstrual patterns in girls are frequent, with worsening at different times of the menstrual cycle common, especially in the peri-pubertal period.

Cognitive symptoms: of inability to concentrate, plan and make decisions, with 'analysis paralysis', have great impact on school attendance, school performance, and the normal enjoyment of movies, team games and hobbies. In a small number of cases these cognitive difficulties move onto alterations in other more fundamental cognitive processes involved with reality testing, such as perception (illusions and hallucinations), ideation and belief (overvalued ideas and delusions) and the coherence of thought itself (thought disorder and fragmentation).

Persistence

While most classifications, such as DSM, use a two-week duration for illness, most young people will only present or be presented for help much later. The rule of 3's is helpful. Almost anyone can be severely depressed for a three-day period and, providing there is no threat to safety or psychosis, most clinicians would wait but be aware that it may signify a vulnerability, depending upon the context. After three weeks most clinicians would expect a warning flag to be raised and begin basic interventions, while recognising that unless there are somatic signs, self-harm or suicidal thoughts, psychological therapies may be sufficient. Once depression has been persistent for a whole school term, say three months, hypothalamic shift (alterations in sleeping, eating, menstrual and physical activity levels) is present, or safety is potentially compromised, medical treatment is warranted. It is, sadly, still not uncommon to find a young person who has had no medical treatment after one or two years of major depression and for whom only psychological therapies have been offered.

Pervasiveness
The greater the impact in different areas of the child or young person's life, the less likely is it to be a 'simple' depression that will remit without help and the more likely it is to have recurrent or chronic features.

Severity
In general:
- the younger the child, the higher the genetic loading and the more severe the depression long term
- the more adversity, the more likely for genetic loading to be expressed and the more likely the illness is to be explained by psychosocial adversity and remain untreated
- the younger the child, the more severe the illness, especially if psychotic symptoms are experienced, the more likely is the conversion to bipolarity.

Prevalence

In pre-puberty, the point prevalence of major depression has been estimated to range from 1.8 to 2.5 per cent, and 'minor' forms of depression at 2.5 per cent. Lifetime pre-pubertal estimates are still not established. Lifetime prevalence estimates major depressive disorder in 13–17 year olds at 17.7 per cent.[7]

Aetiology
Child and adolescent onset depression is a strongly genetic subtype of mood disorder.[8,9] Up to 50 per cent of pre-pubertal children with depression eventually develop bipolar disorder[10] and recurrent, early-onset depression (defined as two or more episodes before age 25) is a malignant form of depression characterised by high genetic loading, frequent recurrence and poor long-term outcome.[11] Using the Family Interview for Genetics Studies, 76 per cent of the subjects (36 out of 47) report at least one first-degree relative with affective disorder, with 87 per cent (41 out of 47) reporting either a first- or second-degree relative affected. The mean age at onset in this group was 15.6 years.[12]

Most evidence at this stage suggests that depression is a disorder of limbic structures interacting with the anterior cingulate gyrus and prefrontal cortex (cognitive symptoms) and basal ganglia (psychomotor agitation and retardation). The limbic system in this formulation would include the amygdala (arousal, anxiety, fear and dread), the nucleus accumbens (anhedonia or lack of enjoyment and motivation), the hypothalamus (sleep, appetite, endocrine and sexual disturbance) and, most centrally, the insula with profound impact on self-loathing, bodily awareness and altered bodily experience.

All the monoamines (dopamine, noradrenalin and serotonin) have been implicated at different times and have provided a basis for treatment. More recently chronobiotics, such as agomelatine, have been shown to be helpful for the sleep disturbance, as well as the depression, without marked sedation.

Course

Shifting the mind-set of the family and the patient to the fact that depression is a long-term disorder and vulnerability, which is manageable, is one of the major tasks of the clinician as time goes on. In depressed children aged 8 to 13, untreated major depression lasted an average of 7.2 months. Subsequent follow-up of these children revealed that a 40 per cent cumulative probability of a recurrence of depression could be expected within two years, reaching 72 per cent within five years. The rate of sub-threshold depression escalating to full depression remained linear for the entire time of follow-up into their early thirties, by which time 67 per cent had presented with a major depressive episode.[13]

Differential diagnosis

Common differentials

- **Bipolar depression:** 10–30 per cent of all depression presenting in children and adolescents will go on to develop into bipolar disorder. The younger the patient, the more affective disorder in the family, the more ADHD comorbidity and the more psychotic symptoms, the greater the likelihood.
- **Generalised anxiety disorder:** Secondary depression associated with chronic anxiety can easily be mistaken for a primary depressive disorder.
- **Post traumatic stress disorder (PTSD):** Secondary depression associated with chronic trauma-related anxiety can easily be mistaken for a primary depressive disorder.
- **Chronic viral infection:** Infections such as hepatitis, infectious mononucleosis and coxsackie viruses may all present as depressive disorders.
- **Bereavement:** May look very similar to depressive illness and merge into it if sustained for too long.
- **Chronic malnutrition:** In Indigenous communities, Third World settings and with anorexia nervosa malnutrition may be present. Depletion of dietary neurotransmitter precursors, glucose for brain metabolism and anaemia secondary to malnutrition, all contribute to depressive pictures that are secondary to a primary medical disorder.

Less common differentials

- Emerging early onset psychosis
- Obsessive–compulsive disorder
- Hypothyroidism
- Primary anaemias.

Rare differentials

- Cerebral systemic lupus erythematosus
- Hyperparathyroidism
- Childhood and adolescent HIV.

Treatment

Practical advice for all depression

1. **Space and time** – giving young people space and time and 'a bit of slack' when they feel bad is good advice.
2. **Activity, diversion and inclusion** – with others who are enjoying themselves, with no expectation that they have to perform.

3. **Focusing on strengths** – and areas of interest and enjoyment while de-emphasising areas of struggle and areas of conflict in their lives, can take the pressure off short term.
4. **Respect** – making a clear distinction between dissatisfaction with what young people do versus our respect and concern for them as individuals and persons, avoids the toxicity of criticism.
5. **Decreased exposure to conflict** – reducing exposure of young people to the conflicts between parents and parents, parents and teachers, and teachers and teachers will reduce their distress even though it does not always take away the conflict.
6. **'It is not you'** – reassuring children and young people that we as adults are adults and that children are not the source of our conflicts.
7. **Depression IS the problem** – helping young people know that sometimes there is no real 'reason' for depression but it does not mean we cannot do anything about it.
8. **Education about basic mental health** – when it is clear that the child or adolescent is not just being a bit self-indulgently glum, explaining what depression is in simple terms, and talking to parents and other relevant teaching staff about what might be happening.
9. **Giving do-able tasks, achievable goals and skills that others admire** – without creating expectations and pressure, is the essence of what teachers and parents do best to help normal depression.
10. **Gathering sympathetic descriptions of the child** – in different settings and with different people, for a recommendation to parents to obtain treatment can be very helpful.

When the depression is major, enduring and severe

1. **Acceptance:** It is worth starting with the fact that we can all only play a part in very difficult-to-treat problems. Teacher conferencing, parent–teacher communication and mental health expert support will all be necessary if empathy fatigue is not going to set in.
2. **More hands:** The school is a big part of the solution but not the only part. Special schools, mental health units for young people and community centres like 'Headspace' (a youth-friendly Australian service for troubled young people) and youth drop-in services may be necessary.
3. **A long time frame for response:** Major, severe depression gets better in months to years, not days to weeks or even weeks to months. When an illness has remained untreated or unresponsive for more than twelve months, it is unusual to be fully resolved before two years.
4. **The person looks better before they are better:** Young people frequently improve in appearance and the way they move and hold themselves before they improve in their mood. Depression gets better from the outside in. This can be confusing for the young person, when everyone begins to tell them they look better but they still feel hopeless and miserable.
5. **Don't confuse garden-variety depression with malignant depression:** Nothing is quite so frustrating for depressed people when others say, 'Oh yes, I get depressed every now and then and I find doing X is helpful'. It is a little like saying you find sunscreen helpful to treat melanomas.
6. **Medication and extreme therapies:** Many people have very definite views on medication for psychological conditions. Telling someone that

they should not be taking their medication, that all psychiatric medications are harmful or avoidable, that herbal products will be sufficient or that they cannot live with psychological 'crutches' may cost a young person their life.

In recent years, there has been a spate of reports in the United Kingdom and Europe about the possibility that selective serotonin re-uptake inhibitors (SSRIs) caused suicide. The effect was that doctors in the United Kingdom and in many parts of Europe stopped prescribing SSRIs as much. Sadly, subsequent studies indicate this effect was minor or non-existent. The association between treatment with SSRIs and suicide in children and adolescents on the individual and ecological level were examined in a nationwide Danish pharmaco-epidemiological register-linkage study[13] including all persons aged 10–17 years treated with antidepressants during the period 1995–1999 (n = 2,569) and a randomly selected control population (n = 50,000). They analysed the relative risk (RR) of suicide according to antidepressant treatment corrected for psychiatric hospital contact to minimise the problem of confounding by indication. The use of SSRIs among children and adolescents increased substantially during the study period, but the suicide rate remained stable. Among 42 suicides nationally aged 10–17 years at death, none was treated with SSRIs within two weeks prior to suicide. The rate of suicide associated with SSRIs (RR = 4.47), however, was not significant when adjusted for severity of illness. Conclusively, they were not able to identify an association between treatment with SSRIs and completed suicide among children and adolescents. Media and public health warnings based upon strongly held ideology rather than scientific wisdom can do great harm in their own right.

When all psychological therapies fail, multiple medications have failed and tormented self-preoccupation with suicide prevails, electroconvulsive therapy may sometimes be needed. It has been consistently shown to work in those rare situations where not much else does and, with modern technologies, does not cause the side-effects that once concerned so many people.[14]

7 **Treatment does not always work straight away, but it does work:** The most prevalent thoughts in a young person's mind are that they will never get better, that life will never get better and that, no matter what they do, the struggle is pointless. All the evidence is that major depression in the young, untreated, is one of the most malignant disorders for quality of life and chronicity of course. Thus it is called major depression for a reason. Depression is one of the most treatable disorders in medicine.

8 **Patience, persistence and predictability:** These are what most depressed people need. Impulsive over-reactions with poorly thought-out solutions rarely help.

9 **Avoid make or break solutions:** High risk interventions that aim at one-off confrontations to resolve long-term depression rarely deliver the desired outcomes and frequently precipitate a crisis which may have very negative consequences.

10 **When everyone is worried it is worth asking for outside help:** The school can act as an effective trigger for a mental health review when concerns are raised about the level of impairment of the young person or their safety.

> **Practice Point**
>
> It is very difficult to deal with chronic, complicated or severe depression without the coordinated care of general practitioners, paediatricians, psychologists and psychiatrists, as well as a coordinated approach with family, school teachers, counselling and support staff. Clinicians in remote regions and poor communities are sometimes forced to provide all these roles as best they can.

Psychological treatments
- **Cognitive behaviour therapy (CBT)** – for mild and moderate depression and to prevent relapse in those who have had effectively treated depressive episodes, cognitive behaviour therapy is usually helpful for those with a mental age greater than 8–10 years. Psychologists are usually highly skilled in this therapy and are able to assist.
- There are **many other forms of psychotherapy** – all may be helpful and most are administered by psychologists and social workers. So long as the patient is not too unwell to engage with treatment and is compliant, most of these therapies are non-specifically helpful.
- **Contextual treatments** – such as family therapy, group therapies and in-patient milieu therapy have shown reasonable results but most have been conducted in naturalistic rather than randomised, placebo-controlled trials. Most clinicians agree that these are good measures to foster family consent and support for the treatment process, reduce isolation and loneliness, and to ensure safety while medical care is being delivered.

Biological treatments
Medication
The more severe the depression, the better medications are found to work against placebo and against other forms of treatment. Noradrenergic medications such as venlafaxine, the tricyclics, reboxetine and mirtazapine are generally less likely to help the younger patient while serotonergic medications such as the SSRIs are more likely to help. The greatest evidence associated with efficacy is with fluoxetine, perhaps because it has been around the longest. It is a non-sedating antidepressant and anxiolytic. However its long half-life makes it especially important to start low and go slow with commencement doses of 0.1 mg/kg/day moving up to 0.6 mg/kg/day over a period of 12 weeks.
- Motor restlessness and agitation are the most common side-effects with sleeplessness, initial anxiety and nausea being frequent.
- Hypomania or frank mania suggest underlying bipolarity, and cross tapering to a mood stabiliser such as valproate should be considered.
- Extrapyramidal side-effects, though uncommon, can be encountered, such as nuchal rigidity with headache and dystonia because of indirect impact on the basal ganglia by serotonin.

- Rare side-effects such as:
  - Serotonergic syndrome should be considered when autonomic and temperature instability are encountered, together with confusion or diaphoresis
  - Syndrome of inappropriate ADH (SIADH) when headaches, confusion, nausea, seizures or hyponatremia are encountered.

Other commonly used SSRIs in childhood include sertraline, fluvoxamine, citalopram and escitalopram. These have more linear kinetics than fluoxetine and are not as subject to CYP 450 2D6 interactions because of metaboliser status. Unlike mood stabilisers or antipsychotics, antidepressants are rarely being used for an acute response and can therefore be subject to the general maxim 'start low and go slow'. Most of these are non-sedating, despite various marketing statements. Therefore if sedation for insomnia, reduction of hyper-arousal, agitation or psychotic symptoms are required, atypical antipsychotics such as quetiapine and olanzapine are helpful acutely and sub-acutely. Benzodiazepines are usually avoided in children and young people, except for acute intramuscular or intravenous sedation to prevent self-harm or aggression, because of behavioural and emotional disinhibition associated with their use. When combinations of psychotropic medications are being considered, it is wise for the paediatrician to consult with a child psychiatrist.

Complications

The most common complications are refusal to seek help, to accept help and to comply with medications. Helping the patients not to give up on themselves is key to recovery. Helping the family not to treat depression as a minor problem that their children will grow out of is equally important. Substance abuse is common to seek relief or oblivion. Inappropriate expectations of rapid recovery by the patient and their family need to be checked by framing the disorder as a longer term problem with initial improvement after 6–12 weeks and a 1–2 year recovery period as a minimum. Fluctuating help acceptance and compliance improves with persistence on the clinician's part.

SUB-THRESHOLD DEPRESSIVE DISORDER

The life-time prevalence of sub-threshold depressive disorder is as high as 26 per cent of all young people under 18 years[15] with approximately two-thirds going on to full threshold depressive syndromes over a 15-year follow-up period. Sub-threshold does not mean sub-clinical. Most of these young people are quite impaired. They just do not reach adult criteria for individual items even though they do for functional impairment. Factors predictive of developing full-blown depressive picture are:
- Being female
- More severe functional impairment
- Comorbid medical symptoms and/or conditions
- Persistent suicidal ideation
- Persistent anxiety symptoms
- Family history loaded for depression.

Sub-threshold disorder should be treated as depressive disorder if the functional impairment, risk factors or consequences of impairment threaten, even where a number of diagnostic items seem to be lacking.

BIPOLAR DISORDER
Defining characteristics
- **Mania:** Those characteristics of mania that do not overlap with ADHD include elation, grandiosity, flight of ideas or racing of thoughts with pressured speech and decreased need for sleep. Those that most commonly overlap with ADHD include distractibility and hyperactivity. The most sensitive but least specific symptom is irritability with major overlap with ODD.
- **Depression:** The more they suffer from the following features, and the more extreme those features are, the more likely the depression will convert into bipolar disorder:[16,17]
  - Increased severity
  - Younger onset
  - Inability to enjoy life (anhedonia)
  - Suicidality
  - Expressing hopelessness
  - Requiring hospitalisation
  - Escalating medication requirements
  - Increased comorbidity including conduct disorder, ADHD, ODD, OCD and alcohol abuse
  - Family history of bipolar disorder
  - Rapid onset of the depressive episode
  - Psychomotor retardation
  - Associated psychotic symptoms
  - Medication (antidepressants and stimulant mainly) associated switching to bipolarity.
- **Mixed:** May have simultaneously sadness, anger, joyful ebullience and driven desperation. This has the effect of seeming insincere, gaming or play-acting, when it is mild, and psychotic or personality-disordered, when severe. Turmoil, volatility and 'driven and desperate', seem appropriate descriptors. These states are more common in adolescents especially.
- **Psychosis:** Visual and 'soft' hallucinations ('are they/aren't they') tend to be more common and delusions less common the younger the child.
- **Rapid or ultradian cycling:** At least four episodes of depression or mania in the same year is rapid cycling. Many young people are ultra-rapid or ultradian cyclers with multiple, extreme mood cycles in the same day.
- **Type I and type II:** These are poorly discriminated in many studies but type 1 includes those with psychosis and frank mania.
- **Bipolar sub-threshold:** See below.
- **Bipolar spectrum disorder:** This includes all varieties of bipolar disorder including sub-threshold disorder so long as they meet criteria for functional impairment and persist sufficiently long to be of clinical concern.
- **Distress:** The deep distress during episodes makes the reality of present help or future cure seem unlikely, or hollow promises. The sudden changes in feeling states make the fear of recurrence a major secondary feature of the disorder. The 'roller-coaster' phenomenon of rapidly changing mood, which drives the young person, rather than being driven by them, makes them hostage to an unpredictable master. Each person has a characteristic signature pattern of mood dysregulation. However the afternoon and early evening tsunami pattern is most characteristic with rising agitation

after about 3 pm and beginning to settle around 8–9 pm. Unalloyed elation and euphoria are less common than mixed states with a driven and desperate quality. Hopelessness and anhedonia (loss of interest and inability to experience pleasure) may be profound but short-lasting only to return again and again. Inability to make a lasting decision because decision making is based upon conviction, and conviction is affected by mood, can lead to profound distress, especially when the decisions involve relationships, vocation or long-term plans.

- **Dysfunction:** The striking feature of children and young people with bipolar disorder is their tendency to perform below their abilities and potential. This is mostly due to concentration and organisational capacities being ravaged by the disorder, despite the preservation of intellect. These cognitive impairments can, and often do, continue in children and young people throughout the inter-episodic periods and are made worse by multiple untreated episodes in the developing period of brain maturation, i.e. childhood and adolescence. They find school difficult and teachers are prone to over-expect and be disappointed. Intensity of emotion and periods of grandiosity or ebullience are mistaken for 'cockyness' and the need to be 'taken down a peg or two'. Substance abuse, self-harm and suicidal ideation, with impulsive sudden attempts and little warning, are common. Parents find themselves following the rollercoaster until they realise what is happening and receive help. When depression and distress are mainly manifested in anger or aggression, the possibility of juvenile offending is increased. Substance and alcohol abuse increase the likelihood of this scenario.

Prevalence

Point prevalence of pre-pubertal bipolar illness is at 0.2–0.4 per cent. Lifetime prevalence of pre-pubertal and early adolescent bipolar disorder remains uncertain.

Life-time prevalence estimates in 13–17 year olds are:[18]
- Bipolar type I disorder 0.5 per cent
- Bipolar type II disorder 1.8 per cent
- Sub-threshold disorder 4.3 per cent.

Therefore the composite category adolescent bipolar spectrum disorder is 6.6 per cent, i.e. around one in 20 adolescents will satisfy the criteria of bipolar spectrum disorder where only one in around 40 will satisfy the narrower criteria. Less than one in 200 children will satisfy the criteria for pre-pubertal and early adolescent bipolar disorder, and perhaps as few as one in 500.

Aetiology

Aetiology of early onset mood disorders[19] and mood disorders at any age cover a great deal of similar territory.[20] Bipolar disorder has extremely strong heritability with links to schizophrenia on the one hand and depression on the other. Heritability increases with decreasing age of onset. Most research at the present time indicates that it is a non-dominant hemisphere disorder of mood regulation involving all the same areas of the brain as depressive disorder but with more widespread disruption to long-term cognitive function (so called hypofrontality) including the executive functions of planning, sequencing, organisation and initiation, together with attention and concentration.[21] Most critically, the profound, chronic, inter-episodic disruption of sleep cycles and diurnal function generally, implicates brainstem and reticular activating systems and the so-called Circadian Locomotor Output Cycles Kaput (CLOCK) genes. Monoamines and gamma amino butyric acid (GABA) are prominent in all causal discussions. Comorbidity with anxiety and obsessionality are common.

Differential diagnosis

Common differentials in pre-pubertal children
- ADHD
- Major depression
- Conduct disorder
- Oppositional defiant disorder
- Complex post-traumatic stress disorder.

Common differentials in adolescence
- Major depression
- Complex post-traumatic stress disorder
- Borderline personality disorder (inappropriate but often used)
- Conduct disorder.

Less common differentials of any age group
- Hyperthyroidism
- Hypoparathyroidism
- Cerebral lupus erythematosus.

Treatment

Practical advice

Some of the suggestions for helping those with bipolar disorder are good for all young people generally. However, in the case of young people with bipolar disorder these suggestions can make the difference between being overwhelmed and ill and being able to have a more normal life.

1. **Routine:** Try to have daily routine.
2. **Reduce the load:** Make sure the routine does not get overloaded. Parents and teachers need to help by monitoring the whole program so that individual demands like sport and academic interests do not provide too much pressure.
3. **Reducing time pressure:** When in doubt as to whether to do something or not, do less and give more time to do it.
4. **Time for sleep and being slack:** Keep regular hours of sleep and relaxation with quiet times timetabled in.
5. **Giving brakes not just accelerators:** Do not push the young person based on their potential but restrain them based on their need for brakes. Even when they resent the restraint they will also often be relieved.
6. **Interpret boredom:** 'I'm bored' can be interpreted as lack of structure and disinterest in schoolwork, as anxious avoidance and difficulty organising themselves. The parts of their brain involved with planning and organising themselves is functioning less well than most adolescents.
7. **Resist the urge to 'put them in their place':** Do not be taken in by bravado and 'life of the party' and 'clown of the classroom' behaviour. Their verbal dexterity is often covering their deep unease with themselves

and their lives. They do not need 'taking down a peg or two' but gently and sympathetically acknowledging their strengths and talking to in a non-public forum.
8. **Achieving personal milestones not public ones:** Keep goals long term and personal, not short term and recognition-oriented. For example, having good friends and being a good friend, enjoying non-competitive activities and looking after their own health and wellbeing. Attempting to be the best, beating others and risk-taking are all very destructive to these young people in the long run. They become anxious, driven, unhappy and are more likely to abuse drugs and alcohol and lose friends.
9. **Making people aware of their own fluctuations in mood:** Help the young person to understand that sometimes feelings change without reasons, and sometimes reasons are sought for mood changes after the fact.
10. **Use alcohol sparingly, if at all, and avoid all illicit substances:** This is often a process of gradual trial and error in coming to accept this because substances and alcohol are so popular in youth culture.

Psychological treatments
- **Cognitive behaviour therapy** – has been modified to address issues of identity around the changes to an individual's life when mood stability finally comes and some of the intensity of life diminishes. This is a more established problem in adulthood.
- **Psycho-education** – the biggest component of treatment is the practical explanation of illness. In particular, encouraging families not to react to all emotional expression as if it is a form of psychopathology and that normal emotions are still possible, even in those with mood disorders.

Contextual treatments
In-patient treatment under mental legislation is often needed to provide the context in which treatment can be reliably provided. Protecting young people from self-harm and suicidal attempts is a priority.

Biological treatments
1. **Acute safety and symptom relief:** Sedating antipsychotics such as olanzapine and quetiapine may be helpful after acute safety has been established. As time goes on moving to less sedating antipsychotics (ziprasidone, amisulpride, aripiprazole) for diurnal periods of agitation, and that cause less weight gain, is essential if young people are to remain compliant with medications. These treatments are to be instituted under the direction of a psychiatrist.
2. **Mood stabilisation:** Use valproate (short term) for ease of use and lithium and lamotrigine (long term) to avoid weight gain and prevent the serious depression and suicidality.
3. **Monitoring:**
    - Lithium levels (trough +/– one hour): 0.6–8 mmols/L with toleration of lower levels if tremor, polyuria or thyroid suppression are a problem. Even levels of 0.4–0.6 mmols/L have been found to be therapeutic in young people, especially those who are aggressive and suicidal. Commencement doses for children of 8–13 years are usually 125 mgs b.d. and those 13 years or over 250 mgs b.d. Levels are usually taken after 48 hours to ensure steady state.

- Valproate levels (trough +/− one hour): 500–600 micromols/L. Young women should be on contraception and folic acid 5 mgms mane to minimise the risk of teratogenic effects on any pregnancy. Levels are usually taken after 5 days of treatment to ensure steady state.
- Lamotrigine: monitoring for Steven Johnson syndrome should be commenced at 12.5 mg mane and elevated by 12.5 mgs/day, each week, in two divided doses after the first week. It is an excellent long-term medication for prevention of depression in bipolar disorder and is weight neutral. Provided the dosing is pursued slowly it is uncommon to encounter a significant rash. The final dose should be 3 mgs/kg/day in two divided doses, mane and nocte. Levels are of little value at this stage.

Complications

Bipolar disorder is a condition that looks different at different times of the day, with different people, in different contexts. Very real and troubling clinical problems with substantial risk of associated suicide, self-injury, harm to others, complications with the law, and breakdown of placement with family or alternate care arrangements are often not seen as having a mood disorder component for many years because the picture looked different to different examiners at different times. In-patient admissions of some weeks are often needed to identify the ultradian mood changes.

Course and prognosis

- **Pre-pubertal bipolar disorder:** This condition despite its apparent 'popularity' has a pernicious and chronic course with reduced inter-episodic recovery, mixed states, ultradian cycling and poor psychosocial adjustment in more than half the children. Executive function is especially impaired with consequent impact on school function, despite adequate intellectual level.[22,23]
- **Adolescent bipolar disorder:** Most adolescent onset disorder is depressive in nature providing a great deal of room for diagnostic confusion. Episode rate of recovery from the index episode is generally high with depressive episodes usually taking around 6 months to recover, while manic episodes take around three months. The recurrence rate means that almost 40 per cent remain chronically impaired, 50 per cent have recurrence within a two-year period and 20 per cent make substantial attempts at suicide with a life-time risk of 19 per cent. Almost a quarter of the time when these young people are followed up they indicate that they are ill and present with the full syndromal picture.[24]

Sub-threshold bipolar disorder

The intermittently, affectively dysregulated young person who does not reach threshold criteria for bipolar disorder may be quite functionally impaired on the one hand, or have no enduring affective disorder beyond adolescence on the other. Sub-threshold does not mean sub-clinical. Most of these young people are quite impaired. They just do not reach adult-derived criteria for individual items even though they do for functional impairment. Where the functional impairment or risks represent clinical thresholds for treatment, the condition should be treated in exactly the same manner as the full threshold disorder. The child, the risks and impairments of the child's quality of life are being treated, not the diagnosis.

CONCLUSION: WHERE IS THE FIELD GOING FROM HERE?

It is likely that there will be ongoing debates about diagnosis of mood disorders in children and young people. Adopting a protective approach to children in general is the sign of a healthy society. If unnecessary exposure of young people to medical treatments is one of those risks, then it is only appropriate that there should be concern about inappropriate medicalisation of 'normal sadness'. At this stage the main danger seems to be predominantly in the opposite direction with the vast majority of children and young people with very substantial disorder ignored, minimised or under-treated, based on quite naïve concepts about childhood.

The consequent danger of young people finding inappropriate solutions in substance abuse or attempting to end their lives remains a threat against which they also need to be protected. It is likely that within five years the emergence of brain-based diagnosis will largely replace the current diagnostic system. However treatments lag behind diagnosis and it is also likely that our current treatments will remain as limited as they are for another decade. Despite these provisos, much can be done to improve quality of life, reduce family and patient uncertainty, and maximise support by providing symptomatic relief and reliable information.

CLINICAL PEARLS

1 **The first clinical question to ask in mood disorders is not 'which diagnosis?' but 'how ill is the child?'**

Functional impairment trumps the type of condition the patient is experiencing. Many disorders in child and adolescent psychiatry are sub-threshold diagnostically within adult-based diagnostic systems, but very real and troubling clinical problems with substantial risk.

2 **When uncertain as to whether depression is unipolar or bipolar depression, stabilise mood before commencing an antidepressant.**

Where the clinical picture is depression but the child is under 14 years, has a bipolar family history and is feeling especially hopeless, consider using a mood stabiliser first rather than moving straight to an antidepressant.

3 **Use sedative medications acutely and weight-neutral medications long term.**

In crisis, use medications that have good anti-agitation properties and will give good sleep (e.g. olanzapine, valproate and quetiapine) and have less tendency to have interactions or CYP P450 metaboliser problems. But if a medication sedates, it usually puts on weight. Switching to non-weight gaining medications as time goes on, such as ziprasidone, amisulpride, aripirazole and lamotrigine, depending on the indications, improves compliance and reduces metabolic syndrome and its consequences.

4 **When in doubt, consult with child psychiatry colleagues.**

Conflict of interest

The author has no received no funding or benefit from any pharmaceutical company and has no financial interest in their welfare.

REFERENCES

1. Kraepelin E. Manic depressive insanity and paranoia. Edinburgh, Scotland: E & S Livingstone; 1921. (Kraepelin's concept of manic depressive illness included almost all depressive conditions of any severity as well as what we refer to as bipolar disorder, with no obvious organic cause.)
2. Joyce PR, Mitchell PB. Mood disorders: recognition and treatment. Sydney: UNSW Press; 2004
3. Harrington R, Fudge H, Rutter M, et al. Adult outcomes of childhood and adolescent depression: II. Links with antisocial disorders. Journal of the American Academy of Child & Adolescent Psychiatry 1991;30(3):434–9
4. Geller B, Delbello M. Bipolar disorder in childhood and early adolescence. New York: Guildford Press; 2005
5. Kessler RC, Avenevoli S, Green J, et al. National comorbidity survey replication adolescent supplement (NCS-A): III. concordance of DSM-IV/CIDI diagnoses with clinical reassessments. Journal of the American Academy of Child & Adolescent Psychiatry 2009;48(4):386–99
6. Pavuluri MN, West A, Hill SK, et al. Neurocognitive function in pediatric bipolar disorder: 3-year follow-up shows cognitive development lagging behind healthy youths. Journal of the American Academy of Child & Adolescent Psychiatry 2009;48(3): 299–307
7. Neuman RJ, Geller B, Rice JP, et al. Increased prevalence and earlier onset of mood disorders among relatives of prepubertal versus adult probands. Journal of the American Academy of Child & Adolescent Psychiatry 1997;36(4):466–73
8. Sullivan PF, Neale MC, Kendler KS. Genetic epidemiology of major depression: review and meta-analysis. American Journal of Psychiatry 2000;157(10):1552
9. Geller B, Zimerman B, Williams M, et al. Bipolar disorder at prospective follow-up of adults who had prepubertal major depressive disorder. American Journal of Psychiatry 2001;158(1):125
10. Zubenko GS, Zubenko WN, Spiker DG, et al. Malignancy of recurrent, early onset major depression: A family study. American Journal of Medical Genetics 2001;105(8): 690–9
11. Smith D, Muir W, Blackwood D. Genetics of early-onset depression. British Journal of Psychiatry: The Journal of Mental Science 2003;182:363; author reply 64
12. Birmaher B, Abelaez C, Brent D. Course and outcome of child and adolescent major depressive disorder. Child Adolesc Psychiatry Clin N Am 2002:11:619–37; Eur Child Adolesc Psychiatry 2006 Jun;15(4):232–40
13. Søndergård L, Kvist K, Andersen PK, et al. Do antidepressants precipitate youth suicide?: A nationwide pharmacoepidemiological study. Eur Child Adolesc Psychiatry 2006 Jun;15(4):232–40
14. Ghaziuddin N, Kutcher SP, Knapp P, et al. Practice parameter for use of electroconvulsive therapy with adolescents. Work Group on Quality Issues; AACAP Am Acad Child Psychiatry 2004 Dec;43(12):1521–39
15. Klein DN, Shankman SA, Lewinsohn PM, et al. Subthreshold depressive disorder in adolescents: Predictors of escalation to full-syndrome depressive disorders. Journal of the American Academy of Child & Adolescent Psychiatry 2009;48(7):703–10
16. Strober M, Carlson G. Bipolar illness in adolescents with major depression: Clinical, genetic, and psychopharmacologic predictors in a three- to four-year prospective follow-up investigation. Archives of General Psychiatry 1982;39(5):549–55
17. Wozniak J, Spencer T, Biederman J, et al. The clinical characteristics of unipolar vs. bipolar major depression in ADHD youth. Journal of Affective Disorders 2004;82(1001):S59–69
18. Kessler RC, Avenevoli S, Green J, et al. National comorbidity survey replication adolescent supplement (NCS-A): III. concordance of DSM-IV/CIDI diagnoses with clinical reassessments. Journal of the American Academy of Child & Adolescent Psychiatry 2009;48(4):386–99
19. Goodwin FK, Jamison KR. Manic-depressive illness: bipolar disorders and recurrent depression. New York: Oxford University Press; 2007

20 Manji HK, Zarate CA, editors. Behavioural neurobiology of bipolar disorder and its treatment. New York: Springer: 2011
21 Biederman J, Faraone SV, Wozniak J, et al. Further evidence of unique developmental phenotypic correlates of pediatric bipolar disorder: findings from a large sample of clinically referred preadolescent children assessed over the last 7 years. Journal of Affective Disorders 2004;82(1001):S45–58
22 Geller B, Tillman R. Prepubertal and early adolescent bipolar 1 disorder: Review of diagnostic validation by Robins and Guze criteria. J Clin Psychiatry 2005;66(Suppl 7):21–8
23 Todd RT, Botteron KN. Etiology and genetics of early-onset mood disorders. Child Adolesc Psychiatric Clin N America 2002;11:499–518
24 Strober M, Schmidt-Lackner S, Freeman R, et al. Recovery and relapse in adolescents with bipolar affective illness: a five-year naturalistic, prospective follow-up. Journal of the American Academy of Child & Adolescent Psychiatry 1995;34(6):724–31

FURTHER READING

Goodwin FK, Jamison KR. Manic-depressive illness: bipolar disorders and recurrent depression. New York: Oxford University Press; 2007 (The definitive guide to mood disorders in the international literature.)

Joyce PR, Mitchell PB. Mood disorders: recognition and treatment. Sydney: UNSW Press; 2004 (The best brief guide to mood disorders but concentrates mainly on adult disorder.)

Manji HK, Zarate CA, editors. Behavioural neurobiology of bipolar disorder and its treatment. New York: Springer; 2011 (The state of the art overview of the neurobiology of bipolar disorder.)

12

Cerebral palsy

Sandra Johnson with
Mary-Clare Waugh

DEFINITIONS

The definition for cerebral palsy (CP) refers to a heterogeneous group of disorders with various aetiologies but all associated with a static motor impairment, and many now refer to the presentation as 'the cerebral palsies'.

An international workshop in 2006 defined CP as 'a group of permanent disorders of the development of movement and posture, causing activity limitation, that are attributed to non-progressive disturbances that occurred in the developing fetal or infant brain'. The motor disorders of cerebral palsy are often accompanied by disturbances of sensation, perception, cognition, communication, behaviour, epilepsy and secondary musculoskeletal problems.[1] The timing of the insult to the developing brain is conventionally under two years of postnatal age.

There are difficulties regarding the definition of CP, which have been addressed by Fiona Stanley et al.[2] While the descriptive term is useful for understanding and managing the condition, it is less useful in research because the definition is not specific and there is heterogeneity in causation. Using classifications based on function are proving to be more useful in clinical and research arenas. A review of the changing inclusion criteria for CP highlights the evolving situation but notes that neurodegenerative conditions, neuromuscular conditions, tumours and neural tube defects are always excluded.[3]

PREVALENCE

Prevalence refers to the number of existing cases in a population and requires large surveys to establish estimates. The overall rate for CP is around 2–2.5 per 1000 live births in developed countries.[4] The rate of CP differs between different geographic areas and over time, and is related to aetiology or causal pathways for the condition.

The prevalence of CP increases with decrease in gestational age at birth, and in extremely low gestational age (<28 weeks) the prevalence is in the order of 100 times that of infants born at term.[4] However, more than half of CP arises in infants of normal birth weight (term or near-term infants) and there has been no reduction in prevalence of CP in this group over recent decades.[5]

CLASSIFICATION

There are several potential classification systems for CP.[6] These can be topographical, functional or based on the motor impairment.

Blair and Stanley proposed that more specific definitions be used for epidemiological studies to allow comparison of results. The great majority of persons with CP (>80 per cent) have spastic cerebral palsy. However the clinical features of spastic CP vary with respect to body distribution, severity of spasticity and the accompanying impairments, depending on the extent and location of brain damage. There have been several attempts to classify this variation but because the underlying disease is not composed of discrete syndromes this has proved difficult. Many people use classifications referring to topography of spasticity that include categories such as monoplegia, paraplegia, diplegia, triplegia, quadriplegia and double hemiplegia. While such categories obviously refer to the number of limbs affected by spasticity, the details of the criteria defining each category vary significantly between observers and may include criteria referring to relative severity of spasticity between body parts and accompanying impairments, as well as how many limbs are affected by spasticity. When seeking classification (for research purposes) or describing a patient (for the clinic), it is advisable to describe clearly the impairments.

An early classification system rarely used today, which provided a physiological and topographical classification, is that of the Nomenclature and Classification Committee of the American Academy for Cerebral Palsy,[7] which divides CP into two main groups:
1   Pyramidal – where spasticity is the prominent feature
2   Extrapyramidal – where chorea, athetosis, dystonia and ataxia are prominent features.

The European network, Surveillance of Cerebral Palsy in Europe (SCPE),[8] conducted population-based surveillance in 14 centres across Europe and used a simple classification, which was adopted by non-European countries, consisting of:
- Unilateral spastic – involves the pyramidal tract, with increased tone and reflexes on one side of body
- Bilateral spastic – as above but involving both sides of body
- Dyskinetic – abnormal movements such as choreoathetosis involving all limbs with facial grimacing and severe oromotor problems; dystonic posturing may also be a feature
- Ataxic – broad-based gait with truncal titubation; unsteady on feet
- Mixed – can include any combination of the above.

Work continues to be done to improve the reliability of this classification system.

Classification using definitions based on motor type, distribution, and functional ability are now routine in the literature and there exists a body of evidence linking the increased risk of comorbidities and prognosis to the subtypes as classified by function.

The classification systems GMFCS, MACS and CFCS are based on function, and are being used in conjunction with typographical and motor impairment descriptors. The FMS is a performance measure of a child's current motor ability and adds to the information of GMFCS.

The Gross Motor Function Classification System (GMFCS) is a five-level classification system that describes the gross motor function of children and young persons with cerebral palsy. The classification is based on their self-initiated movement with emphasis on sitting, walking and wheeled mobility. GMFCS 1 can walk without limitations and GMFCS 5 require a carer-propelled wheelchair for mobility. Distinctions between levels are based on functional abilities, the need for assistive technology including hand-held mobility devices (walkers, crutches or canes) or wheeled mobility. The child can be allocated a GMFCS classification as early as two years of age and this can assist with prognosis about future mobility function as the GMFCS curves indicate. From six years of age a child usually remains in their classification unless other problems emerge.

The original version of 1997 was expanded and revised (GMFCS - E&R) in 2007 to include young people of 12–18 years.

GMFCS

Clinicians can use the GMFCS to prognosticate about function, facilitate clear communication and direct treatment programs. This classification system is used almost ubiquitously in current research in CP.[9–12]
I   Walks without limitations
II   Walks with limitations
III Walks with hand-held mobility device
IV   Self-mobility with limitations, e.g. rolls or crawls; may use powered mobility
V   Transported in a manual wheelchair, carer propelled.

FMS

The functional mobility scale (FMS) is a sensitive and reliable performance measure, which measures how a child mobilises over various distances (5 metres, 50 metres and 500 metres) incorporating the use of aids. The scale was purposely designed and rated in reverse ordering when compared with the GMFCS, i.e. 6 is the most able and 1 the least able.
Rating 6 = independent on all surfaces
Rating 5 = independent on level surfaces
Rating 4 = uses sticks (one or two)
Rating 3 = uses crutches
Rating 2 = uses a walker or frame
Rating 1 = uses a wheelchair

Conventionally, this is written as FMS 5 5 1 indicating that the child walks independently on level surfaces over 5 and 50 metres but requires a wheelchair to mobilise 500 metres.[13]

MACS

The Manual Ability Classification System (MACS) describes how children with cerebral palsy use their hands to handle objects in daily activities. Like the GMFCS, the MACS has five levels with 1 the most able and 5 the least able. The levels are based on the child's self-initiated ability to handle objects and their need for assistance or adaptation to perform manual activities in everyday life.[14]
1   Handles objects easily and successfully
2   Handles most objects but with somewhat reduced quality and or speed of achievement
3   Handles objects with difficulty: needs help to prepare and or modify activities

4   Handles a limited selection of easily managed objects in adapted situations
5   Does not handle objects and has severely limited ability to perform even simple actions.

CFCS

The Communication Functional Classification System (CFCS) is in the process of being validated as a tool to classify communication in CP using similar levels of ability with 1 being the most able communicator and 5 unable to communicate:[15]
1   Effective sender–receiver with unfamiliar and familiar partners
2   Effective but slower sender–receiver with unfamiliar and familiar partners
3   Effective sender–receiver with familiar partners
4   Inconsistent sender and/or receiver with familiar partners
5   Seldom effective sender–receiver even with familiar partners.

Gage classification

The Winters Gage Hick Classification of hemiplegia (unilateral) CP assists with classification and management of the lower limb in hemiplegic CP, and is commonly referred to as the Gage classification.[16]
- Gage type 1 = Equinus in swing only.
- Gage type 2 = Ankle plantar flexion throughout the gait cycle (swing and stance) with fixed or dynamic contracture of the calf, posterior tibial and/or long toe flexors.
- Gage type 3 = As in type 2 plus limited knee flexion in swing. Compensatory gait patterns are vaulting (hip hitching) on the opposite side or circumduction of affected side.
- Gage Type 4 = Involvement as for type 3 plus hip flexors and adductors, so there is hip flexion and adduction in swing. There is a compensatory lumbar lordosis in terminal stance to account for the limited hip motion.

Example

A child can be classified according to function at a number of different levels. One of the advantages of this system is that it allows clear communication between clinicians and researchers about the extent of a child's cerebral palsy regardless of aetiology. For example:
1   Spastic diplegic CP could be described as bilateral spastic CP: GMFCS III, FMS 2 2 1, MACS 2, CFCS 1.
2   Spastic dystonic triplegia CP could be described as bilateral spastic dystonic CP: GMFCS V, MACS 2, CFCS 3.
3   Right hemiplegic CP could be described as right unilateral spastic CP: GMFCS I, FMS 5 5 5, Gage 2, MACS 2, CFCS 1.

Recent approach

A more recent classification system that involves four major dimensions was developed by an executive committee at an international workshop in 2006[1]:
1   Motor abnormalities
    ○   nature and typology – tone and movement disorder: spastic, dyskinetic (including dystonia and choreoathetosis), ataxic. Unilateral or bilateral involvement

    ○ functional motor abilities – extent to which person is limited by the motor function (GMFCS and MACS)
2 Accompanying impairments
    ○ sensory problems, seizures, behaviour, communication (CFCS), cognitive deficits
3 Anatomical and neuroimaging findings
    ○ anatomical distribution
    ○ neuroimaging findings
4 Causation and timing
    ○ whether there is a clearly defined cause/brain malformation
    ○ presumed time frame of injury.

The committee recommended that this classification system be used by researchers and clinicians, although the need for continued development in future years to improve the classification of CP was acknowledged.

Practice Point

Hypotonia is frequently seen in young children with CP, which then evolves into hypertonia. Truncal hypotonia is particularly common with spastic extremities. Isolated hypotonia is usually, but not always, accompanied by intellectual impairment. Some authors exclude all children with isolated hypotonia from the diagnosis of CP and others include only those whose hypotonia cannot be attributed to their intellectual impairment.

AETIOLOGY

The causal pathways leading to CP are numerous and there are many factors associated with increased risk.[2] However, in many cases of CP a satisfactory aetiological pathway cannot be found. Interestingly, about 10 per cent of children with CP in the European Cerebral Palsy Study had no abnormality on brain MRI.[17]

Gestational duration is the strongest predictor of CP risk.[8,18] The rate of CP in neonates born below 33 weeks gestation was found to be 30 times higher than those born at term in one research study.[19]

In relation to neonatal encephalopathy (NE) due to hypoxic ischaemic insult, Cowan et al. found that 80 per cent of term infants with NE had MRI findings consistent with hypoxia in the first two weeks after birth, showing that the use of magnetic resonance imaging (MRI) is becoming more important in recognising injury patterns.[20]

The development of the brain is complex and occurs in a systematic manner where each step has some influence on the next. Neuronal and glial precursors in the germinal zones lining the third and lateral ventricles migrate out to their final locations in the cerebral cortex during the first 20 weeks of gestation.[21] Thereafter rapid growth of all the structures occurs with myelination and synaptogenesis producing the circuits necessary for normal function of the brain after birth. Consequently disruption of the process at any stage of development can lead to dysfunction and abnormality. In CP damage to the developing brain can occur up to two years of age.

Antenatal risk factors for CP include chromosomal and genetic abnormalities, maternal infection (particularly TORCH infections), vascular causes (thrombotic phenomena involving the placenta), Factor V leiden (variant of Factor V which is abnormal and leads to hypercoaguability), causes of intrauterine growth retardation, toxins (e.g. alcohol or methylmercury exposure) and multiple births,[22] especially where there is death of the co-fetus.[23,24] In the past some conditions were labelled as 'cerebral palsy' due to their non-progressive motor status. However, now due to improvements in diagnostic and imaging techniques these children have more specific diagnoses to explain their CP (e.g. some partial trisomies or X-linked hydrocephalus syndrome). These conditions are still labelled as CP, but their CP label should also include the additional information to explain their true underlying diagnosis.[3]

Intrapartum causes include intrapartum asphyxia as the most recognised, where CP is likely to occur in the most severe cases. The International Cerebral Palsy Task Force comprising members from a wide range of clinical and scientific specialties produced the International Consensus Statement in 1999, which allows experts to retrospectively determine whether an intrapartum event was the possible cause of CP.[25] According to the consensus, the outcome of CP is more likely to have had an intrapartum cause in the presence of the following (also refer to the criteria in the referenced article):

- A sentinel obstetric event: ruptured uterus, abruption of the placenta, cord prolapse or massive maternal haemorrhage
- Evidence of metabolic acidosis with arterial cord blood pH <7.00 and base deficit >12 mmol/L
- Apgar scores of 0–6 for longer than 5 minutes
- Early onset of moderate to severe neonatal encephalopathy (NE) in infants >34 weeks gestation. NE is defined as abnormal neurological findings on examination within 12 to 24 hours after birth with signs of cortical dysfunction; which includes lethargy, stupor and seizures in severe cases. In severe cases the signs last for more than 24 hours and ventilation is usually required
- Evidence of multisystem involvement, particularly compromised renal function[26]
- Neuroimaging findings consistent with acute cerebral injury.

Spastic quadriplegic or dyskinetic CP is the type of CP most likely to occur following intrapartum asphyxia. However there is a large body of research to show that in the majority of CP cases the cause is multifactorial, and intrapartum asphyxia as a sole sufficient cause for CP is uncommon.

Postnatal causes of cerebral palsy include kernicterus as a result of severe hyperbiliribinaemia, where athetosis and deafness are common sequelae. Other postnatal aetiologies include acquired brain injuries occurring under the age of two years, such as infections (meningitis and encephalitis), encephalopathies (Reye's syndrome, inherited metabolic disorders with decompensation), cerebrovascular accidents, traumatic brain injury and near drowning.

Acquired hemiplegia in childhood is a form of CP that occurs in early childhood during the period of rapid brain development. This may result from infection, thrombotic phenomenon, vascular accidents or trauma. It may occur following convulsions or might present with only paralysis. The cause of the hemiplegia is unknown in most cases and the onset can be insidious with parents gradually becoming aware of weakness on one side of the infant's body. The condition can also occur acutely and may be associated with a vascular cause.[27] There are many causes of vascular occlusion of the carotid artery and vertebro-basilar system, involving smaller arteries and arterioles, such as Kawasaki's syndrome, disseminated intravascular coagulation, polycythaemia (sickle cell disease) and serious metabolic disorders, to name a few. (See reference for further information and clinical presentation of vascular phenomena.[28])

CLINICAL PRESENTATION

The child with CP primarily presents with motor impairment involving one or more limbs affected by weakness, abnormal muscle tone and postures, abnormal movements (dyskinesias or ataxia), abnormal motor control and brisk reflexes. Ataxia may be present in isolation or in combination with other impairments.

The child's presentation depends on the extent of the underlying brain lesion. Many children with CP have both dystonia and spasticity present. Many CP cases are identified by high risk follow-up for asphyxia, low birth weight and other causes of acquired brain injury in the neonatal period. These children may at first be noted to have delayed motor milestones in early childhood. Usually the infants in this group are given physiotherapy and occupational therapy early, because their development is monitored on a regular basis and therapy support can be very helpful to parents even before the clinician is confident that the baby does have CP.

Hypertonicity (increased muscle tone) can be due to spasticity, dystonia, both spasticity and dystonia, or rigidity. Rigidity is however rarely seen in CP. Spasticity is the velocity dependent increase in stretch reflexes felt as a muscle is moved through its passive range of movement, manifest as a 'spastic catch' when the limb is moved quickly through its expected range of movement. The angle of 'catch' always occurs at the same angle, and after the 'catch' angle the limb can be moved out to its full range of movement, which may be reduced if there is an underlying contracture. Dystonia involves 'involuntary sustained muscle contractions resulting in sustained or intermittent muscle contractions causing twisting and repetitive movements, abnormal postures or both'. Dystonia does not display the consistent 'catch' angle as seen in spasticity when moving the joint quickly through its range of movement.[29–31]

There are a number of impairments and difficulties that accompany the motor deficits in CP including:
- Cognitive impairment – ranging from mild learning difficulties to intellectual impairment (the degree of impairment depends on the extent of the brain damage)
- Sensory deficits – vision and hearing impairments, sensation and proprioception difficulties
- Communication and speech difficulty – related to central processing problems, cognitive impairment and oromotor coordination difficulty
- Behaviour difficulties
- Feeding difficulty
    - due to problems with sucking, swallowing and tongue thrusting often as a result of pseudobulbar palsy
    - drooling
    - regurgitation of food and aspiration
    - gastro-oesophageal reflux
    - inability to feed orally in severe cases, requiring gastrostomy feeds

- Constipation
- Growth impairment – cortical sensory and motor pathways appear to be necessary for normal growth
- Respiratory problems
  - aspiration pneumonia
  - predisposition to chest infections
  - sleep apnoea obstructive and/or central
- Musculoskeletal problems
  - contractures due to increased tone or spasticity preventing muscle stretching
  - joint and boney deformity due to spasticity and/or dystonia and non-weight bearing
  - hip dislocation or subluxation (incidence closely related to GMFCS level)
  - scoliosis
- Seizures – particularly with severe brain damage or injury
- Other problems associated with the underlying condition – e.g. congenital syndromes with major organ involvement.

The frequency of the associated deficits in children with CP was reviewed by Russman, who noted an incidence of intellectual disability at 52 per cent, epilepsy around 45 per cent, visual defects 28 per cent, speech and language problems 38 per cent, and hearing impairment 12 per cent. The review also noted a high overall yield of abnormal neuroimaging findings in children with CP.[32]

CP presentation can be mild, moderate or severe. The clinical presentation also depends on the type of CP (see classifications).

In mild CP, e.g. GMFCS I or II, the child might not have an obvious motor deficit but may have difficulties with speech, communication and learning. Careful examination might reveal subtle weakness with changes in tone in one limb or on one side of the body, but these findings can be difficult to elicit.

In moderate CP, e.g. GMFCS III, there is usually a clearer picture of the motor deficit, with or without speech problems, sensory impairment and cognitive deficits. These children can have intellectual impairment that falls into the mild to moderate range on formal psychometric assessment. However, in some instances children with dystonia or athetosis have average to above-average intelligence, despite the extent of their motor deficits. The degree of physical impairment depends on the extent and location of the brain involvement, while the findings on examination depend on the type of CP.

Severe CP, e.g. GMFCS IV and V, is associated with significant disability including motor impairment and intellectual disability. These children with severe CP are dependent for care and their self-help skills are limited. They may be immobile due to severe spasticity and many are wheelchair dependent. Children with severe to profound CP are more likely to have seizures, and these children are also more likely to have four limb involvement, i.e. spastic double hemiplegia or spastic quadriplegia.

Practice Point

Severe dystonic CP (GMFCS IV and V) can be associated with normal intellect so beware of assuming that the severely physically disabled dystonic child is also severely intellectually disabled.

ASSESSMENT

The assessment of children with CP requires a multidisciplinary approach, as their needs are complex and incorporate intervention with many sub-specialists and allied health professionals. The aim of the doctor on the team is to obtain the medical history, examine the child to determine extent of the disability and to ensure that associated difficulties as discussed above are addressed. Investigations to determine an underlying cause will be needed at the initial assessment, although in the majority of instances no causative agent will be identified. As noted in a useful paper by Horridge 'the clinical judgement of the experienced clinician is more helpful than guidelines in deciding which investigations to do'.[33] This paper also gives a practical approach to assessment and investigation of the child with disability.

The diagnosis of CP is a clinical one, based on the history and physical examination. There is no laboratory investigation to confirm the diagnosis. Please see Text Box 12.1 for investigations that may be required, depending on the child's

---

TEXT BOX 12.1 Investigations for the child with CP

Initial
- Full blood count, creatine kinase, electrolytes (Ca^{2+} and Mg^{2+}): if indicated
- Uric acid: raised in Lesch-Nyhan syndrome
- Chromosome analysis: karyotype, fragile X, microarray comparative genomic hybridisation
- Urine: amino acid and organic acid screening for metabolic conditions
- Tests for thrombotic conditions in unilateral CP, e.g. Factor V Leiden variant
- Formal vision and hearing assessments
- Developmental assessment
- Psychometric and cognitive assessment at around 4 years of age
- Therapy assessment: speech, physiotherapy and OT.

X-ray
- X-ray hips at 12–24 months
- X-ray spine for scoliosis
- Chest X-ray if aspiration suspected
- Skull: thickening of bones, intracranial calcification.

Require neurology opinion
- Neuroimaging: MRI is more specific and sensitive than CT in detecting anatomical abnormalities that may point to causative brain lesions; MRI brain ideally should be done in all cases
- EEG: indicated where clinical seizures are present; may require EEG telemetry and sleep EEG to give more specific information
- Electromyogram: to differentiate myopathy from CP
- Nerve conduction studies to detect presence of neuropathy.

Genetics referral
- Required where there is any suspicion or finding to indicate hereditary or chromosomal disorder.

presentation and the physical findings on examination. All children with CP should have their vision and hearing assessed.

The allied health members of the team will assess the child's fine motor and functional skills (occupational therapist (OT)), speech and communications skills (speech therapist) and gross motor function and mobility skills (physiotherapist). Physiotherapists and OTs provide a program for promoting motor development and, where required, prescribe specific splints and equipment such as walking frames and wheelchairs. Nurses assist with continence, wound care and liaison with clinicians. Specialists in orthotics may also be part of the team to provide orthotics for the upper or lower limb, special boots and specialised braces, e.g. hip abduction brace. The psychologist will assess the child's cognitive and educational skills, and will also provide counselling support for the family as they come to terms with their child's disability. The social worker or clinic nurse often acts as the clinic's case manager or liaison officer for the family and see the child and family on a more regular basis.

Other sub-specialists involved in the assessment process include neurologists (assisting with the diagnosis or management of epilepsy), paediatric rehabilitation specialists (for spasticity and dystonia management), orthopaedic surgeons (to treat contractures and joint dislocations or subluxations), gastroenterologists and general surgeons (particularly where there are feeding difficulties and gastrostomy feeds are required). Genetic specialist involvement is essential where congenital chromosomal disorder or a familial cause is suspected, and they play a valuable role in early assessment even where no clear congenital disorder is identified, as this can be reassuring to the family. Other medical specialists may become involved, especially in severe CP, where there is multisystem involvement or as a result of congenital malformation.

Practice Point

These scenarios should alert the clinician to a diagnosis other than CP:
- Onset of abnormal motor signs in baby who was previously developing normally
- Motor problems in child with family history of motor problems
- Muscle weakness, hypotonia or ataxia as the main findings on examination
- Progressive motor signs or diurnal variation in motor difficulties
- Other systems involved e.g. sensory neural deafness, cataracts, neuropathy, etc to suggest a mitochondrial disorder or a metabolic condition.

DIFFERENTIAL DIAGNOSIS

Please refer to the reading list for more detailed information.
- Variation in normal development should be considered. This is particularly relevant in mild CP where the child presents with motor clumsiness and mild learning difficulty. Bottom shuffling and late walking is often familial and rarely associated with CP.
- Familial spastic paraplegia:[34]
    - Progressive spastic paraplegia

- ○ Variable mode of inheritance (dominant, less often recessive)
- ○ Changes in spinal cord with degeneration of pyramidal tracts, other tracts may also be involved
- ○ Average age of onset 11.5 years (recessive form) and 20 years (dominant form). Some commence prior to 5 years of age
- ○ Usually a positive family history, otherwise diagnosis made by process of exclusion after investigations.
- Spinal cord lesions particularly if there is only lower limb involvement and bowel or bladder problems:
  - ○ Syringomyelia
  - ○ Tethered cord
  - ○ Transverse myelitis
  - ○ Tumours.
- Genetic disorders presenting as CP include:
  - ○ Ataxia telangiectasia
  - ○ Cornelia de Lange
  - ○ Cockayne
  - ○ Incontinentia pigmenti.
- Metabolic disorders:
  - ○ Homocystinuria
  - ○ Lesch-Nyhan syndrome
  - ○ Abetalipoproteinaemia
  - ○ Untreated phenylketonuria
  - ○ Leukodystrophies.
- Metabolic treatable conditions presenting with dystonia:
  - ○ Dopa responsive dystonias
    - – Segawas
    - – Tyrosine hydroxylase deficiency
    - – Aromatic L-amino acid decarboxylase deficiency
  - ○ Methylmalonic aciduria
  - ○ Biotinidase deficiency
  - ○ Glutaric aciduria type 1
  - ○ Glucose transporter 1 deficiency
  - ○ Purine nucleoside phosphorylase deficiency.
- Neurodegenerative disorders:
  - ○ Neuronal ceroid lipofuscinosis (Batten's and Bielschowsky diseases)
  - ○ Gangliosidoses (Tay-Sachs and Sandhoff's diseases)
  - ○ Mucopolysaccharidoses (Hunter's and Hurler's diseases)
  - ○ Pantothenase kinase deficiency (Hallevordan Spatz disease)
  - ○ Infantile Huntington's chorea.
- Tumours of the brain.
- Muscle disorders (Duchenne, Becker, limb–girdle muscular dystrophies).
- Mitochondrial disorders.
- Spinocerebellar ataxias, Friedreich's ataxia,
- Anterior horn cell disease, i.e. spinal muscular atrophy.

MANAGEMENT

Management of the child with CP requires first and foremost support and explanation to the parents. Discovering that the child has a permanent and incurable disorder is devastating for parents, and they will need time and support in coming to terms with the diagnosis. They may show confusion, denial, despair and anger, i.e. all the signs of grieving. Patience, support and continued explanation by the medical and allied health team will slowly aid their process of coming to terms with their child's disorder.

Parents often feel guilty about their child's disability and wonder whether they are to blame in some way. Understanding that this will occur enables the doctor to be prepared with information about prevalence and the fact that in the majority of cases no cause is found for CP. Allowing space and time in the consultation process for parents to experience a range of feelings, while feeling supported, is an invaluable part of working with families and children with disability.

The manner in which information is given to parents at the time of diagnosis is usually remembered by them and has an impact on how they will cope and adjust to their child's disability.[35] Providing parents with information and empowering them to make decisions for their child, rather than a paternalistic professional approach, will ensure a positive partnership between the parents and the professionals on the long road of assisting the child with a disability like CP. See referenced article that provides suggestions for good practice when disclosing the diagnosis of CP to parents.[36]

An approach to management

- If a medical cause is suspected, investigate and refer to specialist colleagues if indicated, e.g. geneticist, neurologist, cardiologist, gastroenterologist.
- Be sure to address investigations as per Text Box 12.1 where indicated. In particular, formal vision and hearing testing is needed and may require repeat assessments through childhood. Consider neuroimaging in all cases (ideally MRI scanning).[17] The growth and nutrition of the child with CP must be monitored and growth charts may assist in early identification of nutritional and metabolic problems.[37]
- Consider medications that may be required:
  ○ Muscle relaxants for generalised spasticity, e.g. baclofen, benzodiazepine, dantrolene (balance with side-effect of increased salivation, drowsiness)
  ○ Botulinum toxin injections for focal spasticity or dystonia
  ○ Dystonia medications, e.g. baclofen, benzhexol and levodopa
  ○ Anticonvulsants usually in consultation with neurologist
  ○ Treatment of oesophageal reflux (marked posture changes and movements can occur in association with pain due to reflux and the painful stimuli of reflux can stimulate muscle spasms (Sandifers syndrome))
  ○ Stool softeners as the vagal stimuli of constipation and straining can aggravate tone
  ○ Medication to assist with sleep, e.g. melatonin
  ○ Other medications depend on associated system dysfunction, e.g. cardiac, endocrine, haematological.
- Involve physical therapists (physiotherapists and occupational therapists) early to assess motor development and to commence strategies to improve positioning, mobility, strength and thus function. Improving strength has a direct effect on function, thus a life-long commitment to strengthening is required. The importance of mobility to allow more active participation must not be underestimated.[38] Use of specialised equipment, splinting of the upper and

lower limbs, serial casting for treatment of contractures and targeted motor learning therapies may be required to improve function, prevent deformity and assist with care.
- Speech therapists assess feeding skills, risk of aspiration and level of communication. A modified barium swallow may be required to assess swallowing in more detail and to determine the consistency of food and fluids required for safe swallowing. Treatments can include strategies to improve swallowing effectively and safely, to improve saliva control, and to improve communication by prescribing communication aides.
- Feeding difficulties:
  - Important in CP as children may have gagging, swallowing problems and tongue thrust
  - Small frequent feeds preferable; feeds may be thickened to facilitate swallowing
  - In severe or profound CP tube feeding via gastrostomy may be required, which greatly reduces the burden of feeding on parents as well as the stress on the child.
- Consider special equipment: usually prescribed by the therapists, but require support from the treating doctor to obtain funding. Mobility aids include orthotics, wheelchairs, walking frames, crutches and sticks. Safe positioning and transfers are assisted by car seats, bath aids, hoists, ramps and up–down beds. Communication aides and specialised computer equipment including touch-screen computers, hand-held computers and smart phones facilitate learning and communication.
- Referral to a paediatric rehabilitation specialist at around 18 months of age for physical assessment regarding treatments for tone management, hip and scoliosis surveillance and orthotic prescriptions. Botulinum toxin injections can be used for focal spasticity or focal dystonia. Intrathecal baclofen is used for generalised spasticity and/or dystonia. A small number of children with pure spasticity might be suitable for selective dorsal rhizotomy.
  - Botulinum toxin injections:
    – This treatment is usually provided in multidisciplinary teams led by paediatric rehabilitation specialists, neurologists or orthopedic surgeons together with physiotherapists, occupational therapists and nurses.
    – Botulinum toxin type A injections are commonly used to treat focal spasticity or dystonia. The evidence recommends that this treatment be combined with therapy to maximise effectiveness and achieve goals.[39,40]
    – Side-effects are usually transient, mild and self-limiting. Severe side-effects can include worsening of dysphagia, generalised weakness and lower respiratory tract infections. They occur in a small number of children usually GMFCS levels IV and V, and as a result some centres in Australia limit the availability of this medication for GMFCS IV and V.[41]
- Intrathecal baclofen (ITB) is used in severe cases of spasticity and or dystonia where other treatments have failed, usually GMFCS IV and V. Suitability for this treatment usually requires a test dose of baclofen delivered via lumbar puncture. ITB therapy involves the surgical placement of a computer-driven battery-powered pump under the skin of the abdomen with a subcutaneous catheter into the intrathecal space to deliver the medication. The pump can

- be programmed to deliver differing doses at different times of the day depending on the child's condition. The treatment is effective but expensive. It requires careful preparation of the families to ensure regular attendance for refills and early detection of withdrawal symptoms, which may indicate a problem with the hardware.[42]
- Orthopaedic surgical treatment might be needed in children with marked deformity or contractures; surgery can include muscle lengthening and transfers, boney de-rotation osteotomy and tendon transfers or lengthening. The timing of a child's orthopaedic surgery is best delayed as long as possible, except in hip subluxation. During periods of rapid growth contractures and boney deformities worsen. Multilevel surgery is usually undertaken at 8–12 years of age.[16]
- Hip surveillance: There is a linear relationship between incidence of hip displacement or subluxation and GMFCS. The amount of displacement is expressed as the migration percentage (MP). MP is a radiographic measure of the amount of ossified femoral head which is not covered by the ossified acetabular roof, i.e. distance A over B in Figure 12.1. The incidence of displacement of the femoral head with MP in excess of 30 per cent is zero per cent for children in GMFCS level I and 90 per cent for children in GMFCS level V.[43] Hip dislocation (MP 100 per cent) is associated with pain and difficulties with seating and posture.

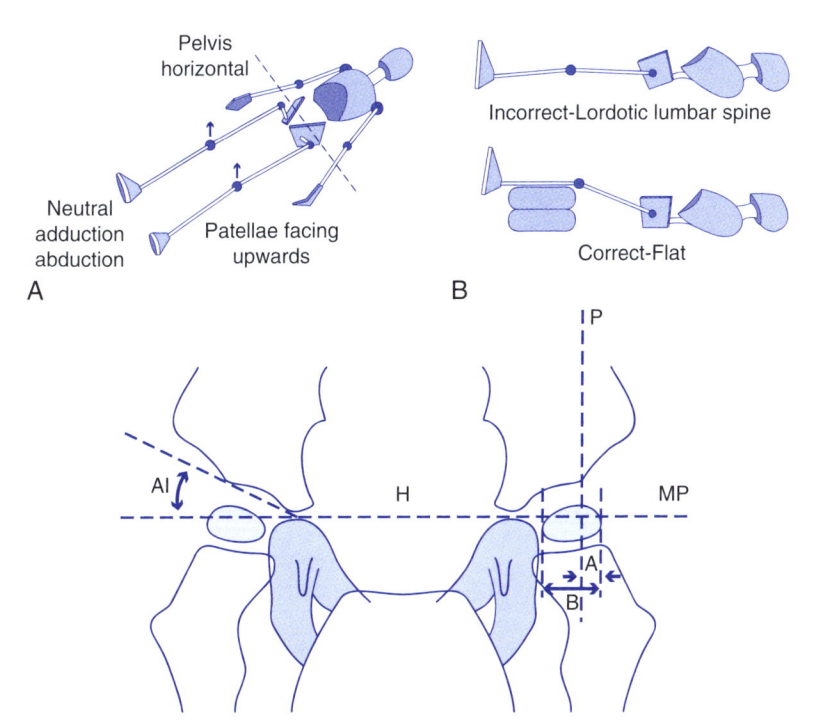

FIGURE 12.1 Position for hip X-ray and measuring hip migration percentage: line H is through the tri-radiate cartilage, line P is perpendicular to H at the edge of the acetabulum, AI is the acetabular index[44] (with permission).

- ○ All children with CP should have a hip X-ray at age 12–24 months of age in a standard position (see Figure 12.1) to determine their hips status and to measure the MPs. Referral to an orthopedic surgeon is recommended when the hip MP exceeds 30 per cent.[44]
- ○ Regular hip surveillance until skeletal maturity is recommended as per the 'Consensus statement on hip surveillance for children with Cerebral Palsy: Australian standards of care 2008'.[45]
- Monitoring of bone health is important particularly in those non-weight-bearing children, those taking anticonvulsants or with poor nutrition. A high index of suspicion for osteoporosis is recommended. Bone density assessments and review by an endocrinologist should occur following a low impact fracture.
- Scoliosis is a serious complication of severe CP.[46] Severe scoliosis impairs physical function and can be the cause of significant pain, pressure sores and difficulties with seating. Spinal orthoses and wheelchair modifications might slow progression of this problem but it needs careful monitoring and management. Surgery may be indicated for some patients.[47]
- Management of drooling or sialorrhoea requires multidisciplinary team management with focus on assessment with appropriate conservative interventions, oral motor training, dental appliances, medical and surgical treatment programs.
  - ○ Medications to alter the production of saliva include anticholinergic agents such as glycopyrolate, benzhexol, benztropine and scopolamine patches.
  - ○ Botulinum toxin injections into the salivary glands or surgical options may also be considered.[48]
- Determine the child's level of cognitive impairment so as to ascertain the interventions required.
  - ○ Occupational and speech therapists together with special education support clinicians may be required to assess cognitive level in very young children to determine the level of subsequent early intervention treatment.
  - ○ Special education teachers work with the child to facilitate school readiness in younger children and to aid learning in school-aged children.
- Preschool child: early intervention therapy and education through special support services, e.g. Cerebral Palsy Foundation, Cerebral Palsy Alliance (formerly the Spastic Centre of NSW), Services for the Deaf and Blind.
- School-aged child: assistance with planning for special school placement, particularly in the child with moderate to severe to profound CP. The child with mild CP is likely to attend a mainstream school but may require special education support for learning difficulties. Many mainstream public schools have special classes such as the IM class (for children with mild intellectual disability) and the IO class (for children with moderate to severe intellectual disability, but who do not have a significant physical impairment).
- Allocate social worker–case worker–specialist nurse as the team member who makes regular contact with the family, visits their home, and liaises with other team members to address the child's specific needs, e.g. OT to assess home or wheelchair modifications in the child who is fully dependent for care; or physiotherapist to arrange walking frame or other mobility aids.

- The team psychologist provides emotional support for the family as needed and behaviour counselling for the child who is non-compliant, frustrated or anxious. Behavioural problems in children with CP require assessment at many levels because pain, frustration and parental stress may play a part.[49,50]
- Respite care should be arranged for parents who need time to spend alone or with the siblings, who often take second place to the child with CP and developmental disability. (See Chapter 13 Developmental and intellectual disability.)
- Application for government financial support through the Carer's Allowance (for children <16 years) and the Disability Support Pension (for those >16 years) via Centrelink needs to done by the doctor involved in management.
- The 'Good Start Program' in Australia as of July 2011 offers substantial funds to assist with early intervention in cerebral palsy, vision impairment, hearing impairment, Down syndrome and fragile X syndrome.
- Encourage parental involvement with support–social groups for persons with CP as this can be enormously helpful to parents as they relate to and learn from other families of children with CP.
- Encourage participation with one of the CP registers available in Australia (also available in North America and Europe). This provides population data collection to calculate incidence and prevalence, to provide prognostic information for parents, and to facilitate investigation into causal pathways and outcomes in CP.[51]
- The general practitioner (GP) is an important partner in the long-term management of children with CP. The GP usually knows the family well, and is the primary support doctor who refers to the developmental paediatrician in the private sector. It is essential that the multidisciplinary hospital team involved in the child's care keep the GP and the paediatrician up to date with the hospital-based management of the child with CP.

Practice Point

Management of the child with CP is a long-term process and regular review is required. Reviewing the diagnosis periodically may reveal a more definitive aetiology in those cases where it is not determined.[52] Problems will need to be addressed as they occur and the team paediatrician or medical officer plays a pivotal role in arranging necessary investigations and referring to other specialists, as well as providing ongoing emotional support for the family. However, the child's parents are the key partners who inform the team through regular feedback about the CP child's progress to enable targeted support and intervention.

ADOLESCENCE AND CP

Adolescence is a challenging time for many young people. Factors impacting on the quality of life for adolescents with CP include health, participation, education, family and CP-specific issues. Parents of adolescents report issues regarding sexuality and relationships, with particular concern about vulnerability of the adolescent. Both adolescents and their parents hold concerns about independence, leaving home and finding a suitable partner.[53]

The development of romantic relationships and sexual activity in young adults with CP was examined in a longitudinal study which showed that they had difficulty establishing steady relationships, despite having similar sexual interest to unaffected persons.[54] Parents and professionals need to be sensitive to the psychosexual development of young individuals with CP.

Professionals who work with CP patients can provide guidance and support for individuals as they move through this transitional period. The case manager or social worker on the team can provide more regular support through home visits. Psychological counselling support may also be required in some circumstances.

PROGNOSIS

CP does not automatically equate with intellectual deficits and parents need to be made aware of this. In the past it was thought that the more severe the CP and the more limbs involved, the worse the prognosis for long-term survival. However with modern medical care and improvements in nutrition, survival of severely disabled CP individuals is longer than was previously thought. The combination of frequent respiratory aspiration resulting in pneumonia, seizures and gastrostomy feeds in children with severe CP reduces life expectancy compared with those who do not have these comorbidities.

Parents might ask whether their child will achieve walking. The prognosis for independent walking in the child with CP was first published by Bleck[55] in 1975. The presence of asymmetric tonic neck reflex, symmetric tonic neck, the Moro reflex, absence of foot placing reaction and absence of parachute reaction at one year of age is associated with poor prognosis for independent walking. The GMFCS classification now provides clear information on prognosis for mobility from as young as two years of age. In general, if the child is unable to sit independently before the age of four years they are unlikely to walk with or without aids, and if the child has not achieved independent walking by six years of age then they are unlikely to ever walk independently.[10]

Spastic quadriplegic (bilateral) CP is associated with intellectual deficits in the majority of cases. In other types of CP prognosis for intellectual development cannot be offered until the child reaches at least two years of age, as language development to some extent reflects cognitive development and therefore waiting until this skill develops is prudent. Many children with CP, particularly those with dystonia or choreoathetosis, have normal intellect even if they do not have normal language development due to oromotor problems.

More than 90 per cent of individuals with CP will live into adulthood. The overall survival rate of all persons with CP in the Western Australian population study is 93 per cent[56] compared with 83 per cent in the Californian data.[57] The difference relates to the fact that the Western Australian database covers everyone with CP including those with mild CP, whereas the Californian database covers the more severely affected cases and includes fewer mild CP cases. Strauss provides an update to his earlier paper on life expectancy in cerebral palsy and describes how it is calculated.[58]

All children with CP, except in very mild cases, require long-term care with intensive medical, therapy, educational and allied health services. Doctors who work with CP children and their families invariably become their advocates in relation to funding services and support for children with disability.

REFERENCES

1. Rosenbaum P, Paneth N, Leviton A, et al. A report: the definition and classification of cerebral palsy, April 2006. Developmental Medicine and Child Neurology 2007;109: 8–14
2. Stanley F, Blair E, Alberman E. What are the cerebral palsies? ch 2. In: Cerebral palsies: Epidemiology and causal pathways. Clinics in Developmental Medicine 151. London: Mac Keith; 2000
3. Badawi N, Watson L, Petterson B, et al. What constitutes cerebral palsy? Dev Med Child Neurology 1998;40:520–7
4. Stanley F, Blair E, Alberman E. How common are the cerebral palsies? ch 4. In: Cerebral palsies: Epidemiology and causal pathways. Clinics in Developmental Medicine 151. London: Mac Keith; 2000
5. Nelson KB. The epidemiology of cerebral palsy in term infants. Mental Retardation and Developmental Disabilities Research Reviews 2002;8:146–50
6. Pakula AT, Van Naarden Braun K, Yeargin-Allsopp M. Cerebral palsy: Classification and epidemiology. Phys Med Rehabil Clin N Am 2009;20(3):425–52
7. Minear WL. A classification of cerebral palsy. Pediatrics 1956;18:841–52
8. Surveillance of Cerebral Palsy in Europe (SCPE). Prevalence and characteristics of children with cerebral palsy in Europe. Dev Med Child Neurol 2002;44:633–40
9. Palisano R, Rosenbaum P, Bartlett D, et al. Content validity of the expanded and revised Gross Motor Function Classification System. Developmental Medicine & Child Neurology 2008;50(10):744–50
10. Rosenbaum P, Walter S, Hanna S, et al. Prognosis for gross motor function in cerebral palsy: Creation of motor development curves. Journal of the American Medical Association 2002;288(11):1357–63
11. Palisano R, Rosenbaum P, Walter S, et al. Development and reliability of a system to classify gross motor function in children with cerebral palsy. Developmental Medicine & Child Neurology 1997;39:214–23
12. Morris C, Galuppi B, Rosenbaum PL. Reliability of family report for the Gross Motor Function Classification System. Dev Med Child Neurol 2006;46(7):455–60
13. Graham HK, Harvey A, Rodda J, et al. The Functional Mobility Scale (FMS). JPO 2004;24(5):514–20
14. Eliasson AC, Krumlinde Sundholm L, et al. The Manual Ability Classification System (MACS) for children with cerebral palsy: scale development and evidence of validity and reliability. Dev Med Child Neurology 2006;48:549–54
15. Hidecker MC, Poole ML, Taylor K, et al. Functional performance profiles of children with cerebral palsy. Developmental Medicine and Child Neurology 2010; poster abstract 52(supp. 5):59–88
16. Gage JR, Schwartz MH, Koop SE, et al. Identification and treatment of gait problems in cerebral palsy, 2nd edn. Clinics in Developmental Medicine. London: Mac Keith: 2009. p. 180–1
17. Bax M, Tydeman C, Flodmark O. Clinical and MRI correlates of cerebral palsy: the European Cerebral Palsy Study. JAMA 2006;296:1602–8
18. Watson L, Blair E, Stanley F. Report of the Western Australia cerebral palsy register to birth year 1999 in Perth. In: TVW Telethon Institute for Child Health Research, Perth, Australia, 2009
19. Stanley FJ. Survival and cerebral palsy in low birth weight infants: Implications for perinatal care. Paediatric and Perinatal Epidemiology 1992;6:298–310
20. Cowan F, Rutherford M, Groenendaal F, et al. Origin and timing of brain lesions in term infants with neonatal encephalopathy. Lancet 2003;361:736–42
21. Barkovich AJ, Gressens P, Evrard P. Formation, maturation and disorders of brain neocortex. American Journal of Neuroradiology 1992;13(2):423–46
22. Pharoah PO. Risk of cerebral palsy in multiple pregnancies. Clinical Perinatology 2006;33(2):301–13
23. Taylor CL, de Groot J, Blair E, Stanley F. The risk of cerebral palsy in survivors of multiple pregnancies with co-fetal loss or death. American Journal of Obstetrics and Gynaecology 2009;201:41, e1–e6

24 Pharoah PO, Dundar Y. Monozygotic twinning, cerebral palsy and congenital anomalies. Human Reproduction Update 2009;15(6):639–48
25 MacLennan A. A template for defining a causal relation between acute intrapartum events and cerebral palsy: international consensus statement. BMJ 1999;319: 1054–9
26 Perlman JM, Tack EC. Renal injury in the asphyxiated newborn infant: relationship to neurological outcome. Journal of Pediatrics 1998;113:875–9
27 Menkes JH. Cerebrovascular disorders, ch 11. In: Textbook of Child Neurology. 3rd ed. Philadelphia: Lea & Febiger; 1985
28 Lenn NJ, Haas RH. Vascular disease, ch 12. In: David RB, editor. Pediatric Neurology for the Clinician. Norwalk, Connecticut: Appleton & Lange; 1992
29 Sanger TD, Delgado MR, Gaebler-Spira D, et al. Task Force on Childhood Motor Disorders. Pediatrics 2003;111(1):e89–97
30 Sanger TD, Chen D, Fehlings DL, et al. Definition and classification of hyperkinetic movements in childhood. Movement Disorders 2010;25(11):1538–49
31 Sanger TD, Chen D, Delgado MR, et al. Taskforce on Childhood Motor Disorders. Pediatrics 2006;118(5):2159–67
32 Russman BS, Ashwal S. Evaluation of the child with cerebral palsy. Seminars in Pediatric Neurology 2004;11(1):47–57
33 Horridge KA. Assessment and investigation of the child with disordered development. Archives Dis Child Educ Pract Ed. Online October 6, 2010. DOI:10.1136/adc.2009. 182436
34 Menkes JH. Heredodegenerative diseases, ch 2. In: Textbook of Child Neurology. 3rd ed. Philadelphia: Lea & Febiger, 1985
35 Davies S, Hall D. 'Contact a family': professionals and parents in partnership. Archives of Disease in Childhood 2005;90:1053–7
36 Baird G, McConachie H, Scrutton D. Parents' perceptions of disclosure of the diagnosis of cerebral palsy. Arch Dis Child 2000;83(6):475–80
37 Day SM, Strauss DJ, et al. Growth patterns in a population of children and adolescents with cerebral palsy. Dev Med Child Neurol 2007;49(3):167–71
38 Bottos M, Gericke C. Ambulatory capacity in cerebral palsy: prognostic criteria and consequences for intervention. Dev Med Child Neurol 2003;45(11):786–90
39 Love SC, Novak I, Kentish M, et al. Botulinum toxin assessment, intervention and aftercare for lower limb spasticity in children with cerebral palsy: international consensus statement. European Journal of Neurology 2010;17(suppl. 2):9–37
40 Fehlings D, Novak I, Berweck S, et al. Botulinum toxin assessment, intervention and follow-up for paediatric upper limb hypertonicity: international consensus statement. European Journal of Neurology 2010;17(suppl. 2):38–56
41 O'Flaherty SJ, Janaman V, Morrow AM, et al. Adverse events and health status following botulinum toxin type A injections in children with cerebral palsy. Developmental Medicine & Child Neurology 2011,53:125–30
42 Deon LL, Gaebler-Spira D. Assessment and treatment of movement disorders in children with cerebral palsy. Orthop Clinics of North America 2010;41:507–17
43 Soo B, Howard JJ, Boyd RN, et al. Hip displacement in cerebral palsy. Journal of Bone and Joint Surgery 2006;88(1):121–9
44 Parrot J, Boyd R, Dobson F, et al. Hip displacement in spastic cerebral palsy: repeatability of radiologic measurement. J Pediatric Orthopedics 2002;22:660–7
45 Wynter M, Gibson N, Kentish M, et al. Consensus Statement on Hip Surveillance for Children with Cerebral Palsy: Australian Standards of Care 2008. Online. Available: http://www.cpaustralia.com.au/ausacpdm; 29 Feb 2012
46 Koop SE. Scoliosis in cerebral palsy. Develop Med Child Neurol 2009;51(Suppl 4):92–8
47 Loeters M, Maathuis C, Hadders-Algra M. Risk factors for emergence and progression of scoliosis in children with severe cerebral palsy: a systematic review. Devel Med Child Neurol 2010;52(7):605–11
48 Fairhurst CBR, Cockerill H. Management of drooling in children. Archives of Disease in Childhood Educ Pract Ed 2011;96:25–30
49 Sipal RF, Schuengel C, et al. Course of behaviour problems of children with cerebral palsy: the role of parental stress and support. Child: Care, Health and Development 2010;36(1):74–84

50 Parkes J, White-Koning M, McCullough N, et al. Psychological problems in children with hemiplegia: a European multicentre survey. Arch Dis Child 2009;94(6):429–33
51 Cans C, Surman G, McManus V, et al. Cerebral palsy registries. Semin Pediatr Neurol 2004;11:18–23
52 Zarrinkalam R, Russo RN, Gibson CS, et al. CP or not CP? A review of diagnoses in a cerebral palsy register. Pediatr Neurol 2010;42:177–80
53 Davis E, Shelly A, Waters E, et al. Quality of life of adolescents with cerebral palsy: perspectives of adolescents and parents. Developmental Medicine Child Neurology 2009;51(3):193–9
54 Wiegerink DJ, Stam HJ, Gorter JW, et al. Development of romantic relationships and sexual activity in young adults with cerebral palsy: a longitudinal study. Arch Phys Med Rehabilitation 2010;91:1423–8
55 Bleck EE. Locomotor prognosis in cerebral palsy. Dev Med Child Neurol 1975;17:18–25
56 Blair E, Watson L, Badawi N, et al. Life expectancy among people with cerebral palsy in Western Australia. Developmental Medicine and Child Neurology 2001;43:508–15
57 Strauss DJ, Shavelle RM, Anderson TW. Life expectancy of children with cerebral palsy. Pediatric Neurology 1998;18:143–9
58 Strauss D, Brooks J, Rosenbloom L, et al. Life expectancy in cerebral palsy: an update. Developmental Medicine Child Neurology 2008;50(7):487–93

FURTHER READING

Scrutton D, Mayston M, Damiano D, editors. Management of the Motor Disorders of Children with Cerebral Palsy, 2nd edn. Clinics in Developmental Medicine. London: Mac Keith; 2004
Gage JR, Schwartz MH, Koop SE, et al. Identification and treatment of gait problems in cerebral palsy, 2nd ed. Clinics in Developmental Medicine. London: Mac Keith; 2009. p. 180–1
Eliasson AC, Burtner PA, editors. Improving Hand Function in Children with Cerebral Palsy. Clinics in Developmental Medicine. London: Mac Keith; Sept 2008
Horstmann HM, Bleck EE, editors. Orthopaedic Management in Cerebral Palsy, 2nd ed. Clinics in Developmental Medicine. London: Mac Keith; Oct 2007. p. 173–4
Morris C, Dias L, editors. Pediatric Orthotics. Clinics in Developmental Medicine. London: Mac Keith; Oct 2007
Russman BS. Disorders of motor execution, ch 19. In: David RB, editor. Pediatric Neurology for the Clinician. Norwalk, Connecticut: Appleton & Lange; 1992
Eicher PS, Batshaw ML. The child with developmental disabilities: Cerebral Palsy. Pediatric Clinics of North America 1993;40(3):537–51

RESOURCES

These websites available 29 Feb 2012.
http://www.cpfoundation.com.au/
http://www.cpaustralia.com.au/
http://www.rch.org.au/emplibrary/cdr/CPBooklet.pdf
http://www.hemihelp.org.uk/hemiplegia/publications/leaflets/
http://www.ninds.nih.gov/disorders/cerebral_palsy/cerebral_palsy.htm
http://www.cpaustralia.com.au/ausacpdm
http://cfcs.us
http://www.macs.nu/
http://motorgrowth.canchild.ca/en/GMFCS/resources/GMFCS-ER.pdf
http://www.wemove.org

13 Developmental and intellectual disability

Jacqueline Small

DEFINITION

Developmental disabilities are a diverse group of severe chronic conditions that are due to mental and/or physical impairments. People with developmental disabilities have problems with major life activities such as language, mobility, learning, self-help, and independent living. Developmental disabilities begin during a person's life before age 18 or 22 years and usually last throughout a person's lifetime.

Intellectual disability (ID) is a particular state of functioning that begins in childhood and is characterised by limitations in both intellectual and adaptive functioning (2 or more standard deviations below the mean). Generally an IQ test score of below 70 or as high as 75 indicates a limitation in intellectual functioning. The onset is before 18 years of age.[1]

PREVALENCE OF INTELLECTUAL DISABILITY

The prevalence of intellectual disability is estimated at 1–4 per cent worldwide. Aetiological factors such as malnutrition, lack of perinatal care, and exposure to toxic and infectious agents, which are more common in low-income and middle-income countries, may contribute to a higher prevalence of intellectual disability in some countries.[2] In some countries, such as China, the prevalence may be higher at 6.68 per cent[3] and in others, such as Scandinavian countries, lower at 0.44–0.70 per cent.[4] In the United Kingdom, it was found that 7.3 per cent of children met the Disability Discrimination Act (DDA) definition (1995 and 2005). Disabled children were more likely to live with low-income, deprivation, debt and poor housing.[5]

World Health Organization (WHO) data suggests that about 10 per cent of the world's population experience some form of disability or impairment and this number is increasing. Eighty per cent of the world's population with ID live in low-income families, most are poor and have limited or no access to basic services.

Practice Points

1. In general, the prevalence of intellectual disability is 1–4 per cent.
2. Factors that influence the prevalence include geographic factors, malnutrition, exposure to toxins, poverty and gender.
3. There remain challenges in defining a 'case' for population-based, epidemiological studies.

AETIOLOGY OF INTELLECTUAL DISABILITY

There are numerous potential causes of intellectual disability including: chromosomal disorders, other genetic defects, inborn errors of metabolism, developmental brain abnormalities, congenital infections, environmental factors, toxins, perinatal problems, trauma, hypothyroidism. Thus any condition that affects the developing brain may result in intellectual disability.

The more likely cause of intellectual disability for any particular child will be influenced by geographic and other local factors. For example, in regions of high alcohol abuse, fetal alcohol syndrome may be common; in regions of iodine deficiency, hypothyroidism may be common; and in regions where HIV or other infections that may affect the growing fetus are common, they may be a leading cause. Thus the search for the cause of intellectual disability should be guided by both professional recommendations as well as local factors.

Identifying the cause of intellectual disability is an important aspect of management of the child with intellectual disability. However, in many cases, perhaps at least 50 per cent, the cause cannot be identified.[6] In general, the more severe the intellectual disability the more likely it is that a specific cause will be found. Mild intellectual disability may be more likely to be secondary to 'familial' and environmental factors. The presence of clinical features can also influence diagnostic yield. Such factors may include: female gender, abnormal prenatal–perinatal history, absence of autistic features, presence of microcephaly, abnormal neurologic examination, and dysmorphic features.[7] Given the numerous possible investigations, it is important to select those more likely to have a positive yield, with a detailed history and examination being paramount in this process.

Up to now, many cases of ID remain undiagnosed even if extensive investigations are undertaken. Conventional karyotyping has been used for many years to investigate intellectual disability with fluorescence in situ hybridisation (FISH) and other genetic testing being added in recent years. However the yield from these tests was probably no greater than 10 per cent.[8] Current recommendations for genetic investigations have been expanded to include comparative genomic hybridisation (CGH) array testing, as this is identifying more causes of the intellectual disability, with widespread support for this being the first line genetic test. Recent studies are suggesting that up to 20 per cent of children with intellectual disability can be identified using these techniques.[9] New research is emerging that suggests strong experimental support for a de novo paradigm for mental retardation. Together with de novo copy number variation, de novo point mutations of large effect could explain the majority of all intellectual disability cases in the population.[10]

There are some genetic syndromes that should be routinely considered in the search for a cause of the intellectual disability. Fragile X syndrome is one such syndrome as it is the most common inherited cause of intellectual disabilities.[11] Fragile X syndrome encompasses a broad phenotype, typified by dysmorphic features, e.g. large ears, long face, enlarged testes, intellectual disability and behavioural problems such as autism. However, 30 per cent of children with fragile X syndrome may not have physical abnormalities and the premutation carrier may have clinical problems such as attention deficit hyperactivity disorder and other learning or cognitive difficulties. Further, the premutation carrier may experience a range of other significant conditions such as fragile X associated tremor and ataxia syndrome (FXTAS), premature ovarian failure, emotional problems such as anxiety, and hypothyroidism. The majority of males and about a third of females have an intellectual disability, the severity of which may vary depending on the level of fragile X mental retardation protein, up to borderline or mild.

Guidelines now exist to assist the practitioner in selecting the appropriate investigation path to be pursued, and these guidelines should be used to inform the selections of investigations made. Maintaining currency of such recommendations is important as new research is emerging about aetiology of intellectual disability. The following recommendations are taken from one such international guideline:[12]

1. Routine metabolic investigations are not recommended as part of an initial evaluation.
2. CGH array testing, replacing karyotype testing, is the current recommendation to investigate for genetic conditions.
3. Fragile X testing is recommended even in the absence of clinical features.
4. Evaluation of serum lead undertaken if clinical risk.
5. Thyroid testing should not be necessary if newborn screening undertaken. However in situations with increased risk of hypothyroidism, e.g. Down syndrome, care must be taken to suspect sub-clinical problems.
6. EEG performed if suspicion of epilepsy.
7. MRI, particularly if neurological abnormalities present.

Practice Points

1. Routine genetic testing should be undertaken for all children with an intellectual disability.
2. There are numerous potential causes of intellectual disability, and so comprehensive physical examination and history should guide selection of targeted investigations.
3. Clinical guidelines exist that can assist the professional in choosing which investigations to perform.
4. Recommendations will continue to change as research progressively identifies the main causes of intellectual disability. Recent recommendations include CGH array to test for multiple genetic defects not previously detected by cytogenetic testing.

THE EARLY TRAJECTORY OF INTELLECTUAL DISABILITY

Some children, who are later confirmed to have a disability, are suspected at or near birth to have a problem that will result in an intellectual disability. Children with significant complications during pregnancy or birth, and children born with a syndrome such as Down syndrome, are some that will be identified during the neonatal period to be at high risk for later developmental problems. Parents of these children will be counselled about this risk and referred to services that can provide monitoring, diagnostic and intervention services for their child. Although the severity of the disability that these children may eventually have will not be certain at or near birth, the early experiences for these parents tend to be more supportive and may result in better adaptation to the disability and its lifetime implications.

For other children, their intellectual disability becomes evident over time with initial parent, and often also professional, concerns likely to be that the child is not reaching developmental milestones. Developmental concerns are quite common and are seen in about 16–18 per cent of children. Of these 90 per cent have language impairment, learning disabilities, or developmental delay. The prevalence of developmental concerns is increased to 22 per cent if behavioural and emotional problems are also included.[13,14] Parents of these children tend to experience a different early course with initial reassurances on recognition of the developmental delay that the child will 'catch up', and diagnosis of the intellectual disability only occurring at a much later age. This gradual evolution of the disability may also affect access to services, which tend to be more readily available for children with more clearly defined developmental conditions. For many of the children for whom early concerns about their development are held, the problems will either resolve or evolve into a condition that may affect only one developmental domain.

Some of the early signs of developmental disability include:
- Delayed sitting, or walking later than other children
- Having trouble talking or not being able to follow directions
- Having trouble understanding social rules, or seeing the consequences of their action
- Not understanding age-appropriate toys or slow to develop interactive play with other children

For all children, even those with a genetic condition associated with developmental or intellectual disability, there is influence on developmental outcome by other factors, e.g. environment. A transactional model, in which the process of development is best considered as an interaction between the child and the environment, is most helpful for understanding the nature of child development and the factors that can adversely affect outcomes.[15] Thus a child may have an underlying predisposition to have an intellectual disability, but factors to which they are exposed influence the expression of this risk. These other factors may include exposure to intervention, socioeconomic status, general family resilience and resources.

Predicting which children with developmental delay will have an intellectual disability is not straightforward. Comprehensive clinical assessment might identify factors that would indicate poorer outcomes and likely ID. Such factors might include more severe degree of developmental delay, global rather than specific developmental delay, epilepsy, structural brain malformation, Down syndrome and cumulative psychosocial adversity. It may be possible at a reasonably young age to predict those children with developmental delay who are most likely to be presenting with the early signs of a developmental disability.[16]

ASSESSMENT AND DIAGNOSIS OF INTELLECTUAL DISABILITY

I think I stopped listening after he said the word (autism/intellectual disability). All I could think about was, will he ever be able to talk or live by himself.

Assessment of intellectual abilities (IQ) can provide important information about the child's capacity for learning and independence, and can be a significant predictor of educational and occupational status at 26 years. Intellectual abilities

Practice Points

1. While some children are identified at or close to birth as being at very high risk of having an intellectual disability, many children present with developmental delay during early childhood as their first sign of intellectual disability.
2. Comprehensive assessment should be undertaken to detect factors, especially identifiable neurological impairments or genetic syndromes, which enable early prediction of a disability.
3. Other health conditions that might compromise developmental outcome, such as untreated chronic health conditions and dietary deficiencies, should specifically be sought. Conditions such as hearing and vision impairment should be excluded by formal assessment.
4. Tools such as developmental screening tests and developmental assessments (see Table 13.1) should be used to accurately assess development, and to obtain a developmental profile that might assist with monitoring progress and predicting the likelihood of intellectual disability.
5. The early experiences of parents of children diagnosed with intellectual disability may have a profound impact on their adaptation to their child's disability. A life-course, family-centred model with close collaboration between agencies and professionals should be implemented from the time developmental delay is suspected.

tend to be more stable when assessed from about 5 years of age, and children tend to retain similar positions relative to their peers.[17] However it is important to consider factors other than IQ that may influence outcome and performance on assessment, as not all IQ tests should be considered valid assessments of long-term intellectual abilities.

In defining and assessing intellectual disability, the American Association on Intellectual and Developmental Disabilities (AAIDD) stresses that professionals must take additional factors into account, such as the community environment typical of the individual's peers and culture, linguistic diversity and cultural differences in the way people communicate, move and behave. Assessments must also assume that limitations in an individual's ability often coexist with strengths, and that a person's level of life functioning will improve if appropriate personalised supports are provided over a sustained period.

Assessment of cognitive or intellectual skills should be undertaken by trained and experienced personnel. Tools such as the Wechsler Scales of Intelligence or Stanford Binet Intelligence Test have been validated and standardised around the world (see Table 13.1). These tools can provide important information about overall IQ as well as a profile that might identify significant strengths and weaknesses; contribute to appropriate developmental expectations for the child; and aid the development of individualised intervention and schooling programs.

Adaptive behaviour refers to those skills that enable a person to function in everyday life within their community. There are tools, such as Vineland Adaptive Behavior Scales, that can measure adaptive skills against those expected for a person of similar age. Adaptive skills include:

TABLE 13.1 Developmental, intellectual and adaptive behaviour assessment tools

Test	Purpose	Notes
Griffiths Mental Developmental Scales	To measure rate of development	Provides a measure of overall development and development in six subscales in children 0–8 yr of age
Bayley Scales of Infant Development	To evaluate facets of development	Provides developmental information in five key domains for children 1–42 mo
Wechsler Preschool and Primary Scale of Intelligence (WPPSI)	To measure overall cognitive ability	Can be used in children aged 2.6–7.3 yr to report overall, verbal and performance IQ
Wechsler Intelligence Scale for Children (WISC)	To measure overall cognitive ability	Can be used in children aged 6.0–16.11 yr and provides information across 4 main domains: verbal comprehension, perceptual reasoning, working memory, processing speed
Stanford Binet Intelligence Scales	To assess intelligence and cognitive abilities	Can be used in children and adults aged 2–85 yr and measures across 4 areas: verbal reasoning, quantitative reasoning, abstract/visual reasoning, short-term memory
Vineland Adaptive Behavior Scales	A measure of adaptive behaviour	A leading measure of personal and social skills needed for everyday living from birth to adulthood
Adaptive Behavior Assessment System (ABAS)	Measures adaptive behaviour	Measures behaviour in different skills areas from birth to adulthood

- conceptual skills, such as language and literacy, money, time, number concepts and self-direction
- social skills, such as interpersonal skills, social responsibility, self-esteem, gullibility, naïveté (i.e. wariness), social problem solving, the ability to follow rules or obey laws and to avoid being victimised
- practical skills, such as activities of daily living (personal care), occupational skills, healthcare, travel–transportation, schedules–routines, safety, use of money, use of the telephone.

Intellectual disability can be categorised according to degree of severity, based on both IQ and assessment of adaptive functioning, which can give a guide as to the degree of independence a person is likely to achieve in daily living and the support needs a person is likely to have. The Better Health Channel describes likely achievements in different areas of daily life according to severity of intellectual disability, and can be a useful resource for families. The DSM-IV defines these categories as given in Table 13.2.

TABLE 13.2 Categories of IQ defined by DSM-IV

Category of ID	Lower IQ limit	Upper IQ limit
Mild	50–55	70
Moderate	35–40	50–55
Severe	20–25	35–40
Profound		20–25

That consultation, when Patrick was officially given a likely diagnosis of …, is one that I'm sure I will never forget. I can remember many things about it – not just what was said, but also the pauses and intonation, the atmosphere in the room, the sounds, and how I felt. It seemed to be happening in a slow motion, like in a movie.

Developmental assessment is more than ascertaining a child's eligibility for services as the family begins a journey into the service systems that hold multiple opportunities for both positive and negative experiences for the family. If parents are to act as spokespersons and advocates for their child with disabilities, it would seem important that they are able to represent accurately the nature of their child's problem, and comprehensive assessment can assist parents in being fully informed about their child's disability and support needs.

Important outcomes of the diagnostic assessment are recommendations about intervention and development of a management plan. How parents perceive their child's disability, understand the recommendations made by professionals, their agreement with the diagnosis, and attitudes and beliefs will strongly influence them and how they assist their child in accessing services.[18] Thus professionals should be aware that sometimes 'hidden' factors will influence compliance with those recommendations and thus access by the child to effective intervention.

Parental perceptions of a child's disability and treatment recommendations are key variables that may determine their use of services. Suggestions to create a diagnostic process that might better meet the family's needs include:[19]

- Build a relationship with family members, collaborate with family through assessment, respect and rely on parents' knowledge
- Do more than a single standardised evaluation and 'discover' what a child can do
- View the child from a framework of competency embedded within a cultural context
- Focus on the parents questions, not your knowledge, demonstrate a good understanding of parental concerns, providing adequate information to address parent concerns
- Diagnosis to be given in direct, realistic, yet sympathetic and positive manner
- Consider the timing of imparting information, attempt to ensure that both parents are seen together in a quiet, private setting with time alone afterwards
- Invite opportunity to meet other parents.

CHAPTER 13   Developmental and intellectual disability   ■   239

Our doctor that diagnosed our son could not have handled our 'bad news' conversation better. She was caring sympathetic (even tears in her eyes), direct, to the point without rushing. She answered our questions 'straight' – no sugar coating, but not total doom and gloom either.

(39-year-old mother of 2-year-old girl)

Practice Points

1   Diagnosis of intellectual disability is based on formal assessment of both intelligence and adaptive behaviour with validated tools.
2   Valid assessment of intelligence at around 5 years of age, and for some children at a younger age, is likely to enable long-term prediction about learning and independence.
3   The process of diagnosis is an important one for parents, and should be built on a high standard of communication skills and delivered in a model that acknowledges and responds to the needs of parents.

INTERVENTION FOR INTELLECTUAL DISABILITY

Intervention for children with intellectual disability should commence as soon as the developmental concerns or risk factors are identified. Comprehensive assessment should identify the pattern of strengths and weaknesses that are to be addressed during intervention, which should be characterised by:[20]

1   Being affordable and delivered in naturalistic environments
2   Building on strengths of child and family
3   Being responsive to cultural and personal priorities
4   Being delivered through research-based practices
5   Assisting family to carry out therapeutic practices in the home
6   Seamless transition between early intervention and public education.

Models of early intervention vary with some characterised by independent practitioners working in relative isolation from others to agencies that provide a range of therapeutic interventions, often including services specifically aimed at supporting parents, to transdisciplinary therapy in which the therapist is multi-skilled and can meet a broad range of the child's needs. There is little evidence that brief, infrequent therapeutic intervention makes much difference for most children with intellectual disability. Services of sufficient intensity and duration should be provided early enough to maximise developmental outcomes and prevent secondary conditions.

Addressing specific areas of difficulty is important. Key areas of focus should include support for:

1   **Communication:** A speech pathologist has expertise in this area. The goal for children should be effective communication of needs and wants to the best of their developmental ability. For some children this may be fluent speech, for others it may be very limited and involve use of objects such as keys to convey needs or wants. Other strategies can be helpful including pictures, e.g. Picture Exchange Communication System, Boardmaker (http://www.spectronicsinoz.com/catalogue/3083) or Makaton, a signing system that emphasises key words (http://www.newcastle.edu.au/research-centre/

special-education/key-word-sign-australia/). Single pictures can be used, e.g. picture for toilet, or several linked to form a story or indicate a sequence of tasks.
2 **Play and general independence skills:** Occupational therapists have specific skills in this area. Adjustment of hand grips may allow writing or drawing skills to progress.
3 **Mobility:** The ability to move freely around the community will have significant influence on independence and development of play skills. Provision of standing equipment may be indicated. Physiotherapists have skills in this domain.
4 **Special education:** Many teachers will have specific training in teaching children with intellectual disability, at least a basic understanding of different communication techniques and skills in working with different professionals.

Children with intellectual disability will continue to have increased need for support once they commence school. In some countries, specific legislation exists to ensure special education support for children with disabilities and special needs. The contemporary approach is to ensure that the child with intellectual disability

Practice Points

1. Early intervention should commence as soon as developmental concerns or risk factors for intellectual disability are identified. This is likely to involve a combination of speech therapy, occupational therapy, physiotherapy, special education and specific family support services such as social work.
2. Intervention is likely to involve a combination of centre- and home-based services, but must include parent education and delivery in naturalistic environments as key components.
3. Services should be delivered in a planned way with parents as the key members of the team that identifies priorities and strategies and involves all key service providers, including educational professionals.
4. Services and support must be delivered in a lifespan model, as key life stages will present their own challenges and issues for parents and the person with intellectual disability.
5. Specialised educational support is likely to be required. This may involve a special class, e.g. in New South Wales: IO for children with moderate intellectual disability, IM for children with mild intellectual disability, SSP Schools for Special Purposes or supplemented teaching in a mainstream class. There are clearly defined eligibility requirements for these services.
6. Transition between services must be planned, e.g. the child with developmental delay (DD) may be eligible for services through community health, while the child with intellectual disability may be eligible for services through disability services.
7. People with intellectual disability will require varying levels of support in their adult life, but with the right support they might be able to participate in many tasks associated with adulthood, such as work and family.

attends the least restrictive schooling option, that is, a mainstream school attended by other children in the community. However for many children, their needs may be better met in a special class or perhaps even a special school. These classes provide smaller student to teacher ratios and more individualised programs. The importance of close collaboration between education, therapeutic, health and other professionals remains paramount to meeting the child and family's complex and ongoing needs.

Transition to post-school adult life is often a challenging time for parents. The significance of the intellectual disability and the limitations on independence may become apparent for the first time, as the contrast with other children who are leaving home, undertaking tertiary studies, entering the workforce or considering marriage is evident. Some adults with an intellectual disability may be able to participate in all of these activities or tasks with support, while others may have mastered few of the daily living skills that are fundamental to independence.

OUTCOMES FOR CHILDREN WITH INTELLECTUAL DISABILITY

He's not going to do anything like you or me ... but we don't rule anything out ... he may never be able to do things ... I don't want to look too far into the future ... We want him to be happy, to interact with his sisters, experience life as best he can ... to laugh and smile.

(Father of a 3-year-old boy with profound DD)

The quality of life for people with ID is influenced by many factors that operate at the individual, family, community and broader society level.[21] IQ is important but not the sole factor in determining outcome and quality of life. Other things that contribute to quality of life include: presence or absence of supportive family and community; opportunities for diverse and enriching experiences; capacity to develop hobbies; and a sense of value for what one can contribute to one's circumstances.

Older teens and adults tend to function at a level of an age equivalent of:[22]
- 8 to 11 years or sixth grade skills in the case of mild intellectual disability
- 5½ to 8 years or second grade skills in moderate ID
- 3 to 5½ years and have difficulty with pre-academic skills in severe ID
- less than 3 years in profound ID.

When I got the diagnosis of intellectual disability, I changed the way I approached intervention. I wanted to focus more on teaching things that would help them through life.

Mother of two young children with ID–autism

A POPULATION PERSPECTIVE

The International Classification of Function (ICF) is a classification of health and health-related domains that describe body functions and structures, activities and participation. Since an individual's functioning and disability occurs within a context, it also includes a list of environmental factors. It is a new guideline to measure health and is conceptually different to past tools, which emphasise disability. It attempts to mainstream the notion of disability and is Complementary to ICD 10.

The United Nations Convention on the Rights of Persons with Disabilities[23] came into force on 3 May 2008. It outlines the civil, cultural, political, social and economic rights of people with disabilities. Member states agree to promote, protect and ensure the full and equal enjoyment of the human rights and fundamental freedoms of people with disabilities and prompt respect for their inherent dignity.

The WHO initiative, launched November 2010,[24] 'Better health better lives: children and young people with intellectual disabilities and their families' aims to ensure that all children and young people with intellectual disabilities are fully participating members of society, living with their families, integrated in the community, and receiving healthcare and support proportional to their needs. In partnership with UNICEF it is a declaration that covers four key objectives and informs future research and policy directions:

1 Promoting and supporting good physical and mental health and wellbeing
2 Eliminating health and other inequalities and preventing other forms of discrimination, neglect and abuse
3 Providing support that prevents family separation and allow parents to care for and protect children and young people with intellectual disabilities
4 Supporting children and young people in the development of their potential and their successful transition through life.

CHALLENGING BEHAVIOURS AND MENTAL HEALTH

Challenging behaviours and mental health or psychological problems, such as outwardly directed aggressive behaviour, may be a significant part of problem behaviours presented by people with IDs. Prevalence rates for behavioural and mental health problems of over 50 per cent have been reported in the literature. Such behaviours often run a long-term course and are a major cause of social exclusion, yet often people with these problems do not access much needed diagnostic and management services.[25] If behavioural and emotional disturbance commence in childhood, they tend to decrease only slowly over time, remaining high into young adulthood.[26]

Although high quality evidence regarding the effectiveness for interventions for children with intellectual disability and challenging behavior is limited, there are many strategies that should be considered and may be useful in reducing the severity and frequency of challenging behaviours.

Principles for managing challenging behaviour

These principles include:
- Thorough and comprehensive assessment, including medical or health factors, of the challenging behavior must be undertaken at the outset
- Observation, where possible, of the behaviour in a setting in which it occurs helps to analyse antecedents, reinforcements and consequences of the behaviour
- Behaviour management by clinical psychologist
- Speech and communication therapy
- Family counselling and support, e.g. respite
- Psycho-pharmacological therapy, e.g. antipsychotics or stimulants, may be considered and guidelines are available to assist this intervention

CHAPTER 13 Developmental and intellectual disability 243

- Reinforcement of principles, e.g. consistency between different environments, positive reward for desired behaviours or limit setting especially where safety for at-risk behaviour is needed
- Review of the environment to ensure it meets the child's needs, e.g. space to play and move around with safety fences
- Formalise behavior recommendations into a plan and disseminate to relevant agencies and people
- Ongoing review by the clinician and team (where available) to ensure that the desired outcome of reduction in problem behaviours occurs.

Practice Points

A critical first stage in management of challenging behaviours is comprehensive evaluation that explores factors such as those noted:

1. What is the level of intellectual disability, in particular communication abilities? Has there been a recent or progressive cognitive decline that might be masquerading as challenging behaviours? Is the child being appropriately supported?
2. Has the cause of the ID been identified and is this associated with a behaviour phenotype that might explain the problematic behaviours?
3. Are there any undetected health problems that might be causing or contributing to the challenging behaviours, e.g. constipation, dental decay, sleep problems, epilepsy, gastro-oesophageal reflux or caused by the behaviours, e.g. low vitamin D due to difficulties taking the child out into sunlight?
4. Are there any comorbid mental health issues, e.g. anxiety or depression, that are commonly found in people with ID?
5. What is the capacity of the family to continue to manage and implement sometimes complex behaviour management plans? How can this be increased, e.g. better utilisation of informal community supports?
6. What services or interventions have been trialled already? What is the parent's experience of these?
7. How can services be brought together to work effectively to ensure best outcomes?
8. What is the nature of the challenging behaviour? What happens before the incident? What is the behaviour like? What happens after the behaviour?

OTHER IMPORTANT ISSUES FOR PEOPLE WITH ID

Community attitudes and practices towards people with ID have varied over time and between cultures. It was not long ago that established practice was to institutionalise young children with ID, effectively separating them from family and community. Some contemporary principles underpinning policy and service delivery for people with ID are as follows:

1. **Family and carers are critically important in the care of people with intellectual disability**.

My subconscious is always focusing on [my son] no matter what I am doing. That kind of vigilance is exhausting.

(Extract from an interview with a mother of an 18-year-old male with intellectual disability).

For most parents of children with ID, their experience is typified by higher levels of stress and demand for care,[27] with the most significant predictors of increased stress being maladaptive behaviours and communication limitations in the child.[28] The impact on a child with ID varies throughout life, with adolescence being one of the most critical phases in the lives of people with ID.[29] There are other factors that influence the degree of stress and possible psychiatric problems for families and carers.[30–32] Identifying parents who are at risk of high levels of stress while the child is young provides an important opportunity for preventative health services.[33] The level of stress experienced by families is a growing concern, with recent data from United States showing that more children are entering out-of-home care placements.[34]

2 **Inclusion.** Organisations in both in Australia and other countries[35] have established policy that children should live and grow up in a family home, enjoying nurturing adult relationships both inside and outside a family home.

3 **Elimination of aversive procedures**[36] which have been used as a means of behaviour management and are characterised by obvious signs of physical pain experienced by the individual, or potential or actual physical side-effects, or dehumanisation of the individual.

4 **Adverse health outcomes.** Substantial health disparities are evident between people with ID and the general population.[37] Obesity has consistently been found to be increased in people with ID compared to the general population[38,39] and increasingly at a very young age. Obesity in people with intellectual disability has been associated with female gender; certain diagnostic subgroups, e.g. Down syndrome; lesser severity of intellectual disability; family living compared to community living compared to institutional living; ethnicity; and socioeconomic status.[40] Optimisation of health outcomes can be assisted by health screening strategies recommended for the general population, as well as for specific groups, e.g. children with Down syndrome.

However a socially and statistically significant proportion of the increased risk of poorer health among children and adolescents with IDs may be attributed to their increased risk of socioeconomic disadvantage, with 31 per cent of the elevated risk for poorer health being accounted for by between-group differences in socioeconomic position and social capital.[41]

REFERENCES

1 American Association Intellectual and Developmental Disability (AAIDD). Definition of Intellectual Disability. Online. Available: http://www.aamr.org/content_100.cfm?navID=21; 25 Feb 2012
2 Mercadante MT, Evans-Lacko S, Paula CS. Perspectives of intellectual disability in Latin American countries: epidemiology, policy, and services for children and adults. Current Opinion in Psychiatry 2009;22(5):469–74
3 Jeevanandam L. Perspectives of intellectual disability in Asia: epidemiology, policy, and services for children and adults. Current Opinion in Psychiatry 2009;22(5): 462–6

CHAPTER 13 Developmental and intellectual disability ■ 245

4. Westerinen H, Kaski M, Virta L, et al. Prevalence of intellectual disability: a comprehensive study based on national registers. Journal of Intellectual Disability Research 2007;51(9):715–25
5. Blackburn CM, Spencer NJ, Read JM. Prevalence of childhood disability and the characteristics and circumstances of disabled children in the UK: secondary analysis of the family resources survey. Pediatrics 2010;10:21
6. Srour M, Mazer B, Shevell MI. Pediatrics 2006;118(1):139–45
7. Shahdadpuri R, Lambert D, Lynch SA. Diagnostic outcome following routine genetics clinic referral for the assessment of global developmental delay. Irish Medical Journal 2009;102(5):146–8
8. De Vries BB, Pfundl R, Leisink M, et al. Diagnostic genome profiling in mental retardation. American Journal Human Genetics 2005;77:606–16
9. Gijsbers AC, Lew JY, Bosch CA, et al. A new diagnostic workflow for patients with mental retardation and/or multiple congenital abnormalities: test arrays first. European Journal of Human Genetics 2009;17(11):1394–402
10. Vissers LELM, de Ligt J, Gilisse C, et al. A de novo paradigm for mental retardation. Nature Genetics 2010;42(12):1109–13
11. Chonchaiya W, Schneider A, Hagerman RJ. Fragile X: A family of disorders. Advances in Pediatrics 2009;56(1):165–86
12. Shevell M, Ashwal S, Donley D, et al. Practice parameter: Evaluation of the child with global developmental delay: Report of the Quality Standards Subcommittee of the American Academy of Neurology and The Practice committee of the Child Neurology Society. Neurology 2003;60:367–80
13. Newacheck PW, Strickland B, Shonkoff JP, et al. An epidemiologic profile of children with special health care needs. Pediatrics 1998;102:117–23
14. Yeargin-Allsopp M, Murphy CC, Oakley GP, et al. A multiple source method for studying the prevalence of developmental disabilities in children: the Metropolitan Atlanta Developmental Disabilities Study Project. Pediatrics 1992;89(4 Pt 1):624–30
15. First LR, Palfrey JS. The infant or young child with developmental delay. New England Journal of Medicine 1994, Feb;330(7):478–83
16. Small Je Van D. Predictive value of the Griffiths Mental Developmental Scale in children with developmental delay. pers. comm
17. Sattler JM, editor. Assessment of children: Cognitive applications. 4th ed. San Diego: Jerome M Sattler; 2001
18. Cadman D, Shurvell B, Davies P, et al. Compliance in the community with consultants' recommendations for developmentally handicapped children. Developmental Medicine & Child Neurology 1984;26(1):40–6
19. Miller LJ, Hanft BE. Building Positive Family Alliances: Partnerships with families as the cornerstone of developmental assessment. Infants and Young Children 1998;11(1):49–60
20. American Association Developmental and Intellectual Disability Early Childhood Services–Position Statement. Online. Available: http://www.aamr.org/; 25 Feb 2012
21. Bronfenbrenner's Ecological System's Theory. Online. Available: http://pt3.nl.edu/paquetteryanwebquest.pdf; 25 Feb 2012
22. American Psychiatry Association. Diagnostic and statistical manual of mental disorders (DSM IV–TR). 4th ed. Washington DC: American Psychiatry Association; 2000
23. United Nations Convention on the Rights of Persons with Disabilities. Online. Available: http://www.un.org/disabilities/; 25 Feb 2012
24. Emerson E, McCulloch A, Graham H, et al. Socioeconomic circumstances and risk of psychiatric disorders among parents of children with early cognitive delay. American Journal on Intellectual & Developmental Disabilities 2010;115(1):30–42
25. Kolaitis G. Young people with intellectual disabilities and mental health needs (Review). Current Opinion in Psychiatry 2008;21(5):469–73
26. Einfeld SL, Piccinin AM, Mackinnon A, et al. Psychopathology in young people with intellectual disability. [Erratum appears in JAMA 2006 Dec 13;296(22):2682] JAMA 2010;296(16):1981–9
27. Haveman M, Van Berkum G, Hölscher P, et al. Needs for services expressed by parents with young intellectually disabled children: a comparison of results in Germany, the Netherlands and Belgium. Journal of Intellectual Disability Research 2000;44(3):310–11

28 Quine L, Pahl J. Stress and coping in mothers caring for a child with severe learning difficulties: a test of Lazarus' transactional model of coping. Journal of Community and Applied Social Psychology 1991;1:57–70
29 Heslop P, Mallett R, Simons K, et al. Bridging the divide at transition: What happens for young people with learning difficulties and their families. Kidderminster: BILD; 2002
30 Lewis P, Abbeduto L, Murphy M, et al. Psychological wellbeing of mothers of youth with fragile X syndrome: syndrome specificity and within syndrome variability. Journal of Intellectual Disability Research 2006;50(12):894–904
31 Hassall R, Rose J, McDonald J. Parenting stress in mothers of children with an Intellectual Disability: The effects of parental cognitions in relation to child characteristics and family support. Journal Intellectual Disability Research 2005;49(6):405–18
32 Leonard BJ, Johnson AL, Brust JD. Preventing mental health problems in children with chronic illness or disability. Children's Health Care 1993;20(3):150–61
33 Trute B, Hiebert-Murphy D. Family adjustment to Childhood Developmental Disability: A measure of parental appraisal of family impacts. Journal of Pediatric Psychology 2002;27(3):271–80
34 Larson SA, Lakin KC, Salmi P, et al. Children and youth with intellectual or developmental disabilities living in congregate care settings (1977–2009): Healthy People 2010 Objective 6.7b Outcomes. Intellectual and Developmental Disabilities 2010;48(5):396–400
35 American Association Intellectual and Developmental Disability – Inclusion Position Statement. Online. Available: http://www.aamr.org/content_161.cfm?navID=31; 25 Feb 2012
36 American Association Intellectual and Developmental Disability – Aversive Procedures Position Statement. Online. Available: http://www.aamr.org/content_169.cfm?navID=31; 25 Feb 2012
37 Walsh PN. Health indicators and intellectual disability [Review]. Current Opinion in Psychiatry 2008;21(5):474–8
38 Rimmer JH, Yamaki K. Obesity and Intellectual Disability [Review]. Mental retardation & developmental disabilities research reviews 2006;12(1):22–7
39 Melville CA, Hamilton S, Hankey CR, et al. The prevalence and determinants of obesity in adults with intellectual disability. Obesity Reviews 2007;8(3):223–30
40 De S, Small J, Baur LA. Obesity and overweight among children with developmental disabilities. Journal of Intellectual & Developmental Disability 2008;33(1):43–7
41 Emerson E, Hatton C. Journal of Intellectual Disability Research 2007;51(Pt 11):866–74

RESOURCES

American Academy Intellectual Developmental Disability http://www.aamr.org/index.cfm
International Society for the Study of Intellectual Disability http://www.iassid.org/
Centre for Developmental Disability Health, Victoria, Menstrual Resources http://www.cddh.monash.org/products-resources.html#menstrual
British Academy of Childhood Disability http://www.bacdis.org.uk/index.htm
Australian Association Developmental Disability Medicine http://ausaddm.wordpress.com/home/
Understanding Intellectual Disability and Health http://www.intellectualdisability.info/
New South Wales Council for Intellectual Disability, Health Information Sheets http://www.nswcid.org.au/health/se-health-pages/standard-fact-sheets.html
Better Health Channel, Intellectual Disability http://www.betterhealth.vic.gov.au/bhcv2/bhcarticles.nsf/pages/Intellectual_disability
The Multicultural Disability Advocacy Association (MDAA) http://www.mdaa.org.au/publications/ethnicity/index.html
International Classification of Diseases and Related Health Problems, 10th edn. World Health Organization http://apps.who.int/classifications/icd10/browse/2010/en
Down Syndrome NSW http://www.dsansw.org.au/index.php?pg=356

14 Child abuse and neglect

Paul Tait

DEFINITION

There are various definitions of child abuse and/or neglect.[1,2] They all derive from a concern that significant harm has occurred to the child as a result of omission or commission by people responsible for the child's care. Implicit is a breach of trust in the relationship between the child and the perpetrator and the resultant psychological harm caused by abuse, as well as the immediate physical harm incurred by the abusive actions. Furthermore, as a society we expect that children have an inherent right to be kept safe and that advocacy for this right should be an essential aspect of the process of recognition and management of children who have been abused.

There are different forms of child abuse. These include neglect, sexual, physical and emotional abuse. The following definitions are derived from the New South Wales Community Services website.[3] There are inherent difficulties in defining what constitutes abusive behaviour and the current definitions reflect a social judgement process that seeks to integrate several social–demographic details with the child's physical and mental status.

Neglect

Child neglect is the continued failure by a parent or caregiver to provide a child with the basic requirements for his or her proper growth and development, such as food, clothing, shelter, medical and dental care and adequate supervision.

Sexual abuse

Sexual abuse is when someone involves a child or young person in a sexual activity by using their power over them or taking advantage of their trust. Often children are bribed or threatened physically and psychologically to coerce them to participate in the activity.

Physical abuse

Physical abuse is a non-accidental injury or pattern of injuries to a child caused by a parent, caregiver or any other person. It includes, but is not limited to, injuries that are caused by excessive discipline, severe beatings or shakings, cigarette burns, attempted strangulation and female genital mutilation. Injuries include bruising, lacerations or welts, burns, fractures or dislocation of joints. Hitting a child around the head or neck and/or using a stick, belt or other object to discipline or punish a child (in a non-trivial way) is a crime in New South Wales.[4]

Psychological abuse or harm

Serious psychological harm can occur where the behaviour of the parent or caregiver damages the confidence and self-esteem of the child or young person, resulting in serious emotional deprivation or trauma. This can include a range of behaviours, such as excessive criticism, withholding affection, exposure to domestic violence, intimidation or threatening behaviour. In other words there is an important family context in which the harm is done.

Although it is possible for 'one-off' incidents to cause serious harm of both a physical and psychological nature, in cases of physical abuse and neglect of young children it is the frequency, persistence and duration of the parental or carer behaviour that is instrumental in defining the consequences for the child.[5,6]

> **Practice Point**
>
> There are medico-legal aspects to management of child abuse cases. This can cause undue concern for clinicians who may unconsciously wish to avoid the issue of abuse as a result of their concerns about losing the trust of the parents or carers, mistakenly accusing parents or carers of wrongdoing or undue worry about the time-consuming nature of being involved with these problems. As clinicians we need to be aware of how these concerns affect the way we deal with such matters, and to be able to recognise our limitations so that we can manage these cases as impartially and professionally as possible. Child abuse is not a problem to be managed in isolation and the resources available to support families and children and clinicians should be accessed readily.

LEGAL ASPECTS AND COMMUNITY SERVICES

It is also helpful to be clear about the distinction between abuse and assault. Abusive behaviour and the various forms of child abuse are perpetrated by a person, usually an adult, who has a caretaker role of the child and is therefore charged with responsibility for the child's wellbeing and safety. Assault may result in similar harmful contact but the perpetrator is not in the caretaker role. An assault is regarded as a criminal offence and much abuse of children will be regarded as offences that require criminal prosecution.

In New South Wales, as in other states and territories, the so-called Child Protection System is enshrined into legislation and the Department of Family and Community Services is the statutory body charged with the responsibility of administering the practical aspects of this legislation. One could argue the merits and shortcomings of an adversarial system based on the need to take punitive action against parents and caregivers who have harmed their children, but the scope of this chapter does not allow such a diversion. Suffice to say that the presence of this legislation emphasises the importance the community places in the safety and wellbeing of children and recognises that child abuse is an important problem that our society needs to address. It is an issue that remains on the political agenda.

The current legislation emphasises the importance of interagency collaboration and cooperation to meet the needs of children coming to attention as a result of concerns of abuse. It also emphasises that child protection is everyone's responsibilty, not just the Community Services officers. Over time there has been an effort to move towards prevention and early intervention, but the reality of case load and managing children already in alternative care impacts on the rate of change that these efforts can instigate.

In New South Wales all suspected cases of abuse are required to be reported to the Community Services call centre, a centralised referral unit, that considers the nature of the report and will prioritise the report according to established criterion. If the report contains information that the child in question has been seriously harmed physically, or if their life is in danger, or there is a sexual assault matter, the case is referred to the Joint Investigation Response Team (JIRT). JIRT comprise members of Community Services and Police and are routinely involved in cases that are of a criminal nature. There are JIRT units strategically placed throughout the state. Matters investigated and prosecuted by JIRT are referred to the criminal courts for prosecution if there is sufficient evidence as determined by the Department of Public Prosecution. The Criminal Court is concerned about whether a crime has been committed and that there is sufficient evidence to convict a person of this crime. It operates on the assumption of innocence and that, based on the information available to the court, a jury can conclude that an accused is responsible of a crime 'beyond reasonable doubt'.

Less serious harm matters are referred to the local Community Service Centres for allocation to a case worker and processing of the matter. Many reports are merely filed as they are not regarded as sufficiently serious to require more intervention. Further action might involve a visit to the family home and gathering of information from the community, such as school or health services.

The Children's Court presides over child care matters that are presented before a magistrate. The Children's Court requires a less rigorous standard of 'evidence' compared with the Criminal Court and the prime concern is the child's safety. The Children's Court process remains formal and has been streamlined such that medical evidence is usually accepted in written form without requiring the author to attend and give evidence in person. In practice it is the venue where applications for a child to be removed from an abusive family situation, either temporarily or permanently, are lodged and processed. Community Services present the case through legal representatives and the child and the parents or carers have separate legal representatives.

Practice Point

The above-mentioned refers to New South Wales legislation. The reader is encouraged to consult guidelines in their particular jurisdiction.

PREVALENCE OF CHILD ABUSE AND NEGLECT

There is no doubt that child abuse is a common and pervasive problem around the world.[7] Over the past 60 years or so much has been written about child abuse. Initially most of the literature reflected on the need to describe and raise awareness of this problem. Subsequently a body of knowledge and literature focused on the diagnosis and appropriate assessment of children who have been abused, and on developing ways of providing therapeutic intervention in support of these children.

In the United States in 2008, the rate of substantiated reports of child maltreatment was approximately 10 per 1,000 children in the age group 0–17 years.

Table 14.1 Primary substantiated maltreatment types in Australian states and territories in 2009–10

	NSW	VIC	QLD	WA	SA	TAS	ACT	NT	Australia
Emotional abuse	8,984	3,137	2,773	346	793	478	330	251	17,092
Neglect	7,999	472	2,230	646	721	286	282	639	13,275
Physical abuse	4,980	2,468	1,505	330	200	122	89	246	9,940
Sexual abuse	4,285	526	414	330	101	77	40	107	5,880
Total	26,248	6,603	6,922	1,652	1,815	963	741	1,243	46,187

Source: AIHW (2011, p. 68)[10]

Younger children are more frequently the victims of child maltreatment than older children. Neglect is the predominant form of abuse for all children and the youngest children are most at risk. In 2008, there were 22 substantiated child maltreatment reports per 1,000 children under age 1, compared with 12 for children aged 1–3 years, 11 for children aged 4–7 years, 9 for children aged 8–11 years, 8 for children aged 12–15 years, and 5.5 for adolescents aged 16–17 years.[8]

In Australia there is no systematic national surveillance of the prevalence of child abuse and neglect. There are variations between individual study prevalence estimates, based on methodological issues. These include the definition used, the way a survey questionnaire is worded, the number of questions asked about abuse and the population surveyed. Each state and territory has its own definition of abuse and the methods for accurate data collection vary.

The Australian Institute of Health and Welfare (AIHW) has compiled figures (see Figure 14.1: reproduced with permission) for child protection activity: in 2009–10 there were 286,437 reports of suspected child abuse and neglect made to state and territory authorities. This figure was a significant decrease from the previous year (16 per cent decrease) and most likely reflects a significant change in the definition of risk of significant harm in New South Wales, being the state with the highest reporting rates of abuse and the largest population.[9] Child neglect (28.7 per cent) and emotional abuse (37 per cent) are the most commonly reported forms of abuse in Australia, followed by physical abuse (22 per cent) and sexual abuse (12.7 per cent).[10] (See Table 14.1: reproduced with permission)

It is highly likely that there is a large percentage of child abuse that is not reported.

IMPACT OF ABUSE

There is general agreement that child maltreatment is common and remains an important source of long-term morbidity in a community.[11–15] Child abuse in general is associated with a number of negative outcomes for children, including lower school achievement, juvenile delinquency, substance abuse, and mental health problems. Certain types of maltreatment can result in long-term physical, social, and emotional problems, and even death. Children who witness domestic

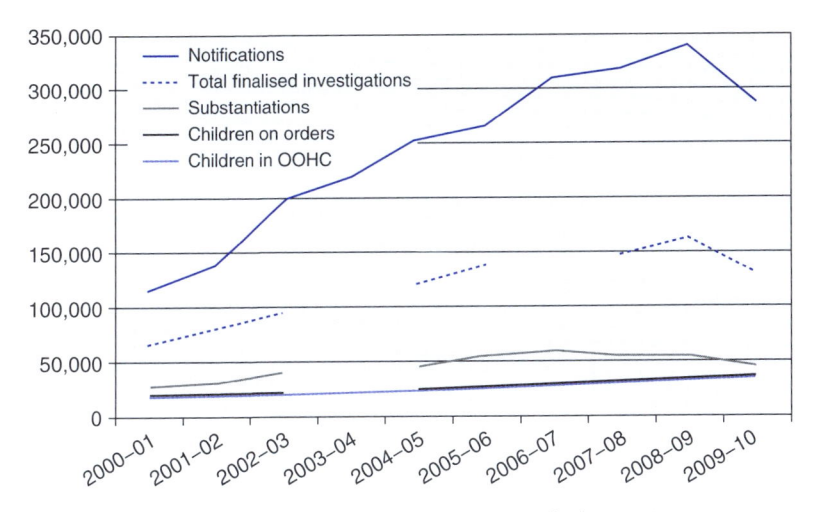

FIGURE 14.1 Total number of notifications, investigations and substantiations across Australia from 2000–01 to 2009–10, and total number of children on orders and in out-of-home care at 30 June 2000 to 2010.

violence are at a greater risk of developing behavioural and emotional problems, and influence their own behaviour in interpersonal relationships, and long-term problems.[16] Early childhood trauma increases the risk of various attachment disorders and post-traumatic stress-related symptomatology.

PHYSICAL ABUSE

Physical abuse represents about 25 per cent of the total reports of child abuse in New South Wales. In the United States about 772,00 children are reported as victims of abuse or neglect and 16 per cent were identified as physically abused. The highest incidence of physical abuse was in children in the first year of life. An estimated 1740 children died as a result of abuse or neglect.[17] There are various manifestations of physical abuse and these are listed in order of frequency of presentation:
- Bruising
- Fractures
- Head injury
- Burns
- Abdominal injury
- Factitious and/or induced illness.

These injuries will vary in severity and frequency, and in the context of an abusive relationship with a carer is unlikely to be a one-off event.

Inflicted physical injuries are more common in younger children with the majority of cases occurring in the child less than 2 years of age. Important indicators of child abuse include:
- Child younger than 2 years
- Several presentations with significant injuries

- Unexplained injuries especially if the injury requires significant medical care
- A significant and unreasonable delay between the injury and the seeking of help or medical assessment
- Injuries of different ages, such as fractures or multiple bruises that are located in unusual locations (see 'bruising' below)
- Injuries explained by parents or carers but where the explanation is incongruous with the child's developmental level
- A history that changes or varies considerably between carers or between interviews.

There is a concern in the community that there is a danger of over-diagnosing physical abuse because it is so easy for children to hurt themself during their day-to-day activities. Alternatively, it is argued that parents are no longer able to discipline their children for fear of being accused of harming them.

The challenge for the clinician is:
- To remain impartial enough to consider the possibility of child abuse when there are sufficient clinical indicators
- To assess the situation appropriately
- To consult with the experts to assist in the assessment process when indicated.

> **Practice Point**
>
> Assessment of injury requires careful consideration of the history of injury, the location and appearance of the injury and the context of the presentation. It is the clinician's role to detect injuries that are suspicious of abuse but not to determine the intention behind the injuries. This decision may ultimately be determined by the legal system.

Bruises

A bruise is caused by an impact that damages blood vessels such that blood escapes into the surrounding dermal or subcutaneous tissues. Bruises are caused by blunt force injury and the extent of bruising depends on a number of factors including:
- Degree of force applied
- Age and sex of the person. The younger the child and female sex increase the likelihood of bruising for the same degree of trauma
- Site of injury
- The rigidity of the object impacting on the body
- General health of the person.

Bruises are said to be the most common presentation for child physical abuse. However it can be difficult to distinguish bruises that occurred as a result of abuse from those that occurred as a result of normal activity or an inadvertent event that was not intentional.

Bruising patterns that may indicate a higher chance of inflicted injury include:[18,19]
- Patterned bruises: e.g. finger imprints, a belt buckle or other implement, bite marks, pinch marks
- Location: it is common to find bruises over bony prominences in toddlers. Bruises are unlikely to occur over padded areas and soft tissue regions such

as abdomen, chest, thighs, face, ears, hands and feet: these sites may be indicative of non-accidental injury
- Symmetrical bruising
- Multiple bruising thought to be of varying ages.

Remember that non-mobile infants rarely bruise in the absence of underlying illness or well documented injury.[20]

Other signs of abuse or neglect such as poor weight gain, developmental delay or unhealthy attachment behaviour must be taken into account.

Documentation of bruises is best performed by using diagrams that are of reasonable size and that represent all planes of the body. Use a tape measure to record the size and location of bruises accurately. Add a description of the colour, shape and degree of swelling or tenderness. Specification of the location of bruises in reference to various bony landmarks can be helpful. Photographs are a very useful way of documenting bruises and other superficial injuries.

Photography

Photographic documentation is a very reliable and accurate means of recording what can be easily missed with the naked eye. It is important to ensure that *consent* has been obtained with an *explanation* as to the reasons for the photographs. Photographs remain part of the medical record and may represent important evidence in a court of law. Careful consideration should be given as to where photographs are stored and who has access to the images.

In order to meet forensic requirements consider the following:
- Take a photograph of the child's details, including name and date of birth.
- A *photograph of the child* for identification purposes is important.
- *Labels* indicating the specific location of bruises being photographed.
- A *measuring tape* placed in proximity to the area photographed to allow appreciation of the size of the bruise in real terms.
- Ensure that a generous number of views are taken with good lighting or flash attachment.
- It is preferable that the photographs are taken professionally but this is not always possible.
- Make an entry in the child's medical notes that photographs have been taken and ensure this is signed and dated.
- Photographs remain part of the medical record and have evidentiary value.
- Photographs are however limited by the quality of the image and readily affected by poor lighting and being out of focus. Care is required in interpreting photographs that are taken by others in the absence of having examined the child.

Differential diagnosis

As with all forms of abuse, careful consideration must be given as to other explanations or medical causes of bruises in young children. While most of these will be self-explanatory they may be overlooked or initially present some confusion for the clinician.[21] The following list refers to some of the most common alternatives:
- Accidental injury
- A bleeding diathesis, congenital or acquired
- Various forms of vasculitis

- Birth marks, especially variations of Mongolian spots
- Alternative medicines or treatments, such as application of hot glass cups in traditional Chinese and Vietnamese treatments
- Self-inflicted injury: for example suction petechii
- Allergic skin reactions
- Paints, dyes or dirt may initially confuse the clinician.

Abusive head trauma

Abusive head trauma, formerly Shaken Baby Syndrome, is an uncommon but important manifestation of child abuse. There is a significant morbidity and mortality associated with this form of abuse. Some studies estimate that death occurs in up to one-third of children and serious morbidity in another third of children injured in this way.[22] It has been estimated that up to 80 per cent of child abuse-related deaths in children under 2 years of age are related to head trauma.[23–25]

The term Shaken Baby Syndrome was originally coined by Caffey, an orthopaedic surgeon, to describe the acceleration–deceleration forces which result in significant brain injury.[26] Classically this type of injury results in the triad of *encephalopathy* as a result of the diffuse nature of the brain injury, *subdural haemorrhage* as a result of the shearing of bridging veins that cross the subdural space[27] and *retinal haemorrhage*, also postulated to be the result of the shearing forces induced by such an injury.

The term Shaken Baby Syndrome has now been superseded. It has been realised that so-called abusive or inflicted head trauma can occur from a number of mechanisms, not just shaking an infant violently. Furthermore, despite a strong body of clinical opinion and circumstantial evidence such as confessions of alleged perpetrators, it has not been convincingly demonstrated through research that abusive head trauma occurs by shaking alone.[28,29] Others argue that some form of impact on the head is required in order to generate the forces needed to injure the infant brain.[30] Finally, the term implies intent and this is not usually something that a clinician is in a position to fully assess even with a confession from the perpetrator.

It is recommended that clinicians move away from the term Shaken Baby Syndrome due to this ongoing controversy, the need for clarity of thinking in regards to this form of child abuse and to avoid confusion in the medico-legal arena. There are authors who question the validity of the concept of brain injury by shaking and have postulated that even minor events or apnoea could result in a similar clinical spectrum.[31,32]

While it is important to be aware of the continued controversy surrounding this phenomenon, the majority of clinicians in the field are in agreement that child abuse is the most common cause of serious head injury in infants and young children.[33,34]

Presentation

The three classic clinical findings of Abusive Head Injury are:
1 encephalopathy
2 retinal haemorrhages
3 subdural haematoma.

The child commonly requires active resuscitation and intensive care.[34] This clinical picture often occurs in the context of an infant and the absence or only vague history of any problems prior to presentation. There is no identifiable underlying medical condition discovered and the outcome is likely to be poor. Spontaneous subdural bleeding in infancy is very rare.[35] The study by Matschke et al.[33] demonstrated the close association between unexplained subdural haemorrhage and abusive head trauma. A recent review article by Chiesa and Duhaime on Abusive Head Trauma is a concise summary of the current clinical and theoretical underpinnings of this condition as well as the areas of contention and uncertainty.[36]

It is common to find injuries in other areas of the child's body, such as bruising, intraabdominal injuries and fractures especially of the posterior ribs just lateral to the costovertebral junction. While there may be external signs of trauma to the scalp, bruising is by no means common and may only be detected at post-mortem on examination of the scalp.[36]

One of the critical points that raise the suspicion of an inflicted head injury is the absence of a history of trauma and relatively trivial or vague description of events leading up to the child's admission. Furthermore, no other medical explanation is forthcoming at the time of admission. When there is a suspicion of abusive head trauma, it is important to exclude other well recognised causes of encephalopathy and shock. These include sepsis (especially meningitis), metabolic disorders, bleeding disorders, other trauma, seizures or other central nervous system disasters, for example a ruptured arterio-venous malformation.

Infants with less serious brain injury can present with subtle findings such as vomiting or non-specific irritability and can be missed clinically.[37] A high index of suspicion is needed. Maguire et al. performed an extensive literature review in an attempt to distinguish inflicted from non-inflicted brain injury. They concluded that apnoea at the time of clinical presentation, retinal haemorrhages and rib fractures were the most important factors supportive of a diagnosis of inflicted brain injury.[38]

Investigations

Young children presenting with significant head injury that is suspicious of being inflicted warrant comprehensive investigations to search for other forms of trauma, including:
- retinal examination by an experienced ophthalmologist
- skeletal survey
- intraabdominal injury.

Investigating the extent of the head injury involves a CT scan initially, as it is more sensitive at detecting acute blood intracranially. An MRI scan is useful some days later as it is more sensitive at detecting intracerebral injuries or ischaemic change. An MRI can also detect blood around the optic nerve sheath.

Consultation with neurosurgery, neurology and rehabilitation teams forms an important component of the ongoing assessment and management.

Fractures

Fractures are a common reason for children being referred with the suspicion of abusive injuries. Reported frequency of fractures in association with child abuse range from 11–55 per cent depending on the study.[39] There are no pathognomonic features of fractures that have been inflicted, though there are some features that should alert the clinician to this possibility including the following:[40]

- Multiple fractures, particularly at various stages of healing
- Metaphyseal corner and bucket-handle fractures, suggesting an avulsion injury
- Fractures of ribs, especially if multiple
- Fractures of the small bones of the hands and feet
- Crush fractures of vertebrae
- Complex skull fracture, defined by Kleinman[41] as more than one fracture line or growing fractures.[42]

Note: Isolated or multiple rib fractures, irrespective of location, have the highest specificity for inflicted injury.[43,44]

As with other forms of physical abuse, the history and context in which the child presents is critical in determining the cause of an injury. All injuries should make some sense to the treating clinician. The younger the child, especially below 12 months of age, the more likely it is that another person is aware of the mechanism of injury or at least should be able to provide a consistent and reliable report of the circumstances at the time of injury.

Mechanisms of injury

Fractures will result when the force applied exceeds the strength and elasticity of the tissue to which the force is applied. This applies as much to biological material, such as bones, as it does to other materials. The direction of the applied force will determine the nature of a fracture. For example, if a person trips and in the ensuing fall their weight-bearing foot is fixed in position and there is a rotation of the body above the ankle, the result is a spiral fracture of the tibia. Spiral fractures are most likely the result of a twisting motion with fixation of one end of the long bone involved.

Torus fractures result when there is compression of long bones, commonly the proximal tibia or distal femur. The direction of force is along the same axis as that of the bone. Transverse fractures mostly result from side-on impact with fixation above and below the site of impact.

This brief account can oversimplify the nature of many injuries under complex and unique situations, but allows some sense to be made of injuries when assessing the relationship between the history provided and the injury seen.

Imaging

Skeletal survey is the investigation of choice for suspected physical abuse in children under 2 years of age. There are two useful reviews of the literature on many aspects of imaging in suspected child physical abuse published recently.[45,46] The skeletal survey should be done with care and using accepted protocols. X-rays are more sensitive for picking up skull and metaphyseal long bone fractures.[47] As mentioned in the American College of Radiology Guidelines oblique views of the ribs can increase the diagnosis of rib fractures. There is less support for routine skeletal surveys in older children, although imaging may be indicated depending on the clinical presentation, such as the presence of brain or intraabdominal injuries.

There is a role for follow-up X-rays two weeks later, especially if the first survey was performed within a few days of the injury as the fracture may not be immediately apparent. A second radiological examination can assist in ageing of fractures, or clarifying an earlier finding of uncertain significance.[48]

Nuclear bone scanning is a useful complementary investigation that requires skill and experience to perform and interpret.[47] The main limitation is its availability.

It is not as useful in detecting skull and metaphyseal fractures but is helpful in rib, pelvic and acromial fractures. It can also detect periosteal trauma without fracture.

Burns

Burns may result from thermal, radiation, chemical and electrical injury. The net result is the disruption of cell membranes and molecular damage or denaturation. Exposure to chemicals; flame; scalds, i.e. contact with hot liquid; friction, such as carpet; contact with objects with extremes of temperature, most commonly excessive heat; and ultraviolet radiation are the most common sources of burn injury. Hot liquid scalding injuries are well described and a relatively common cause of burns in toddlers. Nappy rash is a chemical burn as a result of prolonged exposure to urine or faeces, especially in infancy. Burns, as with many childhood injuries, are often sustained at times of limited parental supervision or times of stress.

Several authors have alluded to the apparent premeditated nature of inflicted burns, but the motivation for this type of abuse is beyond the scope of this chapter. Burn injuries often result in major psychological trauma as well as prolonged physical debilitation.[49]

The severity of a thermal burn is determined by the heat of the agent, usually water; the duration of exposure; the site involved; and the use of first aid measures to minimise injury. There are often quoted graphs defining the temperature and duration of exposure to injury indicating an exponential increase in risk of thermal injury with linear increases in temperature of the contact substance. These data are however based on very limited scientific research but remain the prime reference point on which burn injury is interpreted. The ethics of any scientific research places major restrictions on further research in this area, especially in paediatrics.

Inflicted burn injuries should be suspected when there are certain patterns identified within the distribution of the burn. It is often difficult to distinguish inflicted from accidental burns, but there have been attempts to do so which require validation with more prospective research.[50]

Scald burns cause the greatest injury at the point of contact. As the liquid runs away from the point of contact in the direction of gravity, there will be cooling and less severe injury. This flow away from the point of contact may produce the so-called 'arrow points pattern'. If the child is wearing clothing at the time of contact with the hot liquid, this will affect firstly the distribution, and secondly the severity, as it will retain heat and prolong contact with the skin.

Examples of patterned burns
Immersion burns often occur in younger children and are characterised by clearly demarcated areas of burnt and unburnt skin, such as the glove and stocking type distribution or around the buttock and upper parts of the lower limbs with minimal splash marks evident, possibly with sparing of the buttock or sacral area which may have been in contact with the container. Sparing in skin flexures is usually evident. Several findings may point to a deliberate immersion including:
- Waterline
- Sparing of flexural creases and feet
- Glove and stocking burns
- Doughnut sparing of the buttock.

Cigarette burns are distinguished by their circular shape with the deepest part of the burn being centrally located. They are not uncommonly located on extremities but can be seen on the face and trunk. It is not unusual to see more than one lesion or scarring from previous injuries. The appearance may be confused with impetigo but is usually easily distinguishable by the rapid spread of infective lesion in a centripetal manner with central healing and absence of scarring.

Branding, that is the application of a hot implement against the skin, is also well described. Bar radiators, stove tops, irons and other household items are frequently implicated. These injuries are not always intentional but a careful history is required to establish how they occurred. The application of a heated end of the cigarette lighter is sometimes implicated.

Sunburn is also reasonably common, particularly in Australia. This is usually more as a result of neglect.

As with all injuries a careful history should include details of preceding events leading up to the burn, documentation of people who may have witnessed the event or have been in the vicinity at the time, details of the location of the child in relation to the agent causing the burn, if possible the maximum temperature of the hot water system, and if relevant the height of the bath versus the height of the child. Such information may require a third party, such as police, in order to assist in the investigation.

Other investigations

When abuse is suspected it is important to consider other injuries. A skeletal survey is advised as part of a routine work-up in a child under the age of two with a suspect burn. It has been reported that fractures are relatively uncommon in children with burn injuries, as they tend to be a little older on average. However a recent paper indicated that there was still a significant incidence of occult fractures (14 per cent) in this group of children.[51]

Abdominal trauma

While abdominal trauma as a result of abuse is uncommon, it is said to be the second leading cause of death in young children from abuse-related injuries.[49] Serious abdominal trauma is usually suspected at the time of presentation but may be overlooked in the presence of other injuries, such as a head trauma with loss of consciousness. These injuries are more common in older active children and toddlers due to misadventure or motor vehicle accidents. An earlier study of intraabdominal trauma as a result of abuse identified a mortality rate of up to 50 per cent.[52] Solid and hollow organs are affected with the liver being most commonly injured.

Young children may experience blunt trauma to the abdomen from abuse with blows often localised to the umbilical or epigastric region.[53] The minimum amount of abdominal musculature and subcutaneous fat renders intraabdominal organs more prone to injury. External signs of trauma are often minimal or absent.[54,55]

Practice Point

It is important to have a high index of suspicion for abdominal trauma. Screening for liver enzymes, amylase and lipase, haemoglobin for occult blood loss and even liver and other solid organ imaging should be considered.

FACTITIOUS AND/OR INDUCED ILLNESS (MUNCHAUSEN SYNDROME BY PROXY)

Once again terminology is an important issue to avoid confusion and to satisfy medico-legal requirements. This form of child abuse was first described by Professor Roy Meadow[56,57] when he reported two cases: one where a contaminated urine sample was submitted, and the second where the child was fed large amounts of salt resulting in hypernatraemia. In his cases and in most of the cases subsequently described the perpetrator was the mother, and generally the offending parent had an unusual familiarity with the health system. Donna Rosenberg's excellent review of the literature in 1987[58] highlighted the wide range of presentations from attempted suffocation, seizure disorders or deliberate poisoning to fabrication of medical histories and misleading medical information that resulted in the child being subject to numerous unnecessary tests or admissions to hospital. There was often a lengthy delay between initial presentation and recognition of the abusive pattern. She emphasised the significant mortality rate (9 per cent) and long-term risk of psychological harm in many survivors. Later authors recognised the important role of the medical profession in unwittingly contributing to reinforcing the so-called abnormal illness behaviour in the carers.[59]

The term 'Munchausen syndrome by proxy' was coined in reference to an earlier psychological condition, Munchausen syndrome. The implication was that there was a psychological need in the parent or carer, who was identified as the perpetrator of harm, for special attention that was achieved through contact with the health system. The child was the vector that facilitated ongoing contact with healthcare professionals. The term Munchausen syndrome by proxy is no longer regarded as appropriate as there is no such mental health condition in the DSM, and there is no clear and consistent psychological profile of the perpetrators, nor is there always a well-defined motive. This has led to criticism from legal experts as well as a ground swell of concern from parents who had been implicated in this syndrome that they had been unfairly accused, as it is often a difficult diagnosis to prove.

Factitious or Induced Illness (FII) has presented intriguing and often confounding dilemmas for clinicians dealing with such cases, although it is relatively rare and estimated to be about 2 cases per 10^5 in New Zealand and the United Kingdom with a similar rate in Australia (personal communication APSU data unpublished).[60,61] These cases are often very time-consuming and can be very stressful on individual clinicians, emphasising the importance of a multidisciplinary approach to diagnosis and management. A high index of suspicion is required, and this condition presents challenges for clinicians because the therapeutic relationship assumes a mutual level of trust and honesty with a mutual level of concern for the safety and wellbeing of the child. In the current climate of defensive medical practice it will remain challenging to satisfy the need to exclude reasonable medical problems through careful history and investigation, avoiding the relentless pursuit of more and more elusive medical diagnoses requiring more complex medical management.

The following clues might assist in alerting the busy clinician to the possibility of FII:
- Persistent symptoms in the absence of clinical signs or abnormal tests
- Symptoms that occur only in the presence of a particular carer

- Severe illness or recurrence of illness, e.g. septic episodes, even while in hospital and on appropriate treatment
- Puzzling array of symptoms or presentations that settle under careful observation
- Apparent lack of distress in the parent or carer even in the presence of apparently life-threatening events
- An apparent preoccupation of the parent or carer with the technical aspects of the case, the details of the medical test results or complaints about the quality of care provided
- At the same time the parent or carer might give a superficial impression of attention and concern for the child but careful observation may reveal poor quality interaction and connection with the child.

Case examples

Every case will present its own unique diagnostic dilemmas. The presence of exogenous, that is porcine-derived insulin, in a case of recurrent hypoglycaemia in an infant was only detected after the clinician involved became aware that the older sibling was a victim of FII and requested the appropriate test. A child with several septic episodes while in hospital and already on intravenous antibiotics was diagnosed after an astute microbiologist detected a blood culture positive for three unusual bacteria commonly found in drains. The microbiologist recalled a similar case some years earlier and on review discovered that the earlier case was the current child's sibling. The first child had died of what was thought to be a septic illness and was thought to have an immunodeficiency that was poorly defined.

Practice Point

There was some enthusiasm for covert video-surveillance in detecting FII in certain situations. This is not a practice that is currently recommended, although there have been successful prosecutions as a result of this approach in the past. It is better to gather relevant material, over time if necessary, with which to confront families with the concerns. This confrontation needs careful planning and the involvement of the appropriate child protection statutory authorities. Much background investigation may be warranted to test out the medical and family history, as well as checking the possibility of whether the child has been seen by other medical services that have not been disclosed. In most cases a specialised team is important to assist in the coordination of such investigations and intervention. The involvement of an experienced child psychiatry service can be invaluable in assessing and subsequently working with these families.

CHILD NEGLECT AND EMOTIONAL ABUSE

Child neglect is the most common reason reports are made to statutory authorities. Once again there are problems with definition. This section will focus on a medical perspective, because definitions depend on context and the authors' background, be it legal, social sciences, psychological or medical. There is general agreement that whatever the neglect there is harm as a result. This harm may manifest early with poor growth, as in so-called Failure to Thrive, delayed development in early years, school failure or poor health through to much longer term problems of mental health, poor health in adults and early death. Neglect is regarded as an act of omission rather than one of commission.

Emotional abuse, on the other hand, is a more active form of psychological trauma where the main carers consistently belittle, criticise and undermine the child's sense of self. The overlap with neglect is considerable and the term 'psychological maltreatment' has emerged as a means of standardising and understanding the nature and impact of this abusive behaviour. The American Professional Society on the Abuse of Children (APSAC) define psychological maltreatment as 'a repeated pattern of caregiver behaviour or extreme incident(s) that convey to children that they are worthless, flawed, unloved, unwanted, endangered, or only of value in meeting another's needs'. The APSAC guidelines define six subtypes of psychological maltreatment: spurning, terrorising, isolating, exploiting or corrupting, denying emotional responsiveness, and mental health medical and educational neglect.[62]

Neglect of appropriate care of a child is most closely linked to lower socioeconomic status but is not the same as poverty. Emotional impact of abuse in children should be considered in all forms of abuse. The nature of child abuse is a combination of the exposure to trauma and the disruption or distortion of the healthy, essentially trusting relationship between the parent or carer and the child that maximises normal development physically and psychologically.

Building on Bowlby's original work on attachment,[63] Crittenden's work on attachment behaviour [64] highlights the relevance of attachment behaviour and the importance of the relationship between the primary carer and the child in determining a healthy outcome. Crittenden emphasises that the attachment behaviour is driven by the child in order to secure a safe and nurturing level of care. She argues that a child's behaviour from early infancy is driven to achieve this. Erickson and Egeland refer to the 'psychologically unavailable parent, who overlooks their infant's cues and signals' to highlight the critical nature of this parental function, and the difficulty of measuring this relationship objectively.[65] While there are no readily available clinical tools to assess the quality of interaction between children and their carers, Ainsworth and Crittenden and subsequently Crittenden and her colleagues continue to develop a range of observational and interview-based structured assessment measures that attempt to score the quality of the relationship that has scientific validity and reproducibility.

Medical neglect has become a term that is reflective of the broader phenomenon of neglect but specifically refers to the neglect of medical needs of a child, which as a result causes harm to the child.[66] For example, regular non-attendance for scheduled medical appointments in a child with a chronic medical condition such as diabetes or unstable asthma with resulting repeated hospitalisations. It can be difficult to know where one draws a line between what is acceptable and unacceptable. This decision can be better informed by considering the situation in the context of what is known about the family, how serious are the consequences of non-compliance with medical care, how different is this family's behaviour in regards compliance with that of others, and how much compromise the clinician is having to make with regards to the child's medical care in order to keep the family engaged. It is important to discuss the concerns with colleagues in order to clarify the issues, their chronicity and their seriousness.

In considering the context of the neglect, poverty can play an important part but the focus should remain with the needs of the child. If poverty is the main reason a child is not receiving proper care then this can usually be supported. As with other forms of abuse there are usually other issues that impact on care, such as domestic violence, parental mental health problems, intellectual disability, drug and alcohol dependence, unstable accommodation, access to healthcare services, cultural and religious influences that are poorly understood.

A similar approach is required when assessing an infant who presents with poor weight gain or an older child with undernutrition and, increasingly importantly, obesity. The term organic versus non-organic failure to thrive is no longer used, as it is recognised that there are multiple factors that result in poor weight gain. It is the clinician's role, often in collaboration with other healthcare providers, to uncover the major factors within the child, within the family and the environment in order to address poor weight gain. Clinicians have sufficient skills to be able to ask appropriate questions to allow as complete an understanding of the child's situation as possible.

Assessment

1. **Medical or nutritional:** Growth parameters, especially looking for deviations from an established growth trajectory. Weight in early childhood is the most sensitive to impacts of ill health and emotional and attachment problems. A clinical assessment of the child's nutritional status, including waist and triceps subcutaneous thickness, muscle wasting and a general developmental assessment.
2. **General appearance:** Unkempt appearance and smelly clothes could be judgementally interpreted but may provide a clue as to the level of chaos and disorganisation at home, especially if this is observed on more than one occasion. Information from school or day care may be helpful.
3. **Observation of parent–child interaction:** This can reveal a considerable amount of information and is often overlooked. Careful scrutiny of the quality and nature of a parent's interaction with their child or children and vice versa may offer reassurance, uncertainty or further cause for concern. More obvious things, such as a parent ignoring the child during conversations with the clinician, neglecting to offer safety or comfort when hurt, prop feeding, speaking in derogatory terms to the child, use of unduly coercive or punitive management strategies, should be documented. This information may be helpful both in terms of a diagnostic and also a therapeutic framework.
4. **Medical examination** provides objective information in order to formulate the medical management plan. Include hearing, vision and dental health as they are common problems easily overlooked in this situation that if unattended further compound the child's developmental trajectory.

Management

1. Address immediate medical needs and a clear, simple management plan with follow-up appointments with specified clinicians. The plan should be provided to the parents or carers even if they are illiterate. Copies should be forwarded to other members of the management team.
2. A case conference, including the parents ideally, is a valuable means of developing a practical management plan. It provides an excellent means of

communication to all involved and is effective in ensuring accountability within the team.
3   Regular reviews are important as these cases usually present long-term challenges commensurate with the identified risk factors, many of which will not disappear.
4   Involvement of community-based services that can work with families and enable them to access other services to assist with behaviour management, enriching their parenting skills including nurturing ability. Regular home visiting, for example, in early childhood has been shown to have a protective effect against abusive behaviour.[67,68]

CHILD SEXUAL ABUSE

It is important to be as clear as possible as to what is defined as sexual abuse of children. It is abusive because the actions of the perpetrator are self-centred and harmful to the child–victim. The child is being used for the perpetrator's own needs. It includes any sexual behaviour towards the child and there is a major developmental discrepancy between the perpetrator and the child's capacity to realise and control what is happening. The child usually is aware that something is not right and may often be involved in some degree of coercive behaviour from something as seemingly benign as being friendly and generous through to extreme threats of violence to the child or other family members, or blaming the child for the consequences if anyone finds out. The psychological impact of child sexual abuse follows from these two factors: that is the psychological impact of the breach of trust between an adult and the child, and the trauma from threats that may have been used in the coercion involved.

Child sexual abuse is common although estimates vary depending on the type of population surveyed. It is not possible to accurately quantify the incidence of child sexual abuse. Estimates are that up to 1 in 4 females and 1 in 9 males by age 18 have been involved in sexual activity that was not of their choosing and that they regarded as a traumatic experience.[69]

Swanston et al.[70] studied a cohort of sexually abused children and reviewed the outcomes after a period of nine years comparing them with a control group. They found that the sexually abused young people performed more poorly in a range of measures reflecting a significant negative impact on their emotional wellbeing. This effect appeared to be independent of the therapy provided. They demonstrated that a number of factors impacted on the outcome independent of the abuse, including several adverse family circumstances and child factors such as a sense of despair and hopefulness, the number of adverse events, ratings of their father's care, previous reports of sexual abuse and placement in out-of-home care.

One of the main differences between sexual abuse and other forms of abuse is that the majority of victims are female, with estimates varying between 75–90 per cent, and the perpetrators are almost always male, approximately 95 per cent. Despite considerable research into the motivation of perpetrators and attempts to develop a profile of a typical child sex offender, it is the currently accepted view that there is no typical perpetrator profile and that the dynamics of sexual abuse are complex. There is agreement that the motivation may have some elements of sexual gratification, but more likely this is the powerful reinforcing agent and that the underlying drive is for control and power. It is thought that this offending behaviour often starts in pre-pubertal years and by late adolescence this behaviour has been strongly established and often difficult to treat effectively.[71] Various treatment programs around the world attest to the challenging nature of this offending behaviour and the recidivism rates are significant in many programs but less than with imprisonment alone.[72,73]

Presentation

The most common presentation of child sexual abuse is by way of disclosure. In the past it was not uncommon for disclosures to be minimised or ignored as the nature of the disclosure was so shocking or dangerous in its implications for the family. Now, with the widespread awareness of sexual abuse, children are being heard and the responses appear to be more supportive and appropriate. It is still important to be aware that many children will present with other symptoms that reflect medical or emotional complications of abuse.[74,75]

Common medical indicators include:

- Recurrent urinary tract infections in a school-age child, notably in the absence of a documented congenital disposition
- Recurrent vaginitis, vaginal discharge or genital discomfort for which no medical cause is found
- A change in toileting behaviour, such as the sudden onset of soiling or urinary incontinence in a previously asymptomatic child
- Recurrent abdominal pains and other nonspecific somatic symptoms, especially if there is a clear onset time or pattern
- Presence of sexually transmitted infection, such as genital warts, gonorrhoea or chlamydia.
- Pregnancy.

Children may also present with more obscure symptoms reflecting a degree of emotional distress such as:

- disturbed sleep pattern, onset of nightmares or excessive fearfulness at bedtime that seems uncharacteristic
- Fearfulness when being left with a particular person or situation
- Regression in developmental skills and behaviour
- Unsettled and angry behaviour that is out of character
- Anorexia nervosa and bulimia – it is estimated that up to 50 per cent of bulimic patients have been sexually abused
- Self-harming behaviour and depression in adolescence
- Deteriorating school performance
- Displays of inappropriately explicit sexualised behaviour at a developmental stage where this would not be expected
- Drawings with sexually explicit themes.

None of these behavioural and emotional indicators are specific for abuse, but they should serve as alerts for the astute clinician.

Assessment

The assessment and management of cases of sexual abuse should be managed by appropriately trained clinicians, as there is a high chance that these cases will involve referral to the legal system. All cases of suspected or disclosed sexual abuse require reporting to the appropriate authorities with the jurisdiction to investigate the potential criminal aspects of the matter. All cases of sexual abuse could potentially result in a criminal prosecution.

It is the clinician's role, and indeed responsibility, to be aware of the complex dynamics of child sexual abuse, to be aware that child sexual abuse is common and easily overlooked, and that even when this possibility is entertained it is all too easy to discount this possibility in the hope that a more benign explanation is discovered.

As with any assessment a thorough medical history is required with an emphasis on past history of urinary tract infection, anal or genital trauma or surgical intervention, constipation, soiling or urinary incontinence, previous sexual abuse, consensual sexual activity, menstrual history, possibility of pregnancy and sexually transmitted infections.

The history should also include education achievement, behavioural history and use of illicit drugs or alcohol. Is the child taking medication? Are there any specific allergies? The family history is also important as it enables a clearer understanding of the child's family context. It is quite common to learn that one or other parent has a background of sexual or other abuse and the child's presentation can trigger a major crisis for the adults as memories of their own past trauma are reactivated. Given that the child's recovery is contingent on healthy support from their carers, it is important to be aware of other risk factors that may impact on recovery.

Interviewing children

In most cases of suspected child sexual assault it is not appropriate to interview the child about details of their abuse. This should be left to the statutory authorities, that is Police and Community Services personnel. The medical staff should focus on building a rapport with the child and address any immediate medical concerns that require attention. It is important to clarify with the child what they understand about the assessment and whether they had any particular worries. It is important to explain your role and what will happen, and allow the child some control over what is happening to them. It is equally important to avoid asking leading questions about what has happened.

If the child does volunteer information about what has happened it is important to document this accurately and verbatim. Always keep in mind that the perpetrator may be present or nearby when assessing a child and this will impact on the child's sense of safety and willingness to disclose information.

Examination

Children should be examined by well-trained clinicians, familiar with the process. In an emergency department it makes sense to assess a child to ensure they do not have major injuries that require surgical management or resuscitation. This situation is rare however. Children are examined thoroughly with careful inspection of the whole child for evidence of other injuries, nutritional status and general health.

If the abuse has occurred within 72 hours there is a greater chance of finding offender DNA. Prompt referral to a specialised sexual assault service is essential in such cases. In these cases the child is subjected to a 'forensic assessment' with the view to obtaining relevant swabs for evidence of offender DNA, as well as addressing the child's overall health needs.

In order to examine the genitalia children are usually examined in the supine, frog-leg position. This allows good relaxation and visiblility. A good light source is required. Most centres use a colposcope with videorecording capacity. This equipment provides excellent lighting, magnification and photo-documentation of findings. It is often useful to examine girls in the knee–chest position as well as the supine position as the configuration of the hymen can change considerably with posture. The examination of the genitalia is by inspection only and does not involve the use of instruments or bimanual pelvic examination. The labia majora are separated with gentle traction down and out toward the examiner. This allows a good exposure of the posterior fourchette and hymenal membrane, which are the areas most likely to be injured in cases of penetration of the genital area. There are excellent texts and teaching material as well as review articles on this subject.[76,77]

Much has been written about the genital examination and relevance of findings.[78] It is now well established that the majority of child victims of sexual abuse have normal findings.[79,80] There are various reasons for this fact: the most important is that the nature of sexual abuse uncommonly involves full sexual intercourse in pre-pubertal children. It has also been documented that even significant acute injuries, such as tears to the hymen, heal remarkably well and may be impossible to recognise after some months.[81] Accordingly, there have been attempts at developing algorithms to assist in the decision-making process concerning the likelihood of abuse. Many times it is the statements made by the child alone, possibly with other non-medical corroborative evidence, that influence the outcome of cases in the legal arena.

Anal examination is performed in the left lateral position. It consists of inspection of the area after gentle lateral traction of the buttocks. Prolonged traction will cause distension of perianal veins and sometimes relaxation of the external anal sphincter. It is not uncommon to see pits and relatively thin skin that may have the appearance of scar tissue, in the 6 and 12 o'clock positions of the perianal skin. These are normal variants.

Signs of acute injury to the genital and anal areas are usually readily identified. Bruises, abrasions and even lacerations indicate acute trauma. Diffuse redness, with or without discharge, is a common observation and a nonspecific finding especially in pre-pubertal child.

The signs of chronic penetrating trauma to the anal and genital regions are more difficult to interpret and may vary from normal to complete but healed tears of the hymen, chronic anal fissures, and internal and external anal sphincter dilatation. These findings require careful evaluation and interpretation.

Sexually transmitted diseases

The presence of sexually transmitted diseases in children should arouse suspicion of sexual abuse. The approach to screening for sexually transmitted infections (STIs) in child sexual abuse case should be carried out on a case-by-case basis. Factors that should be taken into account include the age of the child, for example the risks will be different for a sexually active adolescent than a 5-year-old child. Other factors include the perpetrator's background, though this information may not be readily available; the type of abuse, for example fondling of the genitalia versus vaginal intercourse; presence of symptoms such as discharge or dysuria versus asymptomatic.

Human papilloma virus (HPV) is seen rarely in pre-pubertal children, though it is not an unusual reason for suspecting sexual abuse. There are no systematic studies available to estimate incidence in our community. Vertical transmission is described although not common and it can present as genital lesions[82] but this is an unusual explanation beyond the third year of life. HPV is the most common STI in adults. The recent introduction of immunisation of young female adolescents in Australia may have a significant impact on the frequency of this presently common STI.

It is has been assumed, therefore, that sexual transmission is most likely the most common reason for genital or anal HPV in pre-pubertal children. However there remains considerable uncertainty about this assumption as many papilloma viruses are spread by innocuous means, such as via fomites, hands to genital or perianal area with normal child care, even child to child and possibly other skin papilloma viruses not regarded as typical infection of the ano-genital region. There remain many unanswered questions in regards to transmission, incubation periods, behaviour of the viruses in pre-pubertal children and so on. We therefore need to remain circumspect about the significance of the presence of HPV in the ano-genital region, but actively assess each case on its merits.[83]

Treatment requirements vary depending on symptomatology. Radical non-intervention and expectant is the treatment of choice, but topical treatment with podophyllin and other immunomodulators through to diathermy may be required.

Neisseria gonorrhoea can be acquired at birth and is described as endemic in some Aboriginal communities, but in general it is regarded as a strong indicator of sexual abuse. The infection is usually symptomatic, mostly with a florid purulent vaginal discharge. Culture is the gold standard diagnostic test. Nowadays urine screening using PCR testing with DNA specific probes is a very sensitive screening tool and easy to collect.

Treatment with azithromycin 20 mg per kg as a stat dose to a maximum of 1 gm orally or ceftriaxone 125 mg IM single dose with follow-up screening is usually sufficient.

Herpes simplex virus (HSV) either type 1 or 2 are indistinguishable clinically. Any child presenting with genital lesions, testing positive to HSV screening or culture should be investigated for possible sexual abuse. Screening using PCR and culture remain the most accurate diagnostic investigations. Treatment is with acyclovir as early as possible after onset of symptoms.

Trichomonas vaginalis is very uncommon in pre-pubertal children but if present it should be regarded as sexually transmitted. It is more likely to be seen in the adolescent population.

Syphilis, hepatitis B and C as well as HIV infections can all be sexually transmitted, and screening for these infections is often offered to children thought to be at risk even if the risk is very small. Pre-test and post-test counselling is important, especially discussion about the possibility of false positive results. Follow-up medical assessments are important for this reason alone.

Pregnancy and sexual abuse

This is an important consideration in all adolescents who have been sexually assaulted and is easily overlooked in the often emotionally charged atmosphere of the initial assessment. A thorough sexual history and general health enquiry should be routine in these cases. Teenage pregnancy may be the first presentation of sexual abuse with the father being a first-degree relative in many of these cases.[84]

Psychosocial and emotional consequences

Given the common adverse psychological outcomes the management of sexual abuse requires a multidisciplinary approach. Parents as well as the child require support once sexual abuse comes to light. Feelings of guilt, anger and sadness are very common. Complicating these feelings will be the nature of the child's relationship with the perpetrator, possible threats that may have accompanied the abuse, and the implications of disclosure for a family if the perpetrator is within the family. Children can often feel responsible for what has happened and may recant a disclosure for fear of repercussions for themselves or other people. There can be a very strong temptation to let the whole thing go rather than make a fuss. This reaction is not limited to the child and other family members but also those involved in the system set up to deal with these cases.

It is important that clinicians have a clear sense of their personal attitudes towards sexual abuse and are aware of their unconscious reactions that may play out in their dealings with traumatised children and their families. It is also important in clinical practice that there are healthy ways of dealing with these vicariously traumatising experiences.

REFERENCES

1. Feerick MM, Knutson JF, Trickett PK, et al, editors. Child abuse and neglect: Definitions, classifications, and a framework for research. Baltimore: Paul H Brookes Publishing; 2006. p. 29–47
2. Straus M, Kaufman Kantor G. Stress and child abuse. In: Helfer RE, Kempe RS, editors. The Battered Child. 4th ed. Chicago: The University of Chicago Press; 1987. p. 42–59
3. What is Child Abuse? Definition courtesy of Community Services, Department of Family and Community Services NSW. Online. Available: www.community.services.nsw.gov.au; 9 Mar 2012
4. *Crimes Act 1900* (NSW) S.61AA (2)(b)
5. Helfer RE. The developmental basis of child abuse and neglect: an epidemiological approach. In: Helfer RE, Kempe RS, editors. The Battered Child. 4th ed. Chicago: The University of Chicago Press; 1987. p. 60–80
6. Carlson EB, Furby L, Shales JA. Conceptual framework for the long-term psychological effects of traumatic childhood abuse. Child Maltreatment 1997;2(3):272–95
7. Garbarino J. The incidence and prevalence of child maltreatment. In: Ohlin L, Tonry M, editors. Family Violence. Chicago: The University of Chicago Press; 1989. p. 219–61
8. Statement by David Hansell, Principal Deputy Assistant Secretary, Administration for Children and Families, US Department of Health and Human Services (HHS) on The State of the American Child: The Impact of Federal Policies on Children before the Committee on Health, Education, Labor and Pensions Subcommittee on Children and Families United States Senate. July 29, 2010
9. Price-Robertson R, Bromfield L, Vassallo S. The prevalence of child abuse and neglect. National Child Protection Clearinghouse, Australian Institute of Family Studies, Resource sheet, Melbourne: AIFS; Apr 2010
10. Lamont A. Child abuse and neglect statistics. National Child Protection Clearinghouse, Australian Institute of Family Studies, Resource sheet, Melbourne: AIFS, Feb 2011
11. Lieberman AF, Chu A, Van Horn P, et al. Trauma in early childhood: empirical evidence and clinical implications. Development and Psychopathology 2011;23(2):397–410
12. Singer MI, Miller DB, Guo S, et al. The mental health consequences of children's exposure to violence. Mandel School of Applied Social Sciences, Community Health Research Institute, Case Western Reserve University, Cleveland, OH, 1998
13. Scott KM, Smith DR, Ellis PM. Prospectively ascertained Child Maltreatment and its association with DSM-IV mental disorders in young adults. Arch Gen Psychiatry 2010;67:712–19
14. Chen LP, Murad MH, et al. Sexual abuse and lifetime diagnosis of psychiatric disorders: Systematic review and meta-analysis. Mayo Clinic Proc 2010;85:618–29

15 Felitti VJ, Anda RF, Nordenberg D, et al. Relationship of childhood abuse and household dysfunction to many of the leading causes of death in adults. The Adverse Childhood Experiences (ACE) Study. American Journal of Preventive Medicine 1998;14(4):245–58
16 Carpenter GL, Stacks AM. Developmental effects of exposure to intimate partner violence in early childhood: A review of the literature. Children and Youth Services review 2009;31:831–9
17 Reece R. Medical evaluation of physical abuse, ch 11. In: Myers JEB, editor. The American Professional Society on Abuse of Children (APSAC) handbook on child maltreatment. 3rd ed. Thousand Oaks, CA: Sage; 2011
18 S Maguire S, Mann MK, Sibert J, et al. Are there patterns of bruising in childhood which are diagnostic or suggestive of abuse? A systematic review. Arch Dis Child 2005;90: 182–6
19 Pearce MK, Kakzor K, Aldridge S, et al. Bruising characteristics. Discriminating physical child abuse from accidental trauma. Pediatrics 2010;125:67–74
20 Sugar N, Taylor JA, Feldman KW. Bruises in infants and toddlers: those who don't cruise rarely bruise. Arch Pediatr Adolesc Med 1999;153:399–403
21 Ravanfar P, Dinulos JG. Cultural practices affecting the skin of children. Current Opinions in Pediatrics 2010;22:423–31
22 Bonnier C, Nassagone M, Evrard P. Outcome and prognosis of whiplash shaken syndrome; late consequences after a symptom-free interval. Developmental Medicine and Child Neurology 1995;37:9–13
23 Bruce D, Zimmerman R. Shaken Impact Syndrome. Paediatric Annals 1989;340:482–94
24 Case ME, Graham MA, Handy TC, et al, and the National Association of Medical Examiners Ad Hoc Committee on Shaken Baby Syndrome. Position paper on fatal abusive head injuries in infants and young children. American Journal Forensic Medical Pathology 2001;22:112–22
25 Case ME. Abusive head injuries in infants and young children. Legal Medicine 2007;9:83–7
26 Caffey J. On the theory and practice of shaking infants. American Journal of Diseases of Childhood 1972;124:161–9
27 Guthkelch AN. Infantile subdural haematoma and its relationship to whiplash injuries. British Medical Journal 1971;2(5289):430–1
28 Vinchon M, de Foort-Dhellemmes S, Desurmont M, et al. Confessed abuse versus witnessed accidents in infants: comparison of clinical, radiological, and ophthalmological data in corroborated cases. Childs Nerv Syst 2010;26:637–45
29 Adamsbaum C, Grabar S, Mejean N, et al. Abusive Head Trauma: Judicial admissions highlight violent and repetitive shaking. Pediatrics 2010;126:546–55
30 Duhaime AC, Christian CW, Rorke IB, et al. Non-accidental head injury in infants: 'the Shaken Baby Syndrome'. New England Journal of Medicine 1998:1822–9
31 Talbert DG. Shaken baby syndrome: Does it exist? Medical Hypotheses 2009;72: 131–4
32 Geddes JF, Hackshaw AK, Vowles GH, et al. Neuropathology of inflicted head injury in children. I Patterns of brain damage. Brain 2001;124:1290–8
33 Matschke J, Voss J, Obi N, et al. Nonaccidental head injury is the most common cause of subdural bleeding in infants <1 year of age. Pediatrics 2009;124:1587–94
34 Hymel K, Makaroff KL, Laskey AL, et al. Mechanisms, clinical presentations, injuries, and outcomes from inflicted versus non-inflicted head trauma during infancy: results of a prospective multicentered, comparative study. Pediatrics 2007;119:922–9
35 Barlow KM, Minns RA. Annual incidence of Shaken Impact syndrome in young children. Lancet 2000;356(9241):1571–2
36 Chiesa A, Duhaime A-C. Abusive head trauma. Pediatric Clinics North America 2009;317–31
37 Jenny C, Hymel KP, Ritzen A, et al. Analysis of missed cases of abusive head trauma. JAMA 1999;281:621–6
38 Maguire S, Pickerd N, Farewell D, et al. Which clinical features distinguish inflicted from non-inflicted brain injury? A systematic review. Archives of Diseases of Childhood 2009;94:860–7

39 Cooperman DR, Merten DF. Skeletal manifestations of child abuse, ch 7. In: Reece R, Ludwig S, editors. Child abuse, medical diagnosis and management. 2nd ed. Baltimore: Lippincott Williams and Wilkins; 2001
40 Kemp AM, Dunstan F, Harrison S, et al. Patterns of skeletal fractures in child abuse: a systematic review. British Medical Journal 2008;337:a1518
41 Kleinman PK, editor. Diagnostic imaging in child abuse. 2nd ed. St Louis: Mosby; 1998. p. 291
42 Hobbs CJ. Skull fracture and the diagnosis of abuse. Archive of Diseases of Childhood 1984;59:246–52
43 Jayakumar P, Barry M, Ramachandran M. Orthopaedic aspects of paediatric non-accidental injury. J Bone Joint Surg [Br] 2010;92-B:189–95
44 Kemp AM, Dunstan F, Harrison S, et al. Patterns of skeletal fractures in child abuse: systematic review. BMJ 2008;337:a1518
45 Meyer JS, Gunderman R, Coley BD, et al. ACR appropriateness criteria on suspected physical abuse-child. American College of Radiology. Journal of the American College of Radiology 2011;8(2):87–94
46 Diagnostic imaging of child abuse. Section on Radiology. American Academy of Pediatrics. Pediatrics 2009;123:1430–5
47 Mandelstam SA, Cook D, Fitzgerald M, et al. Complementary use of radiological skeletal survey and bone scintigraphy in detection of bony injuries in suspected child abuse. Arch Dis Child. 2003;88:387–90
48 Kleinman PK, Nimkin K, Spevak MR, et al. Follow-up skeletal surveys in suspected child abuse. Am J Radiol. 1996;167:893–6
49 Monteleone JA, Brodeur AE. Child maltreatment: A clinical guide and reference. St Louis: GW Medical Publishing; 1994
50 Maguire S, Moynihan S, Mann M, et al. A systematic review of the features that indicate intentional scalds in children. Burns 2008;34(8):1072–81
51 Hicks RA, Stolfi A. Skeletal surveys in children with burns caused by child abuse. Pediatric Emergency Care 2007;23(5)
52 Touloukian R. Abdominal visceral injuries in battered children. Pediatrics 1968;42(4):642–6
53 Merten DF, Carpenter BL, Becky L. Radiologic imaging of inflicted injury in the child abuse syndrome. Paediatric Clinics of North America 1990;37(4):815–38
54 Gwirtzman LW, Dubowitz H, Langenberg P. Screening for occult abdominal trauma in children with suspected physical abuse. Pediatrics 2009;124(6):1595–602
55 Trokel M, Discala C, Terrin NC, et al. Patient and injury characteristics in abusive abdominal injuries. Pediatric Emergency Care 2006;22(10)
56 Meadow R. Munchausen syndrome by proxy. The hinterland of child abuse. Lancet 1977;2:343–5
57 Meadow R. Munchausen syndrome by proxy. Archives of disease in childhood 1982;57:92–8
58 Rosenberg DA. Web of deceit: A literature review of Munchausen syndrome by proxy. Child Abuse and Neglect 1987;11:547
59 Juredini JN, Shafer AT, Donald TG. 'Munchausen by proxy syndrome': not only pathological parenting but also problematic doctoring? Medical Journal of Australia 2003;178:130–2
60 Denny SJ, Grant CC, Pinnock R. Epidemiology of Munchausen syndrome by proxy in New Zealand. Journal of Paediatrics and Child Health 2001;37:240–3
61 McClure RJ, Davis PM, Meadow SR, et al. Epidemiology of Munchausen by proxy, non-accidental poisoning and non-accidental suffocation. Archives of Diseases of Childhood 1996;75:57–61
62 Hart SN, Brassard MR, Davidson HA, et al. Psychological maltreatment, ch 8. In: Myers JEB, editor. The American Professional Society on Abuse of Children (APSAC) handbook on child maltreatment. 3rd ed. Thousand Oaks, CA: Sage; 2011
63 Bowlby J. Attachment and Loss, vol 1 Attachment. New York: Basic Books; 1969
64 Crittenden PM. Children's strategies for coping with adverse home environments: An interpretation using attachment theory. Child Abuse and Neglect 1992;16(3):329–43

CHAPTER 14 Child abuse and neglect 271

65 Erickson MF, Egeland B, Pianta R. The effects of maltreatment on the development of young children. In: Cicchetti D, Carlson V, editors. Child Maltreatment: Theory and research on the causes and consequences of child abuse and neglect. Cambridge: Cambridge University Press; 1989. p. 647–84
66 Dubowitz H, Black M. Neglect of children's health, ch 14. In: Myers JEB, editor. The American Professional Society on Abuse of Children (APSAC) handbook on child maltreatment. 3rd ed. Thousand Oaks, CA: Sage; 2011. p. 269–92
67 Olds D. The nurse–family partnership: foundations in attachment theory and epidemiology. In: Berlin L, Ziv Y, Amaya-Jackson L, Greenberg M, editors. Enhancing early attachments: theory, research, intervention and policy. New York: Guildford; 2005. p. 217–49
68 International Society for Prevention of Child Abuse and Neglect (ISPCAN). Special Report, Issue 1. preventing physical child abuse and neglect through home visiting. 2006
69 Gorey KM, Leslie DR. The prevalence of child sexual abuse: Integrative review adjustment for potential response and measurement biases. Child Abuse and Neglect 1997;21:391–8
70 Swanston HY, Plunkett AM, O'Toole BI, et al. Nine years after child sexual abuse. Child Abuse and Neglect 2003;27:967–84
71 Vitacco MJ, Caldwell M, Ryba NL, et al. Assessing risk in adolescent sexual offenders: recommendations for clinical practice. Behaviour Science and the Law 2009;27(6): 929–40
72 Woodrow ACB, David A. Effectiveness of a sex offender programme: A risk band analysis. International Journal of Offender Therapy and Comparative Criminology 2011;55(1):43–55
73 Hanson RK, Bloom I, Stephenson M. Evaluating community sex offender treatment programs: a 12-year follow-up of 724 offenders. Canadian Journal of Behavioural Science, Revue canadienne des sciences du comportement 2004;36(2):87–96
74 Hunter RS, Kilstrom N, Loda F. Sexually abused children: identifying masked presentation in a medical setting. Child Abuse and Neglect 1985;9:17–25
75 Kendall-Thackett K, Williams LM, Finkelhor D. Impact of sexual abuse on children. A review and synthesis of recent empirical studies. Psychological Bulletin 1993;13: 164–80
76 Kaplan R, Adams JA, Staring SP, et al. Medical response to child sexual abuse: A resource for professionals working with children and families. St Louis: STM Learning; 2011
77 Heger A, Emans SJ. Evaluation of the sexually abused child. A medical textbook and photographic atlas. New York: Oxford University Press, 1992
78 Adams JA, Kaplan RA, Starling SP, et al. Guidelines for medical care of children who may have been sexually abused. Journal of Paediatric and Adolescent Gynaecology 2007;20:163–72
79 Adams JA, Harper K, Revilla J. Examination findings in legally confirmed child sexual abuse: It's normal to be normal. Pediatrics 1994;94(3):310–7
80 Berenson AB, Chacko MR, Wiemann CM, et al. A case-control study of anatomic changes resulting from sexual abuse. American Journal of Obstetrics and Gynecology 2000;182(4):820–34
81 Finkel MA. Anogenital trauma in sexually abused children. Pediatrics 1989;84: 317–22
82 Watts DH, et al. Low risk of perinatal transmission of human papillomavirus: Results from a prospective cohort study. American Journal of Obstetrics and Gynecology 1998;178:365–73
83 Gutman LT, et al. Cervical-vaginal and intra-anal transmission human papillomavirus infection of young girls with external genital warts. Journal of Infectious Diseases 1994;170:1339–44
84 Holmes MM, et al. Rape-related pregnancy: Estimates and descriptive characteristics from a national sample of women. American Journal of Obstetrics and Gynecology 1996;175: 320–4

FURTHER READING

Myers JEB, editor. The American Professional Society on Abuse of Children (APSAC) handbook on child maltreatment. 3rd ed. Thousand Oaks, CA: Sage; 2011

Monteleone JA, Brodeur AE. Child maltreatment: A clinical guide and reference. 2nd ed. St Louis: GW Medical Publishing; 1998

Frasier L, Rauth-Farley K, Alexander R, et al. Abusive head trauma in infants and children. A medical and forensic reference. St Louis: GW Medical Publishing; 2006

Minns RA, Brown JK. Shaking and other non-accidental head injuries in children. Clinics in Developmental Medicine, No 162. London: MacKeith; 2005

Reece R, Ludwig S. Child abuse, medical diagnosis and management. 2nd ed. Baltimore: Lippincott Williams and Wilkins; 2001

Kleinman PK, editor. Diagnostic imaging in child abuse. 2nd ed. St Louis: Mosby; 1998

Crittenden PM, Ainsworth MDS. Child maltreatment and attachment theory. In: Cicchetti D, Carlson V, editors. Child Maltreatment: Theory and research on the causes and consequences of child abuse and neglect. Cambridge: Cambridge University Press; 1989. p. 432–63

Ainsworth MDS, Blehar M, Waters E, et al. Patterns of attachment. Hillsdale, NJ: Lawrence Erlbaum; 1978

Kaplan R, Adams JA, Staring SP, et al. Medical response to child sexual abuse: A resource for professionals working with children and families. St Louis: STM Learning; 2011

Heger A, Emans SJ. Evaluation of the sexually abused child. A medical textbook and photographic atlas. New York: Oxford University Press; 1992

15 Legal issues

Sandra Johnson

INTRODUCTION

In general doctors do not have training on legal matters in their medical career, yet there are many circumstances where the medical and legal professions interact. It is beneficial to doctors to have an understanding of legal issues, particularly when dealing with children and families. In this chapter the legal principles and rules relate to the State of New South Wales and the Commonwealth of Australia. The reader needs to consider rules that apply within their particular jurisdiction. However the approach and logic is likely to be similar across jurisdictions.

This chapter is not a detailed account of legal medicine, but aims to outline some of the important facts relating to the role of paediatricians when they are expected to deal with legal matters. It may be helpful to refer to Text Box 15.1 for basic legal terminology. More detail about terminology can be found in the *Evidence Act 1995* (Cwlth).[1]

MEDICAL EVIDENCE SOUGHT BY LEGAL TEAMS

When legal teams make contact with doctors they usually seek an opinion about the medical matters of a case. The legal team seeking such opinion might represent the plaintiff or the defence, and the doctor is usually given this information at first contact. The doctor's evidence is based on the facts of the case and should be the same irrespective of which legal party engages the doctor to do the work.

The medical assessment could be regarding a patient under the care of the doctor or regarding a patient unknown to the doctor being consulted and, in either instance, the doctor provides factual and/or opinion evidence. Circumstances where medical assessment is sought include those discussed below.

Factual evidence

The doctor provides facts about the medical findings (diagnosis, treatment and management) of the case. The evidence relates to the facts and findings on history, examination, investigation, diagnosis and treatment, and includes:
- History and physical findings of a case that may allegedly be the result of an injury – accidental, non-accidental or iatrogenic
- Information about diagnosis, treatment and management of a medical condition – where the patient is alleged to have suffered injury resulting in damage or impairment of function of the brain, body, limb or sensory organs
- Assessment of physical function and impairment in relation to long-term care, treatment and support for daily living

TEXT BOX 15.1 Basic legal terminology

Witness – A person who provides evidence to the court.
- Ordinary witness – Any person who gives evidence under oath in a factual manner, based on what they observed first hand. Providing information based on what they were told or heard others say is not factual evidence and instead represents 'hearsay', which is not admissible in court.
- A doctor can be an 'ordinary witness' when they report on facts and findings of a medical assessment without giving expert opinion.
- Expert witness – A person who gives an opinion regarding the facts and findings of the case based on their training, experience and expertise within their field of work. The expert witness gives an opinion based on their knowledge and training, and is expected to give the opinion in order to assist the court in its deliberations.

Tort – A breach of duty of care in civil negligence claims, which renders the individual who is sued to be liable for damages. Tort also includes all civil wrongs such as assault, battery, trespass, defamation.

Plaintiff – The person or party that makes a case against an individual in the court of law. For example, in the case of medical negligence this would be the patient who 'sues' the doctor for damages.

Defence – The legal party that acts in court on behalf of the person/s being sued.

Prosecution – The party or institution that brings about legal proceedings against an individual in relation to a criminal matter.

Civil Law – The division of Common Law that deals with issues arising between individuals or organisations, and is distinct from Criminal Law. In this case the 'burden of proof', which must be established in court and which relates to all the facts and evidence of the case, rests with the plaintiff. The 'standard of proof' is that of 'the balance of probability' where the court decides what constitutes a fair probability, in most instances this is >50 per cent. If the sued party is deemed liable then payment for damages ensues.

Criminal Law – The division of Law that relates to crime, where the safety of the public is at stake and where lives may be endangered. Here the burden of proof rests with the prosecution and the standard of proof is 'beyond reasonable doubt', being a much higher level of proof than in a civil case. A jury (usually consisting of 12 persons) resides over a criminal matter and renders an impartial verdict under oath of guilty or not guilty. If the person is found guilty then punishment ensues, which is directed by the court.

Precedent – A rule or principle established by prior legal cases that have been brought to court and which is used in subsequent cases where the facts are similar. There is a hierarchical system, where a lower court must abide by precedents established in a higher court.

Evidence – The facts of the case, including documents, reports, investigations, statements and inferences drawn based on the facts of the case.

Admissibility – Evidence must be admissible; that is, it must be valid and relevant to the case in order to be acceptable to the court. There are many rules regarding inadmissibility of evidence relating to probative value, relevance, legal privilege, expertise of a witness, hearsay and others, which will not be discussed in this chapter.

- Assessment of mental and cognitive functions in relation to long-term care, treatment and support for daily living
- Findings of the investigations performed on the patient.

Opinion evidence

The doctor is engaged as an expert to give opinion regarding the facts of the case. The doctor's opinion about the medical issues is based on the doctor's clinical training and experience, and is sought by the court regarding the matter under consideration.

The doctor providing opinion evidence is regarded as 'expert witness' to the court. The doctor must provide an unbiased opinion based on knowledge, training and clinical experience with the aim of assisting the court. The doctor is not an advocate for any party irrespective of which legal party engages the doctor to do the assessment. It is important that doctors who provide expert opinion are well versed in court requirements with regards the role of expert witnesses (see Expert Witness Code of Conduct Schedule 7).[2]

Opinion evidence may relate to the doctor's own assessment and findings of the case or the doctor might be asked to give an opinion about another doctor's diagnosis, treatment and management of a case. As mentioned in the Code of Conduct, it is imperative that doctors who give such opinion not stray from their field of expertise (see Expert Witness Code above).

CASES THAT MAY REQUIRE LEGAL MEDICINE ASSESSMENT

The following are types of cases where paediatric opinion might be sought and where factual evidence depends on physical findings:

1. Insurance claims due to injury (non-iatrogenic):
    - Brain damage due to motor vehicle or other accidental injury
    - Injury to limbs resulting in permanent loss of function
    - Loss of sensory function, vision or hearing due to injury.
2. Iatrogenic injury:
    - Cerebral palsy especially in relation to birth injury. There is a large body of research to support the notion that CP is rarely related to obstetric negligence[3,4]
    - Injury following surgery or as a result of medical treatment, e.g. drugs or invasive procedures, where there has been failure to warn about risks and proper consent was not obtained
    - Injury or impairment due to missed diagnosis resulting in failure to treat, e.g. meningitis is the most common
    - Injury due to alleged incorrect treatment as a result of failure to make proper diagnosis.
3. Medical assessment in order for legal team to determine quantum of long-term care, treatment, rehabilitation and support for the individual:
    - To determine the presence of impairment of function
    - To determine whether the functional impairment is in keeping with the alleged injury
    - To determine the extent and degree of impairment/function
    - To give opinion about the type of care, treatment and long-term intervention needs
    - To give opinion about life expectancy in children with disability.

4   Mental state examination:
    This is requested where the accused individual has carried out an act that has harmed another and the cognitive or mental ability of that individual is in question. Forensic psychiatrists are the experts who provide opinion in these circumstances.
5   Child abuse (physical or sexual):
    Where a child has allegedly been abused, the paediatrician might be asked to assess, examine and provide a report for legal medicine purposes. Paediatricians in this role require specialised training and experience in this branch of paediatrics. Their work involves close collaboration with police and other forensic experts. See Chapter 14 Child abuse and neglect.
6   Family court:
    Access arrangements for children when their parents are divorced might be considered in court, particularly when the parties cannot reach agreement. A paediatrician might be asked to provide an opinion about access in relation to the best interest of the child. In this circumstance the paediatrician is acting as an advocate for the needs and wellbeing of the child, but still needs to provide a balanced view based on all the facts of the case. However psychiatrists, psychologists and social workers usually provide these assessments for court.
7   Juvenile court:
    Where a young person breaks the law and as a result faces a civil (causing harm to another) or criminal (breaking the law) charge or causes damages in the civil domain, the paediatrician who has known the child or adolescent over many years might be asked to provide a report about the young person's character or tendencies to aggression, and so on.

> **Practice Point**
>
> For information about the court system in Australia, please consult the reading list at the end of the chapter.

DUTY OF CARE

General

Business owners and people who provide a service to others have a duty of care in the service that they provide. The basis of duty of care within the modern concept of negligence dates back to the alleged adverse effects of a 'snail in a bottle' of ginger beer in *Donoghue v Stevenson 1932 AC 562*. In Australia, duty of care was later described by Judge Mason in the case of *Shaddock & Associates v Parramatta Council*.[5] He indicated that duty of care is applied where a person runs a business where they provide advice or information to another, knowing or ought to know, that the person receiving the advice will rely or act on the advice. In addition, the business owner who provides the advice sets up the business professing to have skills and competence in order to provide advice or information.

Medical

In medicine, it is implicit in the doctor–patient relationship that the doctor owes the patient a duty of care. Dwyer discusses the legal implications of clinical practice guidelines and gives a good description of duty of care for doctors. His well-known statement is that 'the law imposes on a medical practitioner a duty to exercise reasonable care and skill in the provision of professional advice and treatment'. He goes on to say that the duty is 'a single, comprehensive one covering all the ways in which a doctor is called upon to exercises his or her skill and judgement' which 'extends to the examination, diagnosis and treatment of a patient, the provision of information and the processes of obtaining the patient's consent'.[6]

In simple terms, all doctors are required to act in the best interests of their patients and may come under 'breach of duty of care' in relation to: failure to inform; failure to diagnose; failure to treat; failure to warn of material risk of treatment; and failure to obtain proper consent.

CONSENT

Prior to instituting treatment the doctor should obtain informed consent from the patient. This is particularly important where invasive procedures are done during investigations and during medical or surgical treatment of the patient. Consent can also be obtained from a person who is an appointed enduring guardian under various state acts. In New South Wales this is formalised in the *Guardianship Act 1987*.

Physical action to another's body directly, without their permission, could be construed as assault or battery. Assault is where a threat of violence or show of force is made to another, verbal or physical, even if no actual contact occurs with that person's body. Battery refers to direct contact with the body of another person in a threatening and violent manner, without that person's permission. In general, a patient cannot make a claim in battery against a doctor provided that the patient had a broad understanding of the treatment that was to be carried out. It is imperative that doctors obtain consent in any circumstance where a procedure is done on a patient.

Consent must be informed and the characteristics of such consent were described by Ottley in a presentation to the New South Wales Branch of the Australian Medical Association in 1996. The doctor obtaining the consent must be certain that:

- The patient is mentally competent and capable of providing consent; that is, that the patient has the ability to understand the implications of treatment
- The patient is sufficiently informed about the nature of the procedure in order to give consent
- Consent covers details of the procedure and the person who is to perform the procedure
- The consent is given freely, is voluntary and without coercion.

Patients usually find that information given to them in written form aids their understanding of procedures and operations. One group examined what patients wanted to know prior to undergoing surgical treatment.[7] The majority of patients were happy for their doctor to determine their treatment, but they wanted information about their condition, the treatment and side-effects.

In the case of children, consent is provided on their behalf by their parents. The age of consent varies in different jurisdictions and doctors need to be aware of the rules of law in their particular jurisdiction. In Australia, in general, the age of consent is 18 years; and individuals aged 18 years and over have legal capacity if they are cognisant and thus able to give consent to treatment. In the State of NSW the *Minors (Property and Contracts) Act 1970* allows a child aged 14 years and over to give consent to treatment, but the Act also allows parents to consent to treatment for their children who are under 16 years of age.

In United Kingdom the case of *Gillick v West Norfolk and Wisbech Area Health Authority 1986*[8] set a precedent, where it was ruled that parental authority to give consent decreases as the child becomes more competent, so that if a child under 16 years of age is fully capable of understanding the proposed treatment then parental authority ceases. The precedent set in that case was upheld in the decision of the High Court of Australia in *Marion's case* in 1992.[9]

The question of how a paediatrician assesses *Fraser competence* (also known as *Gillick competence*) is an important one as competence requires cognitive ability to understand consequences, to make complex decisions and to make choice based on rational reasoning. Assessments to determine competency need to be developmentally appropriate and may need to be done by an independent third party, such as a child psychologist.[10]

There are many factors that need to be considered when assessing an adolescent's capacity to give consent, including emotional state and anxiety, more so than cognitive ability alone.[11] Assessment of competency is a time-consuming process and it is worth noting that being a minor or having a psychiatric disturbance does not necessarily preclude the ability to give consent.[12] Involvement of children and adolescents in the decision-making process about giving consent for medical treatment is strongly encouraged.[13,14]

MATERIAL RISK

Material risk implies a risk that is relevant and significant to an individual, and that a reasonable person in that individual's situation would want to be told about the risk. This means that it is necessary and imperative for the doctor, carrying out a procedure or providing treatment, to explain the risk to that individual even if the risk is considered to be small. For example, the risk of laryngeal nerve palsy in a singer or actor is highly relevant/significant (and therefore material) to that individual. See cases regarding 'failure to warn'.[15,16]

GUARDIANSHIP

Paediatricians should be familiar with legal guardianship within their jurisdiction, as this might vary across different states and countries.

Parents are the natural legal guardians for children and this applies in most jurisdictions. When children are in out-of-home care, a guardian can be appointed through a government department to look after the wellbeing and interests of the child. In New South Wales, the Children's Guardian is such a government department.[17] The Children's Guardian can also make decisions regarding treatment for children who are in institutional care.

A guardian can be appointed by the court (Guardian Ad Litem: GAL) in order to make recommendations to the court about matters regarding the best interest of the child. An example would be where medical staff have concern that the parents might not be making decisions based on the best interest of the child, where they as Jehovah's Witnesses refuse blood transfusion for their child who has suffered serious blood loss. A court-appointed guardian will consider the child's wishes but needs to make an independent decision about the best interest for the child. The GAL can also act as a tutor or representative for the child in court.

PRIVACY

All doctors are bound by confidentiality regarding their patient's medical information and they should not pass heath information to third parties without the patient's consent. For paediatricians, it is standard practice to send reports to the referring doctor and most doctors also send a copy of their report to the parents in the case of minors.

Privacy laws protect all people from their private information being made available to the public. In Australia, the *National Privacy Act 1988* was legislated and the National Privacy Principles (NPPs) were established.[18]

There are ten NPPs that businesses and organisations need to abide by regarding the collection of information, the use and disclosure of information, data quality, security, openness, access, identifiers, anonymity, transborder data flow and collection of sensitive information. The last covers health information, racial/ethnic origin, political opinion, religious beliefs, membership of professional or trade associations, sexual preferences and criminal record. There are strict rules about privacy in these principles and it is important that doctors (and all businesses) are familiar with them and that the approach recommended be part of their regular practice.

MEDICAL NEGLIGENCE

Civil case

In countries where Common Law is applied, medical negligence usually comes under civil law, where the standard of proof is based on the 'balance of probabilities'. The patient who sues the doctor, together with their legal team, forms the plaintiff and the doctor being sued, together with the legal team from the medical insurance company, forms the defence in court.

In order for the case against the doctor to succeed in court, the plaintiff must prove the following:

- The doctor owed the patient a 'duty of care': if the patient was treated by the doctor, then duty of care is implicit in the doctor–patient relationship.
- There was a breach in duty of care, which might relate to failure to diagnose; failure to treat; or failure to warn of risk. Breach in duty of care might result from acts of omission (failure to do something that should have been done) or acts of commission (doing something incorrectly or inappropriately) which then results in injury.
- As a result of the breach, the patient has suffered an injury, i.e. must establish a causal link between the breach of duty and the harm/injury caused (*Civil Liability Act 2002: Division 3 Section 5D*).
- The injury suffered was foreseeable, the risk of injury was not insignificant and that a reasonable person would have taken steps to avoid the risk of injury (*Civil Liability Act 2002: Division 2 Section 5B*).
- The damage sustained is not too remote from the presumed breach, which again relates to a causal link between the alleged breach and the injury sustained.

This means that it is much more difficult for the plaintiff to sue the doctor if these requirements are not met. However it is unwise to be complacent, and doctors are expected to always act in the best interest of their patients and to be thorough in the service and care that they provide to their patients.

While the number of negligence claims against paediatricians is small, the largest payouts have been for multiply-disabled children with alleged perinatal injury. It is difficult to compare the number of cases across different jurisdictions of different countries because data coding practices vary. In the United Kingdom in an experience over a period of 25 years the most common reasons for paediatricians being sued include:[19]

- Failing to communicate adequately
- Failing to test diagnostic hypotheses
- Inadequate screening, e.g. hip dysplasia
- Lack of guidance in handling rare conditions
- Misunderstanding of fluid balance requirements
- Uncertainty about relevance of vital signs
- Inadequate assessment of neurological status.

Despite the fact that a doctor might not be deemed negligent in providing medical care, and therefore not be liable, there is no doubt that the process of being sued is a very distressing experience which could lead to the doctor giving up medical practice altogether. This is a significant loss to the community because years of training and skills acquired by that doctor are lost.

Criminal case

Criminal medical negligence is rare and in this circumstance the criteria that need to be met are:

- The accused by an act (commission) or omission causes death of a person
- The act or omission falls short of the 'standard of reasonable care' which goes beyond being just a civil wrongdoing, but amounts to a crime (see an example below)
- There is an element of recklessness and gross incompetence.

Case example

An anaesthetist failed to detect endotracheal tube disconnection during an eye operation despite alarms going off to warn that a problem has occurred. The patient subsequently had a cardiac arrest and died.[20] The judge in his deliberations stated that 'if a person holds himself out as possessing special skill and knowledge and he is consulted, as possessing such skill and knowledge, by or on behalf of a patient, he owes a duty to the patient to use due caution in undertaking the treatment'. He went on to say that 'the law requires a fair and reasonable standard of care and competence'. The doctor was found guilty of manslaughter in this case of criminal negligence.

STANDARD OF REASONABLE CARE

In terms of medical treatment the 'standard of reasonable care' is that of an 'ordinary skilled practitioner' who exercises or claims to have the capabilities needed in 'the particular field of medical practice under consideration'.[6] This standard of reasonable care is usually set by college guidelines, training requirements and opinion of the broader population of peers in that field of medicine. This also means that an expert who gives opinion about whether care was reasonable or not must be trained and have expertise in that field of medicine being considered. The expert must not stray into a field in which they have no training and this is clearly stated in the *Expert Witness Code of Conduct* in the *NSW Uniform Civil Procedure Rules 2005* – Schedule 7.[2]

The *Civil Liability Act 2002* Division 6 Section 5O[21] states the 'Standard of Care for professionals' is as follows:

1 'A person practising a profession does not incur a liability in negligence arising from provision of professional service if it can be established that the professional acted in a manner that (at the time the service was provided) was widely accepted in Australia by peer professional opinion as competent professional practice.
2 However, peer professional opinion cannot be relied on … if the court considers that the opinion is irrational.
3 Differing peer professional opinion widely accepted in Australia concerning a matter does not prevent any one or more (or all) of those opinions being relied on …
4 Peer professional opinion does not have to be universally accepted to be considered widely accepted.'

This part of the Act is similar to the rule referred to as the *Bolam Principle*, formulated in the case of *Bolam v Frien Hospital Management Committee*[22] in 1957 where the judge stated that a doctor is not negligent if he acts in accordance with practice accepted at the time as proper practice by a responsible body of medical opinion. This rule has since been challenged in court and consequently statement 2 shows that the court will not abide by medical peer opinion if it is considered irrational.

STANDARDS OF MEDICAL CARE

In medicine, doctors and healthcare organisations consult scientific evidence to inform diagnosis, treatment and management of patients, which is referred to as evidence-based medicine. The evidence is evaluated in rigorous research where *prospective multicentred randomised controlled trials* constitute the optimal approach. Through several stages, including broad consultation with the medical community like colleges and university research departments, the validated evidence is used to formulate recommendations or guidelines for management of disease or disorder.

Before evidence can be used in guidelines that provide 'indicators of the quality of care', it needs to be assessed in study designs like *systematic reviews* where all available data from several research centres is examined and meta-analysis performed so that the level of evidence can be rated from 1 (being of the highest quality) to 8 (lowest quality). The best-practice approach to guide decision making can then be inferred from the highest quality research data.

MEDICAL ERROR

When an error occurs most parents or patients expect an explanation. Open disclosure, where the medical team provides the child and family with an opportunity to ask questions, is encouraged. Most hospitals and private practices have procedures that should be followed when an adverse event has occurred, and doctors need to be familiar with the rules and protocols of the organisation where they work. The early involvement of the medical insurance organisation and their legal team is prudent to guide the doctor or team with the best approach.

One study examined parental attitudes about disclosure of medical errors: it would seem that most families want to be told, although there may be cultural differences about the process and act of disclosure.[23]

Doctors are required to attend continuing education workshops and lectures to ensure that they remain up-to-date in the medical care that they provide to their patients. It is helpful for doctors to consult websites regarding quality care and safety, as well as clinical excellence in healthcare.[24,25] Then the chance of appearing in court is reduced while simultaneously improving patient care.

THE PAEDIATRICIAN AS EXPERT WITNESS

Paediatricians are advocates for children and their rights. The challenge for the paediatrician who appears as an expert witness is that they are in court to assist the court in medical matters relating to the child's case. The paediatrician in this situation is not in court as an advocate for the child. The expert must consult the rules of evidence relevant to their jurisdiction and national state. The aforementioned relates to the Expert Witness Code of Conduct in New South Wales outlined in Schedule 7.[2] The essential points from this rule are:

- The expert's role is to assist the court and to provide information based on clinical practice, experience and training, which is not information that is common knowledge to the court. The opinion provided by the expert must be impartial and must not be influenced by or be under the direction of the legal party that engages the expert; that is the expert is 'not an advocate for a party'. The expert's opinion must be based on independent professional judgement and must relate to the facts of the case.
- In order to assist the court, the expert's report must state the expert's training and qualifications as an expert, must provide the opinion clearly and must state reasons for the opinion given, together with research or other materials consulted in the process of providing the opinion.
- The rule also states that the court can direct experts to reach agreement regarding evidence where there is disparity in opinion, and this important issue avoids wasting court time. The experts must meet and reach agreement, or state why they disagree on important matters if that is the case, in a written report for the court. In this situation again, the experts must be independent and not act under direction of the legal party to withhold or avoid agreement.

As mentioned, the paediatrician, who in most non-court circumstances acts as an advocate for children, must focus on the role of providing impartial evidence to assist the court. By focusing on the facts and by not straying from this role, the paediatrician's evidence and opinion will be admissible in court.

It is worth noting that the traditional immunity previously afforded to expert witnesses has recently been overturned in the highest court in the United Kingdom and further commentary can be read on the referenced link.[26]

Admissibility of expert evidence

Rules that govern expert opinion are found in the *Evidence Act 1995* (Cwlth).[1]

The expert must show the court that they are an expert whose opinion will be valid to the court. The qualifications, training and years of clinical experience will be taken into account and it is usual that the specialist has qualifications in the area of medicine under consideration. It is unwise to appear as an expert in court if the doctor does not have sufficient training and expertise in the particular field, because the doctor's evidence could be deemed inadmissible. In addition, the doctor's training must be from a recognised body of medical knowledge (organisation, college or institution) in order for the training and expertise to be considered valid. This '*expertise rule*' has been open to debate in some circumstances.

The expert is not expected to provide opinion about matters that are regarded as common knowledge and within ordinary human experience; referred to as the '*common knowledge rule*'. In addition the expert's opinion must be based on sound and admissible facts; referred to as the '*basis rule*'. Most importantly, the expert must not encroach on the issue of whether the person is guilty or not guilty because this is a matter for the court, not the expert, to decide; it is referred to as the '*ultimate issue rule*'.

The expert witness' evidence can be deemed inadmissible, where the validity of the opinion or the expert's integrity is called into question, on the basis of the following:

- Lack of qualifications and expertise relevant to the case
- Lack of independence and impartiality
- Acting as an advocate for either party
- Having insufficient basis for giving an opinion; i.e. giving an opinion that is not based on sound, logical, reasonable fact
- Not considering alternatives even when they are presented in a sound, logical fashion; i.e. being biased.

THE PAEDIATRICIAN AS ADVOCATE

Paediatricians advocate for the health and wellbeing of children under their care and in the general community. In this capacity their advice and recommendations inform policy in relation to the needs of children, and this can occur at many levels. The list below is not complete but serves to show that paediatricians play a pivotal role in advocating for children:

- Government policy addressing funding for children's health services
- Policy in relation to advertising and the negative influence of smoking and alcohol in advertising, together with the negative impact on health
- Nutrition, e.g. encouraging folate intake in pregnant women and introduction of folate into bread, intended to reduce the occurrence of neural tube defects;[27] or the sugar content of food in relation to obesity
- Informing policies in relation to child abuse and neglect, particularly noting the negative long-term impact of abuse on children[28,29]
- Children's safety, e.g. safe surfaces in public playgrounds, car safety seats, helmets for bike riders and skiers
- Education of the community about the negative impact on children of domestic violence, smoking within the family home and alcoholism

- Inequity of medical services for children with socioeconomic disadvantage, e.g. Aboriginal and refugee communities
- Advice to health authorities about medical services for children: child-friendly hospitals and clinics; specific medical care for children as opposed to applying adult techniques or approaches to children
- Support for early intervention and educational services for children with disability and other developmental problems to enhance or facilitate optimal development of children.

CONCLUSION

It is advisable for doctors to have basic knowledge of legal principles, particularly in relation to their work. The chapter has provided an overview of legal issues in paediatrics. When doctors give evidence in court, they must have an understanding of the duties of an expert witness and they must recognise the importance of giving impartial evidence.

Further reading and resources for those interested in this subject are provided.

REFERENCES

1. *Evidence Act 1995* (Cwlth). Australian Government Common Law. Online. Available: http://www.comlaw.gov.au/Details/C2011C00207; 5 Mar 2012
2. Expert Witness Code of Conduct Schedule 7. Uniform Civil Procedure Rules: NSW Consolidated Regulations. Online. Available: http://www.austlii.edu.au/au/legis/nsw/consol_reg/ucpr2005305/sch7.html; 5 Mar 2012
3. Johnson SL, Blair E, Stanley FJ. Obstetric malpractice litigation and cerebral palsy in term infants (review). Journal of Forensic and Legal Medicine 2011;18:97–100
4. Johnson SLJ, Hall DMB. Birth injury and the obstetrician (ch 1). In: Bonnar J, editor. Recent advances in Obstetrics and Gynaecology. Edinburgh: Churchill Livingstone; 1993
5. *Shaddock & Associates Pty Ltd v Parramatta City Council* (1981) 150 CLR 225
6. Dwyer P. Legal implications of clinical practice guidelines. MJA 1998;169:292–3
7. Dawes PJD, Davidson P. Informed consent: what do patients want to know? Monash Bioethics Review 1994;13:20–6
8. *Gillick v West Norfolk and Wisbech Area Health Authority* (1986) AC 112
9. *Secretary, Department of Health and Community Services v JWB and SMB (Marion's case)* (1992) 175 CLR 218
10. Larcher V, Hutchinson A. How do paediatricians assess Gillick competence? Archives Disease Childhood 2010;95:307–11
11. Dorn LD, Susman EJ, Fletcher JC. Informed consent in children and adolescents: age, maturation and psychological state. Journal of Adolescent Health 1995;16:185–90
12. Batten DA. Informed consent by children and adolescents to psychiatric treatment. Australian and New Zealand Journal of Psychiatry 1996;30:623–32
13. McCabe MA. Involving children and adolescents in medical decision making: developmental and clinical considerations. Journal of Pediatric Psychology 1996;21(4):505–16
14. Kuther TL. Medical decision-making and minors: Issues of consent and assent. Adolescence 2003;38
15. *Rogers v Whitaker* (1992) 175 CLR 479 Online. Available: http://www.ncbi.nlm.nih.gov/pubmed/11648609; 5 Mar 2012
16. *Chappel v Hart* (1998) 156 ALR 517 Online. Available: http://www.austlii.edu.au/au/journals/UQLJ/1999/13.html; 5 Mar 2012
17. The NSW Children's Guardian. Online. Available: http://www.kidsguardian.nsw.gov.au/; 5 Mar 2012

18. The Privacy Act and National Privacy Principles. Online. Available: http://www.privacy.gov.au/materials/types/infosheets/view/6583; 5 Mar 2012
19. Marcovitch H. When are paediatricians negligent? Archives of Disease in Childhood 2011;96:117–20
20. *R v Adomako* [1995] AC 171. Online. Available: http://www.lawteacher.net/criminal-law/cases/adomako.php; 5 Mar 2012
21. *Civil Liability Act 2002* (NSW). Online. Available: http://www.austlii.edu.au/au/legis/nsw/consol_act/cla2002161/; 5 Mar 2012
22. *Bolam v Friern Hospital Management Committee* (1957) 1 WLR 583
23. Matlow AG, Moody L, Laxer R, et al. Disclosure of medical error to parents and paediatric patients: assessment of parents' attitudes and influencing factors. Archives of Disease in Childhood 2010;95:286–90
24. Australian Commission on Quality and Safety in Healthcare. Online. Available: http://www.aihw.gov.au/safety-and-quality-of-health-care/; 5 Mar 2012
25. Clinical Excellence Commission. Online. Available: http://www.cec.health.nsw.gov.au/; 5 Mar 2012
26. Should expert witnesses and barristers be safe from being sued? Online. Available: http://www.abc.net.au/rn/lawreport/stories/2011/3209941.htm; 5 Mar 2012
27. Maberly G, Stanley F. Mandatory fortification of flour with folic acid: an overdue public health opportunity. Med J Aust 2005;183:342–3
28. Bross D, Krugman R. Child Maltreatment Law and Policy as a Foundation for Child Advocacy. Pediatric Clinics of North America 2009;56(2)
29. Moeller J. The combination effects of physical, sexual and emotional abuse during childhood: Long-term health consequences for women. Child Abuse & Neglect 1993;17:623–40

FURTHER READING

Skene L. Law and Medical Practice: rights, duties, claims and defences. 2nd ed. Chatswood, NSW: Lexis Nexis Butterworths; 2004
Branthwaite M, Beresford N. Law for doctors: Principles and practicalities. 2nd ed. London: Royal Society of Medicine Press; 2003
Carvan J. Understanding the Australian legal system. 5th ed. Pyrmont, NSW: Thomson Lawbook; 2005
Eike-Henner K. Informed consent by children: The new reality. Canadian Med Association Journal 1995;152:1495–7
Miller VA. Parent–child collaborative decision making for the management of chronic illness: a qualitative analysis. Families, Systems and Health 2009;27(3):249–66

RESOURCES

Australasian College of Legal Medicine (ACLM). Online. Available: http://www.legalmedicine.com.au/; 5 Mar 2012
Medicolegal Society of NSW. Online. Available: http://www.medicolegal.org.au/; 5 Mar 2012

Index

Page numbers followed by 'f' indicate figures, 't' indicate tables, and 'b' indicate boxes.

A
ABA. *see* applied behavioural analysis
ABAS. *see* Adaptive Behavior Assessment System
ABC. *see* Autism Behavior Checklist
abdominal trauma, 258
ABR. *see* auditory brainstem evoked response
abusive head trauma, 254–255
   investigations in, 255
   presentation of, 254–255
acoustic neuroma, 57
acoustic reflex, 66
acquired aphasia, 129t
acquired hemiplegia, 217–218
activation likelihood estimation (ALE), 147
Adaptive Behavior Assessment System (ABAS), 37, 237t
adaptive behaviour, assessment tools for, 237t
adaptive functioning, 37
ADEC. *see* Autism Detection in Early Childhood
ADHD. *see* attention deficit hyperactivity disorder
ADI-R. *see* Autism Diagnostic Interview-Revised
admissibility, 274b
adolescence
   ADHD in, 166–167
   bipolar disorder in, 208
   CP and, 227–228
   mood disorders in, 195–196
ADOS. *see* Autism Diagnostic Observation Schedule
ADST. *see* Australian Developmental Screening Test
adulthood transition
   ADHD in, 167
   ASD in, 109
Ages and Stages Questionnaire, 3rd edition, 29t
agnosia, verbal auditory, 132
Ainsworth, Mary, 3
albinism, 71–72

alcohol, 5, 207
ALE. *see* activation likelihood estimation
amblyopia, 74
American Association on Intellectual and Developmental Disabilities, 236
ANSD. *see* auditory neuropathy spectrum disorder
antipsychotics, 207
anxiety
   maternal, 5
   separation, 196
anxiety disorders, 98, 199
APD. *see* auditory processing disorder
aphasia, 142
   acquired, 129t
   developmental, 128
   Wernicke's, 130
applied behavioural analysis (ABA), 106
arcuate fasciculus, 129
ASAS. *see* Australian Scale for Asperger's Syndrome
ASD. *see* autism spectrum disorder
Asperger's syndrome, 89–91
   coordination problems with, 45
   diagnostic criteria for, 91b
asphyxia, 56
   birth, 56
   intrapartum, 217
assault, 248
assessment. *see* developmental assessment; *specific disorder*
ASSQ. *see* Autism Spectrum Screening Questionnaire
astigmatism, 74
asymmetric tonic neck reflex (ATNR), 16
atomoxetine (Strattera), 159–161, 160t, 183t
Attenta. *see* methylphenidate
attention, 28
   in-, 149
   joint, 95
attention deficit hyperactivity disorder (ADHD), 98, 145
   adolescent patients with, 166–167
   adulthood transition with, 167
   aetiology of, 146–147

environment in, 146–147
epigenetics in, 147
genetics in, 146
assessment of, 152–153
diagnostic tools for, 156
differential diagnosis in, 157
educational, 157
history in, 153–154
learning skills, 155–156
physical examination in, 155
psychiatric, 158
psychometric, 157–158
social skills, 153–154
therapy, 158
clinical presentation of, 151–152
comorbidities with, 151
diagnostic criteria for, 148–150, 149b
executive dysfunction and, 150
management of, 157–161
classroom-based, 162
follow-up in, 158–159
home-based, 162
medical, 157
medications for, 159–161, 160t, 166–167
ongoing, 164–166
parental concerns with, 161
preschool, 161–163
school involvement in, 159
school-aged, 163
treatment approach in, 161–166
working memory approach in, 159
mood disorders and, 196
neurobiology of, 147–148
outcomes of, 168
preschool child with, 155
prevalence of, 145
rating scales of, 150b
school-aged child with, 155–156
types of, 145, 152
auditory brainstem evoked response (ABR), 64–65
auditory neuropathy spectrum disorder (ANSD), 50, 60–61
auditory processing disorder (APD), 115
Australian Developmental Screening Test (ADST), 33t
Australian Scale for Asperger's Syndrome (ASAS), 100t
Autism Behavior Checklist (ABC), 100t
Autism Detection in Early Childhood (ADEC), 100t
Autism Diagnostic Interview-Revised (ADI-R), 99–102, 101t

Autism Diagnostic Observation Schedule (ADOS), 101t, 102
autism spectrum disorder (ASD)
adulthood transition with, 109
aetiology of, 93–95
cognitive theories of, 94–95
environmental risks in, 93
genetics in, 93
neuropathology in, 94
classification of, DMS-IV-TR, 89–92
clinical presentation of, 95–97
communication skills in, 96
play skills in, 96
savant skills in, 97
social skills in, 95–96
stereotypical behaviours in, 96–97
coordination problems with, 45
diagnosis of
diagnostic tools for, 99–102, 100t
differential diagnosis of, 97–98
early, 98–99
genetic counselling in, 105
history in, 103–104
investigations in, 104
multidisciplinary assessment in, 102–105
physical examination in, 104
family support and, 105b
history of, 88–89
intervention for, 105–106
behavioural, 106
biological, 107–109
combined, 107
complimentary and alternative medicine in, 108–109
developmental, 106
dietary, 108–109
family-based, 107
medication in, 107–108
models of, 106–109
therapy-based, 106
in preschool children, 98
prevalence of, 92–93
prognosis with, 109–110
screening for, 99
strengths with, 97
types of, 89–92
Autism Spectrum Screening Questionnaire (ASSQ), 100t
autistic disorder, 89, 90b
autosomal dominant optic atrophy, 72

B
babble, 19
baclofen, 224–225

Index 289

BAP. *see* broader autism phenotype
Battelle Developmental Inventory
  Screening test (BDIST), 33t
Bayley Infant Neurodevelopmental
  Screener (BINS), 33t, 237t
BDIST. *see* Battelle Developmental
  Inventory Screening test
behaviour, 28. *see also* cognitive behaviour
  techniques; cognitive behaviour
  therapy
  adaptive, 237t
  ASD and, 106
  boundaries of, 177
  expectations of, 177
  with ID, 242–243
  management of, 181
  neurological examination and, 16
  stereotypic, 96–97
behaviour difficulties, 173
  causes of, 178
  child's point of view with, 176–177
  classification of, 174–175
  clinical approach to, 175–178
  communication and, 180b
  examination of, 177–178
  history with, 175, 176t
  management of, 179–182
    activity-based support in,
      181–182
    counselling in, 181
    medication, 182, 183t
    parent training and support in,
      179–181
  prevalence of, 174
bereavement, 199
bilingualism, 133–134
bilirubin, 18
BINS. *see* Bayley Infant
  Neurodevelopmental Screener
biopsychosocial model, 7
bipolar disorder, 195–196, 204–208
  adolescent, 208
  aetiology of, 205–206
  defining characteristics of, 204–205
  depression in, 204
  differential diagnosis of, 199, 206
  over-diagnosis of, 194
  pre-pubertal, 208
  prevalence of, 205
  prognosis of, 208
  sub-threshold, 208
  treatment of, 206–208
    biological, 207–208
    complications with, 208
    contextual, 207

  practical advice in, 206–207
  psychological, 207
birth asphyxia, 56
birth weight, 4
blindness
  legal, 70
  total, 70
block assessment tool, 34, 34f
boredom, 206
BOTMP. *see* Bruininks–Oseretsky Test of
  Motor Proficiency
brain. *see also* auditory brainstem evoked
  response
  development of, 9–10
  minimal dysfunction of, 41
  plasticity of, 9–10
branding, 258
Brigance Screens, 29t
broader autism phenotype (BAP), 92
Broca's area, 129
Bruininks–Oseretsky Test of Motor
  Proficiency (BOTMP), 42–43
bruises, 252–254
burns, 257–258

C

care. *see also* duty of care
  standard of medical, 281
  standard of reasonable, 280–281
CARS2. *see* Childhood Autism Rating
  Scale, 2nd edition
cataracts, 73
CBCL. *see* Child Behaviour Checklist
CBT. *see* cognitive behaviour therapy
central coherence theory, 94
cerebral palsy (CP), 212
  adolescence and, 227–228
  aetiology of, 216–218
  assessment of, 220–221
    differential diagnosis in, 221–222
    initial, 220
    neurological, 220
    X-ray, 220
  classification of, 212–216
    CFCS, 215
    FMS, 214
    Gage classification, 215
    GMCFS, 214
    MACS, 214–215
  clinical presentation of, 218–219
  impairments with, 218–219
  management of, 222–227
    approach to, 223–227
  prevalence of, 212
  prognosis of, 228

CFCS. *see* Communication Functional Classification System
CGH. *see* comparative genomic hybridisation
Charcot-Marie-Tooth disease (CMT), 44t
Checklist for Autism in Toddler-23 (CHAT-23), 100t
child abuse, 247–248. *see also* neglect; physical abuse; sexual abuse
assault's distinction from, 248
community services and, 248–249
emotional, 250t, 260–263
factitious or induced illness as, 259–260
impact of, 250–251
legal aspects of, 248–249, 276
prevalence of, 249–250, 250t, 251f
psychological, 248
Child and Youth Mental Health Services (CYMHS), 181
Child Behaviour Checklist (CBCL), 174
Child Protection System, 248
Childhood Autism Rating Scale, 2nd edition (CARS2), 99, 100t
childhood disintegrative disorder, 92
children's court, 249
chromosomal abnormalities, 93
cigarette burns, 258
Civil Law, 274b
civil unrest, 6–7
clonidine, 183t
clumsy child syndrome, 41
CMT. *see* Charcot-Marie-Tooth disease
CMV. *see* cytomegalovirus
CNV. *see* copy number variants
cognition, 197
cognitive behaviour techniques, 181
cognitive behaviour therapy (CBT), 202, 207
Cognitive Orientation to Daily Occupational Performance program (CO-OP), 46
cognitive skills, 27
cognitive theories, 94–95
common knowledge rule, 283
communication, 26–27
with ASD, 96
behaviour difficulties and, 180b
functional training in, 106
non-verbal, 26–27
positive, 180b
verbal, 26
Communication Functional Classification System (CFCS), 215

comparative genomic hybridisation (CGH), 233
competence, 278
complimentary and alternative medicine, 108–109
Concerta. *see* dexamphetamine
conductive hearing loss, 50, 57–60
acquired, 58
hereditary, 57–58
autosomal dominant, 57–58
non-Mendelian malformation syndromes in, 58
X-linked dominant, 58
OME and, 58
congenital abnormalities, 4
congenital deafness, 18
congenital muscular dystrophies, 44t
congenital myasthenic syndromes, 44t
congenital myopathies, 44t
congenital rubella syndrome (CRS), 54
consent, 277–278
contextual treatment, 202, 207
CO-OP. *see* Cognitive Orientation to Daily Occupational Performance program
coordination, 40. *see also* developmental coordination disorder
hand–eye, 27
problems with, 45
copy number variants (CNV), 93, 146
cornea, irregularities of, 74
cortical or cerebral visual impairment (CVI), 75–76
cortical under connectivity theory, 94–95
counselling
behaviour difficulties management with, 181
genetic, 105
CP. *see* cerebral palsy
creatine kinase, 20
Criminal Law, 274b
CRS. *see* congenital rubella syndrome
culture, 7, 15–16
CVI. *see* cortical or cerebral visual impairment
CYMHS. *see* Child and Youth Mental Health Services
cytomegalovirus (CMV), 55, 71

D
DAS. *see* Differential Ability Scales
DCD. *see* developmental coordination disorder

Index   291

deafness, 4
  congenital, 18
  drugs and, 18
  from infections, 18
  from toxins, 18
  word, 132
defence, 274b
delayed development, 1, 25–26, 97
Denver II, 28b
deoxyribonucleic acid (DNA), 7–8
depression, 195–203
  aetiology of, 198
  in bipolar disorder, 204
  course of, 199
  defining characteristics of, 196–198
    distress in, 196–197
    dysfunction in, 197
    persistence in, 197–198
    pervasiveness, 198
    severity in, 198
  differential diagnosis of, 199
  maternal, 5
  prevalence of, 198
  sub-threshold, 203
  treatment of, 199–203
    biological, 202–203
    complications with, 203
    general advice for, 199–200
    medication for, 202–203
    psychological, 202
    strategies for major depression in, 200–201
development, 25–26
  assessment tool, 237t
  brain, 9–10
  delayed, 1, 25–26, 97
  disordered, 25–26
  domains of, 26–28
  influences on, 3–8
    conditions as, 4
    cultural, 7
    environmental, 4–7
    extrinsic, 4–7
    gender, 4
    genetic, 3–4
    hereditary, 3
    intrinsic, 3–4
    postnatal, 5–7
    prenatal, 4–5
  language, 5–6, 135t
  normal, 1
    hearing in, 11t–13t
    milestones in, 10–14
    motor skills in, 11t–13t
    social skills, 11t–13t
    stages of, 10–14, 11t–13t
    vision in, 11t–13t
  theories of, 2–3
  zone of proximal, 3
developmental aphasia, 128
developmental assessment, 1–2, 26–28
  follow-up and review after, 38
  history in, 30–31
  multidisciplinary, 36–38
  observation in, 31–32
  office-based, 28–38
    block assessment tool in, 34, 34f
    Goodenough–Harris Drawing Test in, 35
    informal tools for, 34–35
    questions for, 28–30
    screening tools for, 28
  paediatrician's role in, 2
  psychometric, 37
  stage setting for, 30
  standardised, 37–38
developmental coordination disorder (DCD), 40
  assessment of, 42–43
  clinical presentation of, 41–42
  comorbidities with, 41
  management of, 45–46
    functional skills approach to, 46
    process deficit approach to, 46
  motor skills and, 41–42
  neuromuscular disorders and, 43–45
  outcomes with, 42
  prevalence of, 41
  social interaction with, 42
developmental disability, 1, 232
developmental language disorder (DLD), 128
developmental surveillance, 99
developmental verbal dyspraxia, 132
dexamphetamine (Ritalin LA, Concerta), 159–161, 160t
Diagnostic and Statistical Manual of Mental Disorders, 4th edition (DSM-IV)
  IQ categories of, 238t
  language disorder classification, 131
Diagnostic Interview for Social and Communication Disorders (DISCO), 101t, 102
diet
  ASD treatment with, 108–109
  gluten- and casein-free, 109
Differential Ability Scales (DAS), 37
disability. *see* developmental disability; intellectual disability

DISCO. *see* Diagnostic Interview for Social and Communication Disorders
disintegrative disorder, 92
disordered development, 25–26
distress, 196–197, 204–205
DLD. *see* developmental language disorder
DMD. *see* Duchenne and Becker muscular dystrophy
DNA methylation, 7–8
Donoghue v Stenson 1932 AC 562, 276
Down syndrome, 45, 60
drawing skills
   Goodenough–Harris test of, 35
   with SLD, 121
drugs, deafness and, 18. *see also* medication
DSM-IV. *see* Diagnostic and Statistical Manual of Mental Disorders, 4th edition
Duchenne and Becker muscular dystrophy (DMD), 44t
duty of care, 276–277
   general, 276
   medical, 276–277
dysarthria, 142
dyscalculia, 114
dysfluency, 19
dysfunction, 205
   brain, 41
   in depression, 197
   executive
      ADHD and, 150
      theory of, 94
dysgraphia, 114–115
dyslexia, 114
dyspraxia, 142
   developmental verbal, 132
   motor, 40
dysrhythmia, 142
dystrophies, 44t

E

Ecological Intervention (EI), 46
education
   ADHD and, 157
   psycho-, 207
   SES and, 6
EI. *see* Ecological Intervention
emotion
   language disorders and, 138
   sexual abuse and, 267–268
emotional abuse, 250t, 260–263
emotional disturbance, 175
environment. *see also* sensorineural hearing loss
   ADHD and, 146–147
   ASD and, 93
   development influenced by, 4–7
   family, 186
   learning, 186–187
   prenatal, 4–5
   school, 186
   social, 187
epigenetics, 7–8, 147
error
   medical, 281–282
   refractive, 74
esotropia, 75
evidence, 274b
   medical, 273–275
   factual, 273–275
   opinion, 275
Evidence Act 1995, 273, 283
examination, 14–15. *see also* neurological examination; *specific disorder*
   physical, 32–33
   tests in, 33t
   red flags in, 17–20
executive dysfunction
   ADHD and, 150
   theory, 94
exotropia, 75
experiences, early, 8–10
Expert Witness Code of Conduct, 282
expertise rule, 283
eye
   hand–eye coordination, 27
   injury to, 75
   movement of, 17–18

F

factitious or induced illness (FII), 259–260
family
   ASD intervention based in, 107
   environment of, 186
   support from, 38, 105b
family court, 276
farsightedness, 74
FII. *see* factitious or induced illness
fluorescence in situ hybridisation (FISH), 233
FMS. *see* functional mobility scale
fractures, 255–257
   imaging of, 256–257
   injury mechanisms of, 256
   skull, 57

fragile X associated tremor and ataxia syndrome (FXTAS), 233–234
fragile X syndrome, 233–234
Fraser competence, 278
Freud, Sigmund, 2
functional communication training, 106
functional mobility scale (FMS), 214
functional neuroanatomy, 129–130
FXTAS. *see* fragile X associated tremor and ataxia syndrome

G
Gage classification. *see* Winters Gage Hick Classification of hemiplegia
gender, development influenced by, 4
gene
   disorders of, 93
   expression of, 7–8
generalised anxiety disorder, 199
genetics. *see also* epigenetics; sensorineural hearing loss
   ADHD and, 146
   ASD and, 93
   counselling, 105
   development influenced by, 3
   twin studies and, 3
   vision loss and, 71–72
genome map, 3
Gesell figures, 35f
GFCF diet. *see* gluten- and casein-free diet
Gillick competence, 278
Gillick v West Norfolk and Wisbech Area Health Authority 1986, 278
glaucoma, 73
global developmental delay, 97
glue ear, 18, 58
gluten- and casein-free diet (GFCF diet), 109
GMDS. *see* Griffiths Mental Development Scales
GMFCS. *see* Gross Motor Function Classification System
gonorrhea, 267
Goodenough–Harris Drawing Test, 35
grasp reflex, 16
Griffiths Mental Development Scales (GMDS), 37, 42–43, 237t
Gross Motor Function Classification System (GMFCS), 213–214
guardianship, 278–279

H
hallucinations, 204
handedness, 20

hand–eye coordination, 27
head control, 17
head trauma, 254–255
   investigations in, 255
   presentation of, 254–255
hearing
   assessment of, 32, 65–66
      diagnostic ABR for, 65
      SSEP testing in, 65
      tympanometry for, 66
      visual reinforcement audiometry for, 66
   impairment of, 18
   in normal development, 11t–13t
   processing problems, 118t
   screening of, 64–65
      ABR for, 64
      oto-acoustic emissions for, 64
      pure tone audiometry for, 65
hearing loss, 50. *see also* conductive hearing loss; deafness; sensorineural hearing loss
   aetiology of, 51–58
   ANSD and, 60–61
   classification of, 59–61
      degree of loss in, 59, 60t
      time of onset in, 61
   clinical presentation of, 61–63, 62b
   early intervention for, 67–68
   language disorders and, 137
   management of, 66–67
   mixed, 50, 60
   prevalence of, 51
   prognosis of, 68–69
   risk factors for, 51–58, 63b
   types of, 50, 59–61
hemiplegia
   acquired, 217–218
   Gage classification of, 215
hepatitis, 267
herpes simplex virus (HSV), 55, 267
hip
   displacement of, 225–226
   X-ray of, 225f
histone modification, 7–8
HIV. *see* human immunodeficiency virus
homelessness, 186
HPV. *see* human papilloma virus
HSV. *see* herpes simplex virus
human immunodeficiency virus (HIV), 267
human papilloma virus (HPV), 266–267
Hurricane Katrina, 187
hyperactivity, 149
hyperbilirubinemia, 55

Index

hyperopia, 74
hypertropia, 75
hypotropia, 75
hypoxia, 56

I
iatrogenic injury, 275
ICF. *see* International Classification of Function
ID. *see* intellectual disability
imaging
  of fractures, 256–257
  neuro-, 94
immersion burns, 257
inattention, 149
infants
  premature, 4, 55–56
  toy tests for, 66
infections
  CP from, 217
  deafness from, 18
  viral, 199
  vision loss caused by, 70–71
    acquired, 71
    congenital, 70–71
informed consent, 277–278
insurance claims, 275
intellectual disability (ID), 232
  aetiology of, 233–234
  assessment of, 235–239
    differential diagnosis in, 97
    tools for, 237t
  behaviour challenges with, 242–243
  community attitudes towards, 243–244
  early trajectory of, 234–235
  intervention for, 239–241
  IQ categories in, 238t
  mental health with, 242–243
  outcomes for, 241
  population perspective on, 241–242
  prevalence of, 232
  principles for, 243–244
intelligence quotient (IQ), 238t
International Classification of Function (ICF), 241
intrapartum asphyxia, 217
intrathecal baclofen (ITB), 224–225
IQ. *see* intelligence quotient
ITB. *see* intrathecal baclofen

J
JIRT. *see* Joint Investigation Response Team
joint attention, 95

Joint Investigation Response Team (JIRT), 249
juvenile court, 276
juvenile myasthenia gravis, 44t

K
KABC. *see* Kaufman Assessment Battery for Children
Kanner, Leo, 88
karyotyping, 233
Kaufman Assessment Battery for Children (KABC), 37
Klein, Melanie, 2–3
Klinefelter's syndrome, 45

L
lamotrigine, 208
language, 15–16
  assessment of, 32
  delay of, 133b
  development of, 5–6, 135t
  functional neuroanatomy of, 129–130
  problems with, 19
  skills, 121
language disorders, 115, 127–128. *see also* developmental language disorder; specific language impairment
  aetiology of, 131–134
  assessment of, 136–138, 138t–139t
  classification of, 130–131
  clinical presentation of, 134–136
  comorbidity with, 136
  emotional causes of, 138
  factors associated with, 133b
  hearing impairment and, 137
  management of, 139–141
  medical causes of, 137
  neurological disorders and, 137
  preschool child with, 134–136
  prevalence of, 130
  prognosis of, 141
  school-aged child with, 136
  terminology of, 141–142
  types of, 132b
law, 273
  child abuse and, 248–249
  terminology of, 274b
lead, 147
learning. *see also* specific learning disorder
  environment, 186–187
  skills, 155–156
Leber's optic atrophy, 72
legal medical assessment, 275–276
lexical–syntactic deficit, 132

limb–girdle dystrophies, 44t
lithium, 207–208

M

MACS. *see* Manual Ability Classification System
malnutrition, 199
mania, 204
Manual Ability Classification System (MACS), 214–215
material risk, 278
mathematical ability, 121
measles, 71
medical care standards, 281
medical error, 281–282
medical evidence, 273–275
  factual, 273–275
  opinion, 275
medical investigation, 33–34
medical negligence, 279–280
medication
  for ADHD, 159–161, 160t, 166–167
  for ASD treatment, 107–108
  for behaviour difficulties, 182, 183t
  for depression, 202–203
meningitis, 18, 56
mental state examination, 276
mercury, 147
methylphenidate (Ritalin, Attenta), 159–161, 160t
mindfulness, 181
minimal brain dysfunction, 41
minor neurological dysfunction, 41
Minors (Property and Contracts) Act 1970, 277–278
mixed hearing loss, 50, 60
mood
  movement's relationship with, 197
  ultradian variation in, 196
mood disorders, 194–196, 209, 209b
  adult–adolescent differences in, 195–196
  child–adolescent differences in, 195–196
  disorders associated with, 196
Moro reflex, 16
mother, anxiety, depression, and stress in, 5
motor dysfunction, 41
motor dyspraxia, 40. *see also* developmental coordination disorder
motor impairment, 4, 40
motor proficiency, 42–43
motor skills
  DCD and, 41–42
  fine, 19–20, 27
    assessment of, 32
  gross, 20, 27
    assessment of, 32
  in normal development, 11t–13t
  SLD and, 121, 123t
motor system, 40
motor tone, 17
movement
  eye, 17–18
  mood's relation with, 197
mumps, 18
Münchausen syndrome by proxy, 259–260
muscular disorders. *see* neuromuscular disorders
muscular dystrophies, 44t
mutism, selective, 128
myasthenia gravis, 44t
myopathies, 44t
myopia, 74
myotonic dystrophy, 44t

N

National Health and Nutritional Examination Survey (NHANES), 51
natural disasters, 187
NE. *see* neonatal encephalopathy
nearsightedness, 74
neglect, 247, 260–263
  assessment of, 262
  management of, 262–263
  prevalence of, 249–250, 250t
negligence, medical, 279–280
Neisseria gonorrhoeae, 267
neonatal encephalopathy (NE), 216
neonatal intensive care unit (NICU), 55
neuroanatomy, functional, 129–130
neuroimaging, 94
neurological disorders, 137
neurological dysfunction, 41
neurological examination, 16–17
  appearance in, 16
  behaviour in, 16
  reflexes in, 16
  tone in, 17
neuroma, acoustic, 57
neuromuscular disorders
  DCD and, 43–45
  inherited, 44t
neuroplasticity, 9–10
NHANES. *see* National Health and Nutritional Examination Survey

NICU. *see* neonatal intensive care unit
non-Mendelian malformation syndromes, 53, 58
non-verbal communication, 26–27
normal development, 1
   hearing in, 11t–13t
   milestones in, 10–14
   motor skills in, 11t–13t
   social skills, 11t–13t
   stages of, 10–14, 11t–13t
   vision in, 11t–13t
nutrition, 5–6, 51, 199

O

OAE. *see* oto-acoustic emission
observation, 31–32
occupational therapist (OT), 45–46
ODD. *see* oppositional defiant disorder
OME. *see* otitis media with effusion
omega-3, 183t
OPD. *see* otopalatodigital syndrome
oppositional defiant disorder (ODD), 196
optic atrophy, 72
organs, diseases of, 4
OT. *see* occupational therapist
otitis media, 18
otitis media with effusion (OME), 58
oto-acoustic emission (OAE), 64
otopalatodigital syndrome (OPD), 58
ototoxins, 56

P

paediatrician
   as advocate, 283–284
   as expert witness, 282–283
   role of, 2
parachute reflex, 17
parents
   ADHD treatment concerns of, 161
   involvement of, 186
   training of, 179–181
PDD. *see* pervasive developmental disorder
Peabody Developmental Motor Scales (PDMS), 42–43
pencil, 35
perceptio-motor dysfunction, 41
personal–social skills, 27
pervasive developmental disorder (PDD), 91–92
phonologic production deficit, 132
phonologic–syntactic deficit, 132
phonology, 141
phoria, 75

photography, of physical abuse, 253
physical abuse, 247, 250t, 251–258
   abdominal trauma in, 258
   abusive head trauma in, 254–255
   bruises in, 252–254
   burns in, 257–258
   differential diagnosis of, 253–254
   fractures in, 255–257
   photography of, 253
   physical examination, 32–33, 33t. *see also specific disorder*
Piaget, Jean, 3
placing reflex, 16
plaintiff, 274b
play
   associative, 28
   parallel, 27
   solitary, 27
   spectator, 28
play skills, 27–28
   ASD and, 96
   functional, 28
   social, 27–28
polychlorinated biphenyl, 147
positive parenting programs, 181
post traumatic stress disorder (PTSD), 199
poverty, 186
pragmatics, 141
pregnancy, 154, 267
premature infant, 4, 55–56
prenatal environment, 4–5
presbyopia, 74
preschool child
   ADHD in, 155
      management of, 161–163
   language disorders of, 134–136
primary congenital glaucoma, 73
primitive reflex, 16
privacy, 279
prosecution, 274b
psychoanalysis, 2
psycho-education, 207
psychological abuse, 248
psychometric assessment, 37
psychosis, 199, 204
PTSD. *see* post traumatic stress disorder
pure tone audiometry (PTA), 65–66

R

reactive attachment disorder of infancy and early childhood, 98
reading ability, 121, 123t
red flags, 17–18
red reflex, 17–18

reflex
  acoustic, 66
  ATNR, 16
  grasp, 16
  Moro, 16
  in neurological examination, 16
  parachute, 17
  placing/stepping, 16
  primitive, 16
  red, 17–18
  side protective, 17
refractive errors, 74
resilience, 9
retinal degeneration, 73
retinopathy of prematurity (ROP), 72–73
Rett's disorder, 92
risk, material, 278
risperidone, 107
Ritalin. *see* methylphenidate
Ritalin LA. *see* dexamphetamine
ROP. *see* retinopathy of prematurity
routine, 206
rubella, 54, 71

S
savant skills, 97
school. *see also* preschool child
  ADHD and, 159
  environment, 186
school failure, 119b
school phobia, 185
school refusal, 185
  assessment of, 189–191
  clinical investigations of, 190
  clinical presentation of, 188
  comorbid psychiatric symptoms and disorders with, 189
  family environment and, 186
  functions of, 187–188, 188b
  learning environment and, 186–187
  management of, 189–191
  prognosis of, 192
  risk factors for, 186–187
  school environment and, 186
  social environment and, 187
  treatment of, 191–192
School Refusal Assessment Scale (SRAS), 187–188
school-aged child
  ADHD in, 155–156
    management in, 163
  with language disorders, 136
scoliosis, 226
SCQ. *see* Social Communication Questionnaire
screening tools, 28, 29t. *see also specific test or questionnaire*
selective mutism, 128
selective serotonin reuptake inhibitors (SSRIs), 200
self-help skills, 32
semantic–pragmatic deficit, 132
semantics, 141
sensorineural hearing loss (SNHL), 50–57, 59
  environmental, 53–57
    birth asphyxia in, 56
    CMV in, 55
    hyperbilirubinemia in, 55
    hypoxia in, 56
    injuries in, 57
    meningitis in, 56
    noise in, 57
    ototoxins in, 56
    perinatal, 55–56
    postnatal, 56–57
    prematurity in, 55–56
    prenatal causes of, 53–55
    rubella in, 54
    toxoplasmosis in, 54
    tumours in, 57
  genetics of, 51–53
    autosomal dominant, 51–52
    autosomal recessive, 52–53
    mitochondrial, 53
    non-Mendelian malformation syndromes in, 53
    X-linked, 53
sensory impairments, 4
Sensory Integration Therapy (SIT), 46
sensory motor dysfunction, 41
separation anxiety, 196
serous otitis media, 18
SES. *see* socioeconomic status
sexual abuse, 247, 250t, 263–268
  assessment of, 264–265
  emotional consequences of, 267–268
  examination for, 265–266
  interviewing children about, 265
  pregnancy and, 267
  presentation of, 264–266
  psychosocial consequences of, 267–268
  STDs from, 266–267
sexually transmitted disease (STD), 266–267
Shaddock & Associates v Parramatta Council, 276
Shaken Baby Syndrome, 254–255
siblings, 6
side protective reflex, 17

single gene disorders, 93
SIT. *see* Sensory Integration Therapy
skull fractures, 57
SLD. *see* specific learning disorder
sleep, 197, 206
SLI. *see* specific language impairment
SNHL. *see* sensorineural hearing loss
Social Communication Questionnaire (SCQ), 100t
social environment, 187
social interaction
 DCD and, 42
 problems with, 19
social skills
 ADHD and, 153–154
 ASD and, 95–96
 depression and, 197
 in normal development, 11t–13t
 personal–, 27
 SLD and, 121, 123t
socioeconomic status (SES), 6
specific language impairment (SLI), 98, 127–128
specific learning disorder (SLD), 113
 aetiology of, 116
  acquired, 116
  congenital, 116
 assessment of, 118–121
  differential diagnosis in, 118, 119b
  history in, 120b
  medical investigations in, 122t
  physical examination in, 120b
  skills, 121, 123t
  tests used in, 123t
 classification of, 114–115
 clinical presentation of, 117
  auditory processing problems in, 118t
  visual processing problems in, 117t
 comorbidity with, 116, 125
 management of, 121–125, 124b
 medical reports and, 125
 types of, 114–115
speech
 functional neuroanatomy of, 129–130
 problems with, 19
speech discrimination tests, 66
spinal muscular atrophy, 44t
spondyloepiphyseal dysplasia, 45
squint, 17–18
SRAS. *see* School Refusal Assessment Scale
SSEP. *see* steady state evoked potential
SSRIs. *see* selective serotonin reuptake inhibitors

standard of reasonable care, 280–281
standards of medical care, 281
Stanford–Binet Intelligence Scale, 37, 237t
STD. *see* sexually transmitted disease
steady state evoked potential (SSEP), 65
stepping reflex, 16
stereotypic behaviours, 96–97
STG. *see* superior temporal gyrus
stimulants, 161b, 183t
strabismus, 75
Strattera. *see* atomoxetine
stress
 maternal, 5
 post traumatic, 199
suicide
 attempts, 196
 SSRIs and, 200
sunburn, 258
superior temporal gyrus (STG), 130
supervision, 186
syntax, 141
syphilis, 267

T
TEACCH. *see* Treatment and Education of Autistic and Related Communication Handicapped Children
temperament, 177
theory of mind (ToM), 94
tone, 17
tort, 274b
toxins, 147
 deafness from, 18
 oto–, 56
toxoplasmosis, 54
toys, 6, 66
trachoma, 71
transactional model, 7
Treacher-Collins syndrome, 57–58
Treatment and Education of Autistic and Related Communication Handicapped Children (TEACCH), 107
trichomonas vaginalis, 267
tropia, 75
truancy, 185–186
 assessment of, 189–191
 clinical investigations of, 190
 clinical presentation of, 189
 comorbid psychiatric symptoms and disorders with, 189
 family environment and, 186

learning environment and, 186–187
management of, 189–191
prognosis of, 192
risk factors for, 186–187
school environment and, 186
social environment and, 187
treatment of, 191–192
tsunami, of 2004, 187
tumours
  SNHL with, 57
  vision loss from, 76
twin studies, 3
tympanometry, 66

U

ultimate issue rule, 283
ultradian cycling, 204
ultradian mood variation, 196
Universal Nonverbal Intelligence Test (UNIT), 15–16
uveitis, 75

V

valproate, 207–208
verbal auditory agnosia, 132
verbal communication, 26
Vineland Adaptive Behavior Scales, 37, 237t
viral infection, 199. *see also specific virus*
vision. *see also* eye
  assessment of, 32, 78–81
  in normal development, 11t–13t
  processing problems, 117t
  screening tests for, 78, 79t–80t
vision loss, 17–18, 70–82
  aetiology of, 70–76
  from amblyopia, 74
  assessment of, 78–81
  from cataracts, 73
  classification of, 76–77
  clinical presentation of, 77–78
  from cortical or cerebral visual impairment, 75–76
  from eye injury, 75
  genetic, 71–72
  from glaucoma, 73
  infections causing, 70–71
    acquired, 71
    congenital, 70–71
  management of, 81–82
  prevalence of, 70
  prognosis of, 82
  from retinal degeneration, 73
  from retinopathy of prematurity, 72–73
  risk factors for, 70–76
  screening tests for, 78, 79t–80t
  from strabismus, 75
  from tumour, 76
  types of, 76–77
  from uveitis, 75
  from vitamin A deficiency, 73
visual reinforcement audiometry (VRA), 66
vitamin A, 73
VRA. *see* visual reinforcement audiometry
Vygotsky, Lev, 3

W

Waardenburg's syndrome, 51–52
war, 6–7
Wechsler Intelligence Scale for Children (WISC), 237t
Wechsler Preschool and Primary Scale of Intelligence (WPPSI), 37, 237t
weight gain/loss, 197
Wernicke's aphasia, 130
Wernicke's area, 129
Winters Gage Hick Classification of hemiplegia (Gage classification), 215
WISC. *see* Wechsler Intelligence Scale for Children
witness, 274b
  admissibility of, 274b
  code of conduct of, 282
  paediatrician as, 282–283
word deafness, 132
working memory, 159
WPPSI. *see* Wechsler Preschool and Primary Scale of Intelligence

X

X-linked Alport's syndrome (XLAS), 53
X-rays
  CP assessment with, 220
  of hip, 225f

Z

zone of proximal development (ZPD), 3